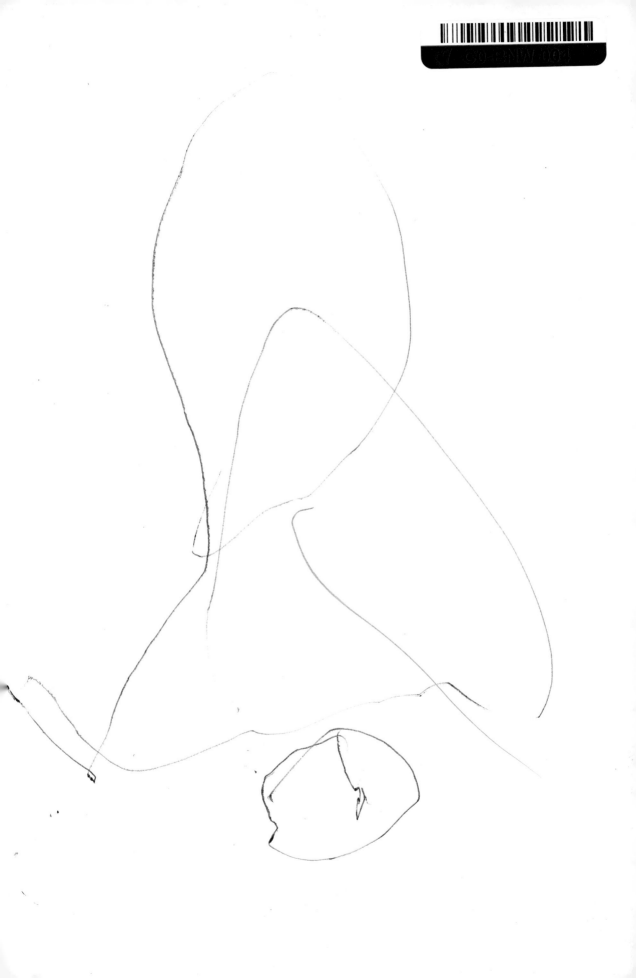

NORMAL AND ABNORMAL DEVELOPMENT OF THE HUMAN NERVOUS SYSTEM

ILLUSTRATIONS BY
Phyllis J. Wood

PHOTOGRAPHIC ASSISTANCE BY
Warren R. Criss

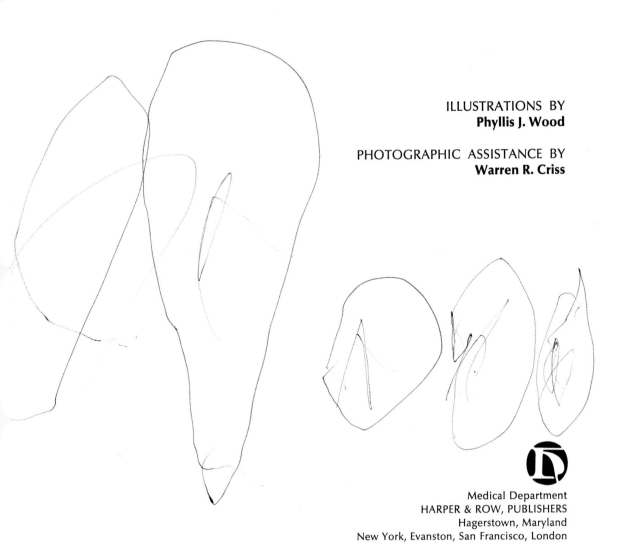

Medical Department
HARPER & ROW, PUBLISHERS
Hagerstown, Maryland
New York, Evanston, San Francisco, London

Library of Congress Cataloging in Publication Data

Main entry under title:

Normal and abnormal development of the human nervous
system.

Includes Bibliographies
and Index.
1. Developmental neurology.   2.   Nervous system—
Abnormalities and deformities.   I.   Lemire, Ronald J.,
1933–   [DNLM: 1.   Central nervous system—Abnormalities.   2.   Central nervous system—Embryology.   WL101
N842]
RJ252.N6   618.3′2   75-8711
ISBN 0-06-141530-8

CONTENTS

PREFACE

While the literature on the normal and abnormal development of the brain is abundant, it appears in multiple journals published over many years. The numerous investigations have not been brought together in any comprehensive text that directs itself to specific sequential discussion, thus making retrieval both time-consuming and difficult—and impractical for the busy practitioner. NORMAL AND ABNORMAL DEVELOPMENT OF THE HUMAN NERVOUS SYSTEM consolidates as much as possible of the currently available information on the normal development of various components of the human nervous system and analyzes the various diseases of the developing nervous system in terms of their possible causes and the times at which these etiologic factors could exert the effects which result in abnormal development. This information is presented in a standardized graphic manner which the authors—a pediatrician, a neurosurgeon, and two neuropathologists—have refined over the past several years.[1-6]

The book begins with brief considerations of the patterns of general embryonic and fetal development (Section I) necessary to an understanding of the more detailed descriptions of the patterns of neural development, in which the closure and early differentiation of the neural tube (Section 2) play most important roles. The subsequent analyses of nervous system development are generally along gross anatomic lines, beginning with the more primitive segmental structures of the spinal cord and brain stem (Section 3) and continuing through the phylogenetically more recently acquired suprasegmental structures (cerebellum, colliculi and forebrain in Section 4). This neuroanatomic concept of Adolf Meyer and Louis Hausman is introduced in Chapter 2, which students of the more usual cross-sectional neuroanatomy may wish to digest before reading further. Discussions of the development of the nonneural tissues surrounding and related to the nervous system and of diseases affecting the nervous system as a part of their more generalized nature (Section 5) conclude the book. In the discussion of neural neoplasms occurring in infants and children (Chapter 22), a deliberate attempt is made to emphasize the basic biologic features of cytokinetics and tumor growth—specifically several examples where the data warrant subscription to the hypothesis of constant expotential doubling times—and to point out that the traditional generalizations based on histopathologic grading of neoplasms is fraught with danger if one ignores specific types and sites of tumors.

In general, most chapters begin with an analysis of of the normal development and end with an analysis of abnormal development. This presentation of major features of development of each part of the nervous system allows ready cross reference to the development of other parts of the nervous system and of other organs as collated with body size and gestational age. Extensions to postnatal growth and development are made where pertinent since a very significant part of human nervous system development occurs after birth. Indeed, one can only deplore the past isolation of embryologists from pediatric pathologists and neuropathologists whose interest has overemphasized the adult and who have failed to see the continuity expressed most easily in a graphic analysis using a logarithmic time scale, the "biological time" of Lecomte du Nouy.[7, 8] Although these graphic presentations are supplemented by the text, the reader will quickly find that there are many blank spaces in the graphs where future studies will add interesting and important information—the field is by no means complete.

In addition to pediatricians, neurosurgeons, and neuropathologists—the specialists represented by the authors—it is hoped that the book will be useful to embryologists, geneticists, pathologists, neurologists, and others interested in mental retardation and interaction between environmental and genetic factors as they affect the developing nervous system.

Beyond the information from previously published studies by other investigators, we have included many unpublished observations based on material taken from many sources to whom we are greatly indebted. Normal and abnormal embryos and fetuses have been made available to us through Dr. Thomas H. Shepard, Director of the Central Laboratory for Human Embryology at the University of Washington. Illustrations of most of the gross and microscopic anomalies have been selected from the files of the Laboratory of Neuropathology, formerly supported by a Training Grant in Neuropathology (NS-5231-15) from the National Institute of Neurological Diseases and Stroke, U.S. Public Health Service. Since 1960 over 14,000 cases have been examined in the half-dozen hospitals affiliated with the University of Washington. Over 4,400 of these cases have been studied by many trainees and other faculty members and about 10% of these contained malformations of the nervous system. Most of the cases have come from the Children's Orthopedic Hospital and Medical Center (Dr. J. Bruce Beckwith, Director of Laboratories) and the University Hospital (Dr. H. Thomas Norris, Director of the Pathology Laboratory). Other cases have been obtained through Harborview Medical Center (formerly King County Hospital), Seattle Veterans Administration Hospital, U.S. Public Health Service Hospital, Swedish Hospital, Virginia Mason Hospital, and Fircrest and Rainier Schools for the mentally handicapped.

Numerous colleagues have generously contributed to the book in many ways. In addition to the case material mentioned above, Drs. J. Bruce Beckwith and Thomas H. Shepard have provided us with a background of extremely interested general support and specific detailed information. Drs. Cheng-Mei Shaw, S. Mark Sumi, and Robert M. Shuman have performed detailed neuropathologic examinations on many of the cases illustrated and have provided expert assistance in reviewing parts of the text. Special acknowledgment is made to Dr. David B. Shurtleff, who has contributed in ways too numerous to name. While several typists contributed to the early drafts of the manuscript, we are specifically grateful to Alice J. Pope who took such a personal interest in its completion and checked much of it for accuracy. Needless to say, however, the authors take full responsibility for any mistakes or omissions. We also want to thank the National Foundation–March of Dimes who generously funded the entire cost of the illustrations. Finally, the personal attention of the staff of the Medical Department of Harper and Row, Publishers, has made the conclusion of our project most enjoyable.

REFERENCES

1. Dennis JP, Rosenberg HS, Alvord EC Jr: Megalencephaly, internal hydrocephalus and other neurological aspects of achondroplasia. Brain 84:427–445, 1961
2. Du Noüy L: Human Destiny. New York, Longmans, Green & Co, 1947
3. Du Noüy L: Biological Time. New York, Macmillan, 1937
4. Lemire RJ: Embryology of the central nervous system. Scientific Foundations of Paediatrics. Edited by JA Davis and J Dobbing. London, Heinemann, 1974, pp 547–564
5. Lemire RJ: Variation in development of the caudal neural tube in human embryos (Horizons XIV–XXI). Teratology 2:361–370, 1969
6. Lemire RJ, Shurtleff DB: Malformations of the skull. In Brennemann–Kelley Practice of Pediatrics. Vol. IV. Edited by VC Kelley. Hagerstown, Harper and Row, 1971
7. Loeser JD, Alvord EC Jr: Agenesis of the corpus callosum. Brain 91:553–570, 1968
8. Loeser JD, Lemire RJ, Alvord EC Jr: The development of the folia in the human cerebellar vermis. Anat Rec 173:109–114, 1972

GENERAL EMBRYONIC AND FETAL DEVELOPMENTAL FEATURES

1

STAGES OF EMBRYONIC DEVELOPMENT; GROWTH OF FETAL STRUCTURES AND ORGANS

Normal and abnormal growth of the embryo and fetus* has been a focus of scientific interest for centuries. Since a knowledge of the normal parameters of general growth is important for anyone studying a specific system, such as the central nervous system (CNS), it seems appropriate to begin this book with a brief chapter on the general aspects of human prenatal growth.

DEVELOPMENTAL STAGES IN HUMAN EMBRYOS

Streeter[12] selected the word *horizon* to discuss embryonic development believing it to be consistent with usage in other scientific disciplines: "in the present instance the term is used to emphasize the importance of thinking of the embryo as a living organism which in its time takes on many guises, always progressing from the smaller and simpler to the larger and more complex." He proposed that embryonic growth be divided into 23 separate phases,† each identified by specific morphologic features. Before his

death he published three separate articles dealing with horizons XI–XVIII.[12, 13, 14] Work which he had nearly completed on horizons XIX–XXIII was later compiled by Heuser and Corner,[17] who in addition described horizon X.[2] Horizons XI–XXIII were then combined into a single volume[16] that included a previously published study on cartilage and bone.[15] Although Streeter[12] proposed the formats for horizons I–IX, they have only recently been described in detail.[7]

O'Rahilly[7] found it necessary to make some modifications in the earlier classification of horizons proposed by Streeter. There is thus some overlapping between O'Rahilly's and Streeter's systems until horizon XI is reached (Table 1-1). Another change is the use of the word "stage" instead of "horizon," and we will adopt this system in the present book. O'Rahilly also proposed that Arabic numerals be substituted for the Roman numerals used by Streeter, but we have chosen to retain the latter to avoid confusion with the Arabic numerals used for crown–rump (CR) length and gestational age.

Although it is difficult to condense the details of the embryonic stages, a few general comments will clarify our reasons for utilizing this system. If one analyzes the two other measurements by which embryonic development can be staged, *i.e.*, size and gestational age, a marked variability becomes apparent. If all embryos of a given gestational age are compared, there is marked variability in size. Likewise, embryos at a given size have marked variability in gestational age. The reason is not that such a discrepancy really exists in the development

---

*An embryo is defined as "an animal in the early stages of growth and differentiation that is characterized by cleavage, the laying down of fundamental tissues and the formation of primitive organs and organ systems";[20] a fetus is an animal from the end of the embryonic period until birth.

† Streeter originally decided on 25 embryonic horizons that would end when the eyelids came together, but he later changed this to 23 so that the fetal stages would begin with marrow formation in the humerus. He credited Franklin P. Mall with first suggesting that embryos be classified in stages.

TABLE 1–1. COMPARISON BETWEEN O'RAHILLY'S "CARNEGIE" STAGING SYSTEM AND STREETER'S "DEVELOPMENTAL HORIZONS"[7]

Developmental horizon	Carnegie stage	Streeter's (1942) criteria
I	1	Unicellular
II	2	Segmentation
III	3	Free blastocyst
IV	4–5	Implanting
V	5	Implanted but avillous
VI		Chorionic villi
		Distinct yolk sac
VII		Branching villi
	6	Axis of germ disc defined
		Primitive groove
VIII		
		Primitive node
	7	
		Notochordal process
IX		Neural folds
	8	
	9	1–3 pairs of somites
X	10	4–12 pairs of somites
XI	11	13–20 pairs of somites
XII	12	21–29 pairs of somites

of the embryo but that differing types of measurements and imprecise menstrual cycle data are frequently introduced. By contrast, there are common landmarks in embryos staged primarily according to morphology, with size and gestational age being secondary factors. Table 1–2 gives the relationships of these three factors, and Figures 1–1a to 1–1d provide various growth curves to which features of development can be related.

Correlations of size and gestational age are continuously being revised, and those presented in Table 1–2 and in the growth curves throughout the text are only representative. Selected features of general embryonic growth are presented by organ system in Figures 1–2 to 1–6. These should provide the reader with some comparative index of the development of other organs with the more detailed development of the nervous system which will be presented in subsequent chapters. It should be noted that some of these features are also used in the assignment of certain embryos to a given stage.

FETAL GROWTH

Streeter arbitrarily defined the onset of the fetal period by the appearance of marrow formation in the humerus but unfortunately the fetal stages of growth have not been morphologically staged in the detail of the embryonic period. Therefore, one must rely on the rather imprecise crown–rump (CR) and crown–heel (CH) lengths. There is some variation in fetal size at each gestational age, and the growth lines in Figures 1–1a to 1–1d are only suggestive of the means.

Most fetuses retain a sitting posture. A measurement of the CR length is thus more convenient and sometimes more accurate than the CH length. Most embryologists have used the CR length as representative of fetal size, whereas some neonatologists[6] prefer CH length or body weight during the "premature period." Another measurement worth mentioning is the foot length (FL),[11, 19] which is easily and accurately

TABLE 1–2. RELATIONSHIP OF STAGES OF EMBRYONIC DEVELOPMENT TO SIZE AND AGE OF THE EMBRYO

Stage	Crown–rump length (mm)	Gestational age (days)*
I	—	0–1 (1)
II	—	1–4 (2–3)
III	—	4–5 (4–5)
IV	—	6–9 (5–6)
V	0.1–0.2	10–12 (7–12)
VI	0.2	13–15 (13–15)
VII	0.4	16–17 (15–17)
VIII	1.0–1.5	18 (17–19)
IX	1.5–2.5	20 (19–21)
X	2–3.5	22 (22–23)
XI	2.5–4.5	24 (23–26)
XII	3–5	26 (26–30)
XIII	4–6	28 (28–32)
XIV	5–7	32 (31–35)
XV	7–9	34.5 (35–38)
XVI	8–11	37 (37–42)
XVII	11–14	40 (42–44)
XVIII	13–17	43 (44–48)
XIX	16–18	45 (48–51)
XX	18–22	47 (51–53)
XXI	22–24	48.5 (53–54)
XXII	23–28	50 (54–56)
XXIII	27–31	52 (56–60)

* Gestational ages and CR lengths are from O'Rahilly,[7] Iffy et al.[3] and Shepard.[10] Numbers appearing in parentheses are the data of Jirasek[4] on the therapeutic abortions.

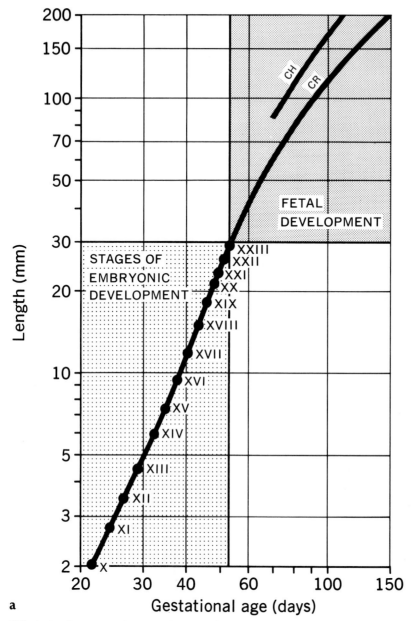

a

FIG. 1–1.   Representative growth curves for crown–rump (CR) and crown–heel (CH) lengths during part of the embryonic, fetal and early postnatal periods. The Roman numerals designate the embryonic stages. Stage X was chosen as the lower limit on the graphs to be used throughout much of the book since most morphologic landmarks in the development of the nervous system occur after this stage, with the exception of onset of neurulation. Figures 1–1a through 1–1d provide a continuum of growth from stage X of the embryonic period through the fifth postnatal year. Developmental landmarks of most structures in the central nervous system (CNS) in this book have been related to one or more of these curves.

taken and correlates well with other fetal indices of development. Its greatest value has been on specimens that are not intact for one reason or another (*e.g.*, curettage).

Scammon and Calkins[9] made a comprehensive study of human fetal growth. Beginning in most cases with 30-mm CR length (equal to embryos of stage XXIII), they correlated   numerous   anthropometric measurements of the fetus throughout gesta-

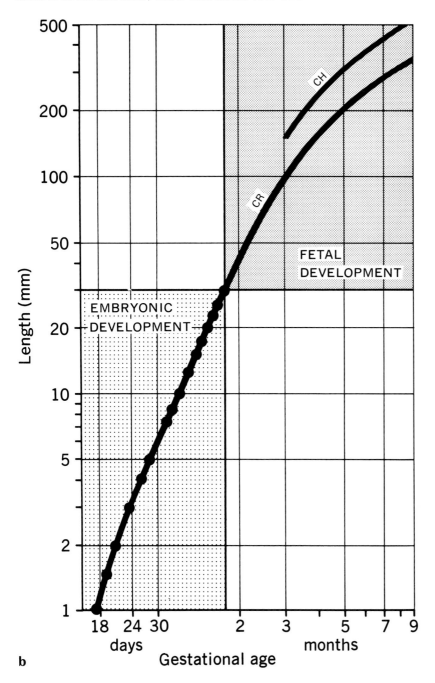

b

tion. Their studies are particularly useful for comparing the growth of one part of the body with that of another part. Additional information is found in a subsequent publication by Scammon,[8] who constructed nomographs of growth utilizing many common measurements. The growth figures used in the present book are in part derived from those of Scammon and Calkins[9] and in part from Lubchenco et al.[5]

FETAL ORGAN WEIGHTS

An additional parameter by which fetal growth can be measured is the weight of individual organs. Tanimura et al.[18] provide

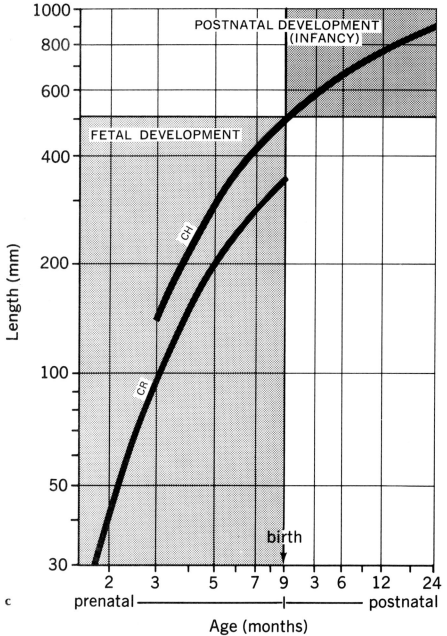

FIG. 1–1   (continued)

weight standards for organs in fetuses from the end of the embryonic period to a body weight of 500 g. For body weights over 500 g until birth the standards of Gruenwald and Minh[1] are useful. The weights of other organs will not be presented in this book, but those of the brain can be found in Chapter 3.

SUMMARY

The material presented in this chapter is intended to provide the background for information of more-general aspects of embryonic and fetal growth. The landmarks of development used throughout the remainder of the book and the various growth curves

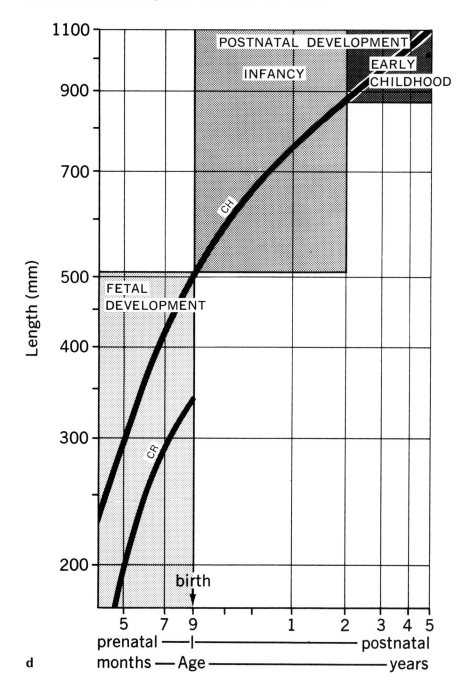

presented in our graphs are only representative of much more comprehensive studies carried out by the individuals cited above. The Streeter stages will be our basis for making embryologic comparisons; we will use a system employing two lengths, crown-rump (CR) and/or crown-heel (CH), for the remainder of fetal and postnatal life. In doing so, we are aware of certain limitations that this places on those readers more accustomed to thinking of development in terms of body weight, but hopefully the correlations with gestational age will be an adequate compromise.

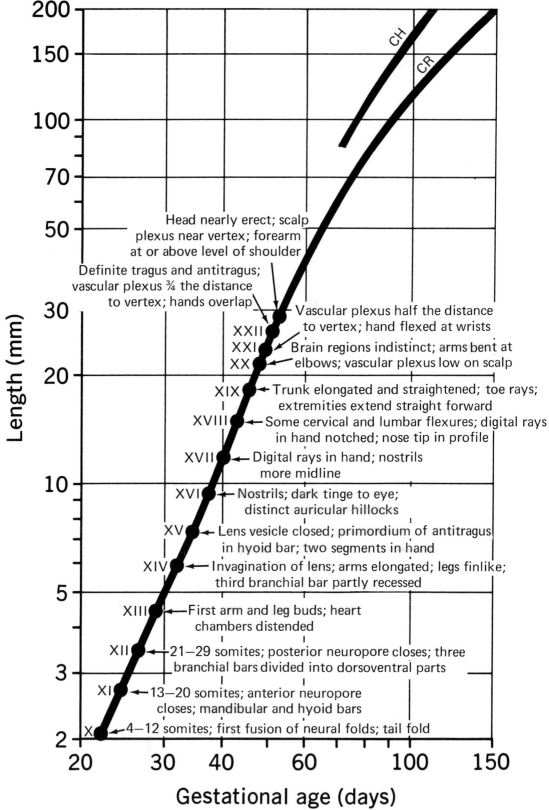

FIG. 1–2. External features exhibited by human embryos correlated with CR length and gestational age.

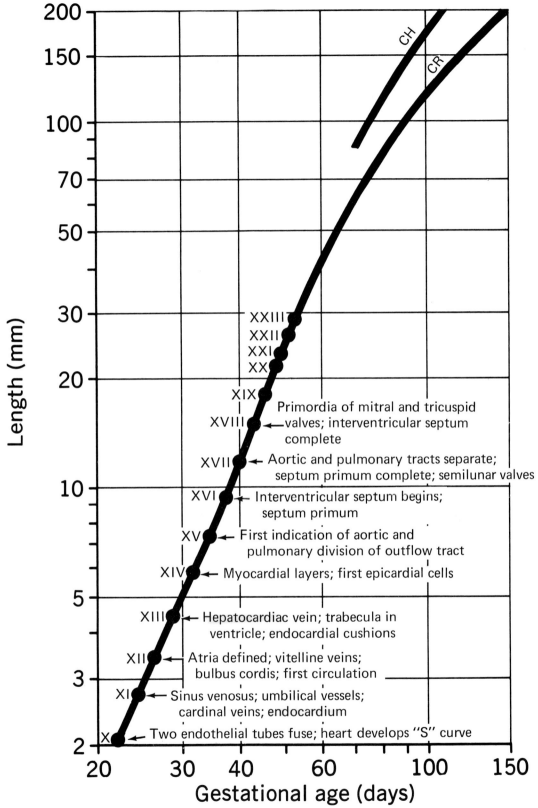

FIG. 1–3. Development of the human heart during the middle portion of the embryonic period.

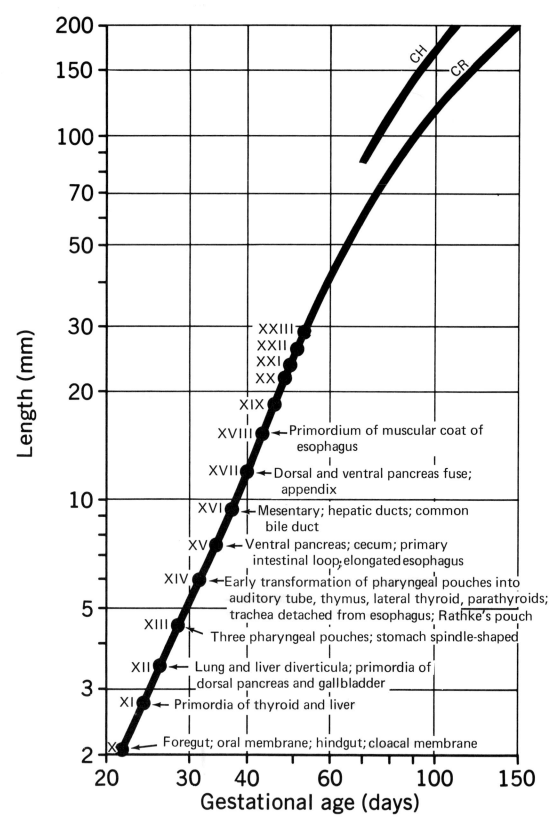

FIG. 1–4. Development of the human gastrointestinal tract correlated with CR length and gestational age.

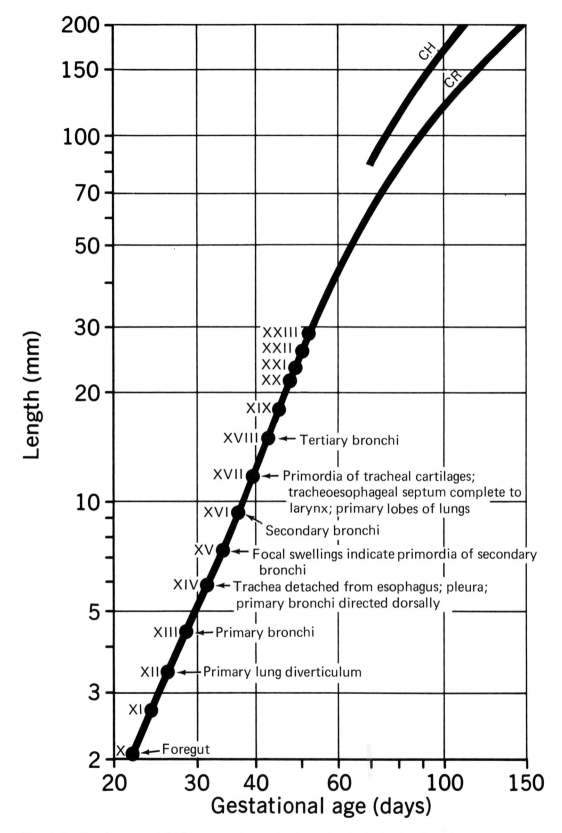

FIG. 1–5. Development of the human respiratory tract correlated with CR length and gestational age.

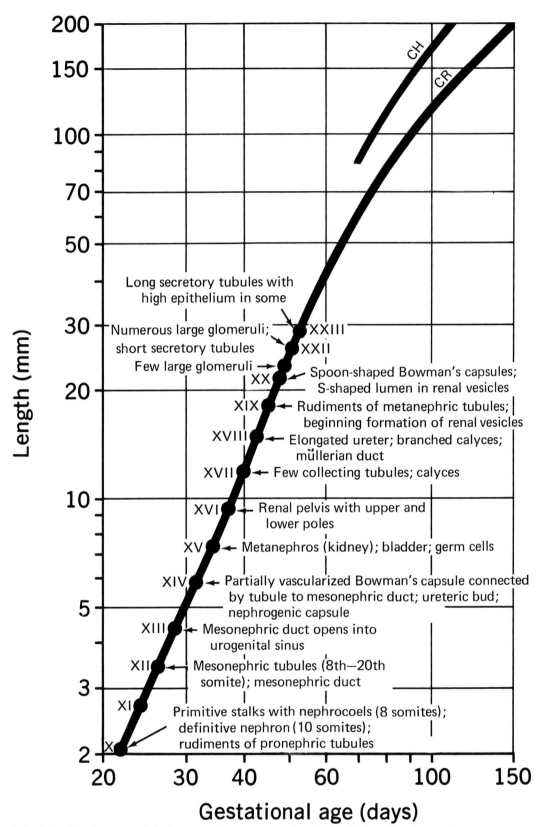

FIG. 1–6. Development of the human urinary tract correlated with CR length and gestational age.

REFERENCES

1. Gruenwald P, Minh HN: Evaluation of body and organ weights in perinatal pathology: I. Normal standards derived from autopsies. Am J Clin Pathol 34:247–253, 1960

2. Heuser CH, Corner GW: Developmental horizons in human embryos. Description of age group X, 4 to 12 somites. Contrib Embryol 36:29–39, 1957

3. Iffy L, Shepard TH, Jakobovits A, Lemire RJ, Kerner P: The rate of growth in young human embryos of Streeter's Horizons XIII–XXIII. Acta Anat (Basel) 66:178–186, 1967

4. Jirásek JE: Development of the Genital System and Male Pseudohermaphroditism. Edited by MM Cohen, Jr. Baltimore, Johns Hopkins Press, 1971

5. Lubchenco LO, Hansman C, Boyd E: Intrauterine growth in length and head circumference from live births at gestational ages from 26 to 42 weeks. Pediatrics 37:403–408, 1966

6. Lubchenco LO, Hansman C, Dressler M, Boyd E: Intrauterine growth as estimated from liveborn birth–weight data at 24 to 42 weeks of gestation. Pediatrics 32:793–800, 1963

7. O'Rahilly R: Developmental Stages in Human Embryos, Part A: Embryos of the First Three Weeks (Stages 1 to 9). Washington DC, Carnegie Inst Wash, 1973

8. Scammon RE: Two simple nomographs for estimating the age and some of the major external dimensions of the human fetus. Anat Rec 68:221–225, 1937

9. Scammon RE, Calkins LA: The Development and Growth of the External Dimensions of the Human Body in the Fetal Period. Minneapolis, Univ Minnesota Press, 1929

10. Shepard TH: Growth and development of the human embryo and fetus. Endocrine and Genetic Diseases of Childhood. Edited by LI Gardner. Philadelphia, WB Saunders, 1969, pp. 1–6

11. Streeter GL: Weight, sitting height, head size, foot length and menstrual age of the human embryo. Contrib Embryol 11:143–170, 1920

12. Streeter GL: Developmental horizons in human embryos. Description of age group XI, 13 to 20 somites, and age group XII, 21 to 29 somites. Contrib Embryol 30:211–245, 1942

13. Streeter GL: Developmental horizons in human embryos. Description of age group XIII, embryos about 4 or 5 millimeters long, and age group XIV, period of indentation of the lens vesicle. Contrib Embryol 31:27–63, 1945

14. Streeter GL: Developmental horizons in human embryos. Description of age groups XV, XVI, XVII and XVIII, being the third issue of a survey of the Carnegie collection. Contrib Embryol 32:133–203, 1948

15. Streeter GL: Developmental horizons in human embryos (fourth issue). A review of the histogenesis of bone and cartilage. Contrib Embryol 33:149–167, 1949

16. Streeter GL: Developmental Horizons in Human Embryos. Age Groups XI–XXIII. Embryology Reprint, vol II. Washington DC, Carnegie Inst Wash, 1951

17. Streeter GL, Heuser CH, Corner GW: Developmental horizons in human embryos. Description of age groups XIX, XX, XXI, XXII and XXIII, being the fifth issue of a survey of the Carnegie collection. Contrib Embryol 34:165–196, 1951

18. Tanimura T, Nelson T, Hollingsworth RR, Shepard TH: Weight standards for organs from early human fetuses. Anat Rec 171:227–236, 1971

19. Trolle D: Age of foetus determined from its measures. Acta Obstet Gynecol Scand 27:327–337, 1948

20. Webster's Seventh New Collegiate Dictionary. Springfield, G&C Merriam Company, 1967

2

FUNCTIONAL AND STRUCTURAL ORGANIZATION OF THE CNS

GENERAL FEATURES

One must understand the overall functional and structural organization of the nervous system if one is to understand the principles on which diagnoses are made in the living patient. Fortunately for the patient, but unfortunately for the diagnostician, the nervous system is a continuously growing organ that can adapt to lesions. As it does so, however, it modifies the clinical appearance of the patient as a function of his age when the disease began and of the amount of time he has survived subsequently. These modifications will be considered in detail in subsequent chapters; the general principles will be presented in this chapter.

SEGMENTATION OF THE NERVOUS SYSTEM

Perhaps the simplest scheme is that developed by Adolf Meyer and elaborated by Louis Hausman,[3,4] whose ontogenetic and phylogenetic studies permit one to divide the nervous system into segmental and intra-, inter- and suprasegmental parts. The segmental nature of even the adult spinal cord is readily appreciated, and one can see that the adult brain stem (Fig. 2–1) and even more obviously the embryonic brain stem (Fig. 2–2) are also divided in a segmental manner. Each segment (Fig. 2–3) develops from neuroectoderm and consists of primary afferent neurons (*receptor plate*) and motor neurons (*motor plate*) with interneurons or second-order sensory neurons (*association plate*). This last group of association plate elements is especially important, since some of its neurons give rise not only to intrasegmental connections between primary afferent and final motor neurons but also to intersegmental nerve fibers connecting to adjacent or distant segments. Other neurons of the association plate give rise to ascending suprasegmental tracts to the suprasegmental organs, *i.e.*, the cerebellum, colliculi and forebrain.

Finally, the association plate neurons as well as the motor plate neurons receive synaptic connections from the descending suprasegmental tracts which connect the suprasegmental organs with the segmental apparatus. Thus, one can appreciate that the labels *receptor* (or *sensory*) and *effector* (or *motor*) can be meaningfully attached only to the receptor and motor plate neurons; to use such labels for any of the association plate functions is to adopt a clinicophysiologic slang which, though it may be useful most times, is at least potentially misleading at other times.

The above divisions easily accommodate the more classic anatomic approach in which the central nervous system (CNS) is divided into spinal cord and brain, which can be subdivided into cerebral hemispheres (forebrain), brain stem (midbrain and hindbrain, including the pons and medulla oblongata) and cerebellum. These gross subdivisions can be related to certain major landmarks in the skull (Figs. 2–4 and 2–5).

The tentorium cerebelli is a fold of dura that divides the cranial cavity into supratentorial and infratentorial compartments; the cerebral hemispheres are above and the cerebellum and most of the brain stem be-

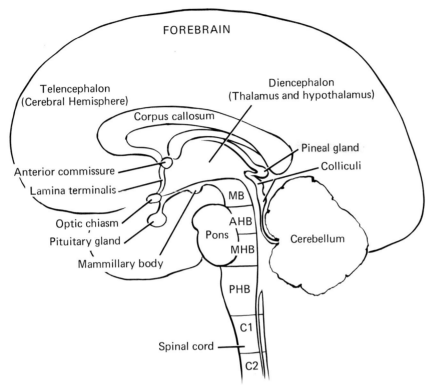

FIG. 2–1. Midsagittal diagram of the brain and upper cervical cord showing the relationship of spinal and brain stem segments to suprasegmental organs (cerebellum, colliculi and forebrain). *MB,* midbrain; *AHB,* anterior hindbrain; *MHB,* middle hindbrain; *PHB,* posterior hindbrain. (Adapted from Hausman, 1961)

FIG. 2–2. Midsagittal diagram of stage XV human embryo. The receptor plate ganglia have been displaced ventrally to avoid superposition on the motor plate. (Adapted from Streeter, 1948)

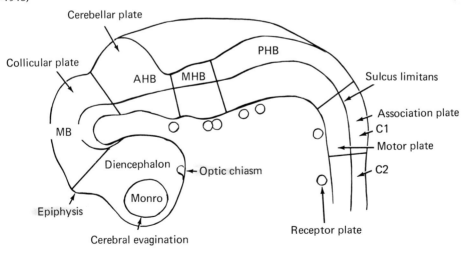

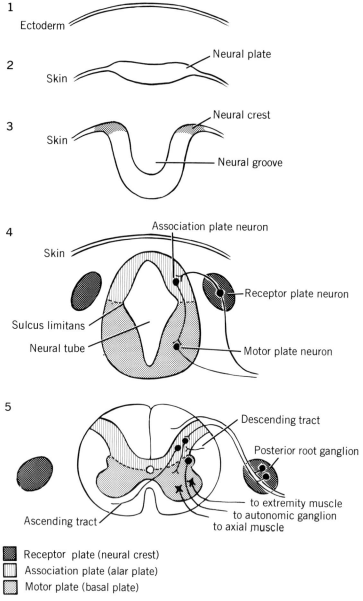

1

Ectoderm

2

Skin

Neural plate

3

Skin

Neural crest

Neural groove

4

Association plate neuron

Skin

Receptor plate neuron

Sulcus limitans

Neural tube

Motor plate neuron

5

Descending tract

Posterior root ganglion

to extremity muscle
to autonomic ganglion
to axial muscle

Ascending tract

▓ Receptor plate (neural crest)
▓ Association plate (alar plate)
▓ Motor plate (basal plate)

FIG. 2–3. Stages in the development of a spinal cord segment. Developmental and synaptic relationships between receptor, motor and association plates are shown.

low the tentorium (in the posterior fossa). The brain stem consists of the midbrain, which lies at the level of the tentorium (within the tentorial notch or incisura tentorii), and the hindbrain in the posterior fossa. The hindbrain is continuous with the spinal cord through the foramen magnum. Since the cerebellum is derived from the hindbrain, one can see even in the adult the persistence of the fundamental embryologic divisions of the nervous system: forebrain, midbrain, hindbrain and spinal cord.

When correlated with a few major neurologic structures, these major landmarks (incisura tentorii and foramen magnum) provide a basis for rapid localization of most

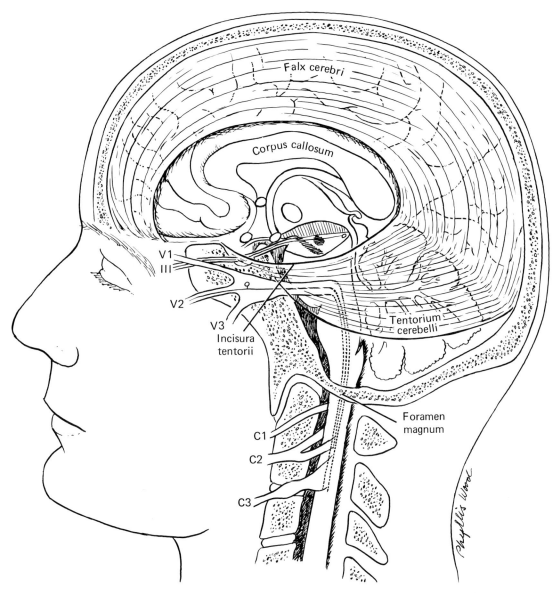

FIG. 2–4. Lateral view of the partially dissected skull and brain, showing the falx cerebri and tentorium cerebelli as dural folds and the foramen magnum bounded by its bony rim. The incisura tentorii and the oculomotor (III) and the trigeminal (V) cranial nerves are emphasized, especially the descending tract of the trigeminal nerve.

lesions depending on a few relatively simple patterns of sensory and motor deficits. These major neurologic structures are the oculomotor nerve (exiting from the midbrain at the level of the incisura tentorii), the trigeminal nerve (entering in the upper part of the hindbrain), the ascending spinothalamic tract (subserving pain and temperature sensation) and the descending corticospinal or pyramidal tract (subserving voluntary motor activity).

FOUR CLASSIC SYNDROMES PRODUCED BY DISEASE

The involvement of these major neurologic structures at various levels of the nervous system with diseases of any type produces

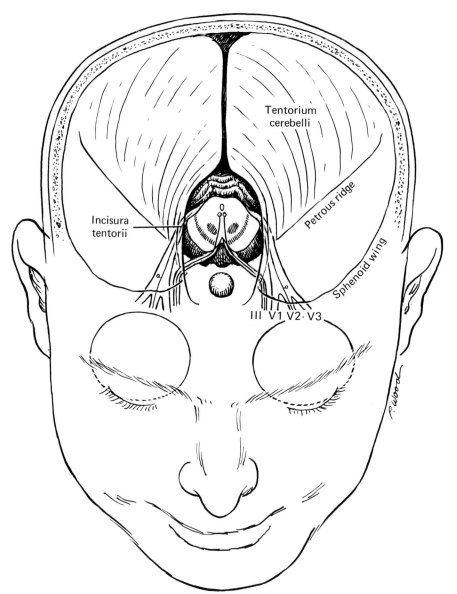

FIG. 2–5. Frontal view of the partially dissected skull and brain, showing the incisura tentorii surrounding the midbrain and separated from it by the subarachnoid space (cisterna ambiens).

one of four classic syndromes (Fig. 2–6): 1) the ordinary, predominantly motor hemiplegia characteristic of contralateral forebrain lesions involving cerebral cortex or internal capsule, 2) its midbrain variant with an added ipsilateral oculomotor palsy, 3) Wallenberg's syndrome with cruciate hemihypalgesia and dysfunction of one or more of the lower cranial nerves, and 4) Brown-

Sequard's syndrome of more or less complete hemisection of the spinal cord.

Although these syndromes rarely result from purely congenital malformations and have been classically defined in adults, they occur in varying degrees of completeness even in infants with acquired disease. Of course, the more developed the infant's nervous system before the disease starts, and

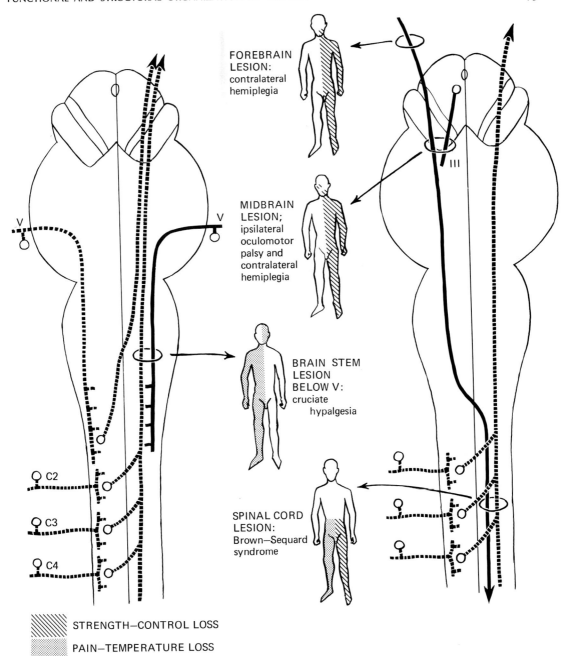

STRENGTH—CONTROL LOSS

PAIN—TEMPERATURE LOSS

FIG. 2–6. The sites of lesions responsible for the major clinical findings in the four classic neurologic syndromes. In addition to the labeled segmental nerves, note the descending corticospinal tract (solid line) and the ascending spinothalamic and trigeminothalamic tracts (interrupted lines).

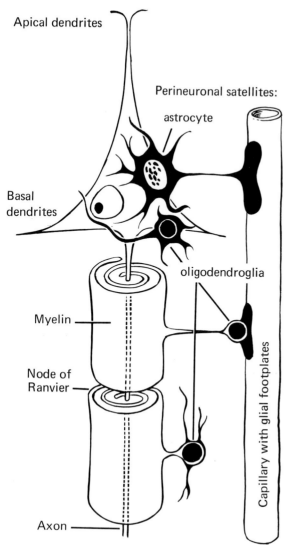

FIG. 2–7. Relationships between capillaries, glia (astrocytes and oligodendroglia) and neurons.

interconnections of the nervous system being by the nerve cells (neurons). Each neuron typically has many dendrites, a cell body receiving synaptic endings from other neurons and a single axon that may branch extensively to provide synaptic connections to other neurons. The neurons are supported physically and metabolically by interstitial cells (glia centrally, Schwann cells peripherally) and blood vessels (Fig. 2–7). Nerve fibers (axons) are the communicating links within and between segmental and suprasegmental elements.

Most of the nervous system develops from the ectoderm by the proliferation of cells in the midsagittal line to form the neural plate (Fig. 2–3). Continued proliferation transforms the plate into the neural groove, the sides of which are the neural folds, whose dorsal-most parts are the neural crests. This process, and the subsequent closure of the neural groove into a tubular structure, is referred to as neurulation and is further discussed in Chapters 4 and 5, where the exceptional development (*canalization* and *regression*) of the lumbar, sacral and coccygeal segments beneath the ectoderm will be described. The resultant neural tube provides the fundamental outline of the hollow adult CNS; *i.e.*, the brain and spinal cord develop from cells comprising the wall surrounding this primitive central canal or ventricle. Migrations of cells from the wall (ependymal zone) form two major parts of the CNS separated by a longitudinal sulcus limitans: 1) the dorsal, alar or association plate and 2) the ventral, basal or motor plate (Figs. 2–2 and 2–3). In addition, migrations of cells from the neural crests lead to discrete segmental ganglia comprising the third component of each neural segment, the receptor plate, whose peripheral dendrites end in specific sensory transducers (end organs) and whose central axons generally project upon and establish synaptic contacts with the cells of the segmental association plate (also known as secondary sensory or internuncial neurons).

As noted above, the association cells (Fig. 2–8) may either connect synaptically directly with cells of the motor plate of the same segment (intrasegmental fibers) or project to one or more of the three major expansions of the association plate known as the suprasegmental organs (forebrain, colliculi or tec-

the more rapid the onset of the disease process, the more typical will be the resulting syndrome. Finally, although analyzing variations of these themes constitutes one of the most interesting features of neurologic practice, one should not become lost in a maze of greater details (such as will shortly be presented) and misdiagnose any of these classic patterns due to treatable diseases.

COMPONENTS OF THE CNS

The nervous system contains neurons, glia and blood vessels, the major functional

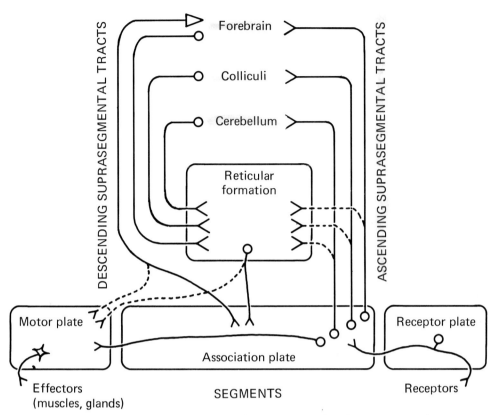

FIG. 2–8. Major interconnections of segmental, intersegmental and suprasegmental portions of the nervous system. (Adapted from Hausman, 1961)

tum and cerebellum). These suprasegmental organs make up over 90% of the bulk of the adult CNS. They are widely interconnected and project back down upon the segmental association plate for further modulation of the activity of the motor and association plate elements. In general, the long ascending and descending tracts connecting the segments and suprasegmental organs are known as afferent (ascending) and efferent (descending) suprasegmental tracts to and from each specific suprasegmental organ. Since there are three major suprasegmental organs, we may expect at least three such pairs of tracts for each segment, one afferent and efferent pair related to each of the three suprasegmental organs. Although the commonly used names may vary, one can expect to find one or more examples of *spinocerebellar* and *cerebellospinal* tracts, *spinocollicular* and *colliculospinal* tracts, and *spino-*

cerebral and *cerebrospinal* tracts, and corresponding tracts related to the brain stem segments. To anticipate what will eventually follow, these tracts do exist and are commonly known as spinocerebellar, dentatorubrospinal, spinotectal, tectospinal, spinothalamic and corticospinal tracts.

THE SEGMENTAL NERVOUS SYSTEM

Looked at as a rostrocaudal stack (Fig. 2–1), the brain stem and spinal segments correspond exactly to the body segments if one allows for the various migrations of cells which occur in embryogenesis. For simplicity and completeness, one may also allow for two rostral evaginations from the forebrain for the olfactory and visual systems to supplement the purely segmental nervous system, as follows:

Forebrain (FB): Cranial nerves I and II: olfactory and visual sensory and hypothalamic motor (control of autonomic and endocrine systems)

Midbrain (MB): Cranial nerves III and IV: intraocular and most extraocular muscles

Anterior hindbrain (AHB): Cranial nerve V: face sensation and jaw muscles

Middle hindbrain (MHB): Cranial nerves VI, VII and VIII: auditory, vestibular and taste sensations and facial muscles (plus lateral rectus muscle of the eye)

Posterior hindbrain (PHB): Cranial nerves IX, X and XII: respiratory, cardiovascular and gastrointestinal sensations and mouth, pharyngeal and laryngeal muscles

Cervical nerves I–IV, including Cranial nerve XI: neck sensory and motor functions, including the diaphragm

Cervical nerve V–Thoracic nerve I: upper extremity sensory and motor functions

Thoracic nerve I–Lumbar nerve II: chest and abdomen sensory and motor functions, sympathetics to the whole body

Lumbar nerve II–Sacral nerve II: lower extremity sensory and motor functions

Sacral nerves III–V: bladder, bowel and genital sensory and motor functions (including sacral parasympathetics)

This segmental arrangement permits a logical method of testing the intactness of sensory and motor functions of the body and of deducing the site of a lesion in the nervous system to account for deficits in or modifications of these functions. It should be obvious that without primary sensory or final motor units available for testing one cannot evaluate the association units, especially the suprasegmental organs and their connections with the segmental apparatus.

COMPONENTS OF THE SEGMENTAL NERVOUS SYSTEM

Each neural segment consists of three parts (Figs. 2–3 and 2–8): receptor, association and motor plates, and each of these plates is in turn composed of three parts.

The Receptor Plate

The receptor plate is composed of neurons whose cell bodies lie in discrete ganglia,

generally one to each side of each segment, lying outside the CNS and containing 3 sizes of neurons, small, medium and large. Their proportionately sized peripheral branches (dendrites) course in peripheral nerves and end as three types of sensory end organs: 1) free nerve nets, 2) expanded nerve tips amongst relatively simple encapsulating cells and 3) more complicated and encapsulated sensory elements that occur in various concentrations in localized regions of the skin, subcutaneous tissue, muscle and other deep tissues and organs. These end organs act as transducers for specific sensory stimuli (see below), and special sensory transducers exist for olfactory, visual, auditory, vestibular, taste, cardiopulmonary, chemical and pressure receptors. In general, each sensory neuron has a centrally directed axon, which enters the CNS though a dorsal root (or its equivalent in special situations). Each primary afferent axon branches centrally into rostral and caudal primary branches, from which secondary collaterals establish synaptic connections with the second-sensory (association) neurons.

Although there is still considerable argument about the specific functions of these three sizes of neurons, it is at least schematically simplest to consider that the small cells subserve pain and temperature sensations, the large cells subserve muscle spindle afferents, and the medium-size cells subserve a wide variety of other sensory (afferent) transducers and neural messages. In some segments of the brain stem special sensory systems are added (auditory, vestibular, taste, respiratory, cardiac and gastrointestinal), and two special sensory systems (olfactory and visual) directly enter the forebrain (a suprasegmental organ) without traversing any specific segment.

The Association Plate

Since each of the receptor plate elements projects upon the segmental association plate, we may expect each segment to have three such association nuclei (i.e., groups of related cells within the CNS receiving more or less specifically each of the three receptor plate elements).

PAIN-TEMPERATURE FIBERS. The small pain–temperature fibers (Fig. 2–9) project upon a laminated complex of three neuronal nuclei (*marginalis*, *gelatinosa* and *proprius*—layers 1, 2 and 3 of Rexed's scheme) in the posterior horn of the spinal cord and in the related caudal part of the similarly laminated nucleus of the descending (spinal) tract of the trigeminal nerve. These association plate cells are just beneath the primary sensory fibers that enter Lissauer's tract (in each of the spinal segments) and the spinal tract of the trigeminal nerve (for the brain stem segments). Intra- and intersegmental connections of these association plate elements with the motor plate establish polysynaptic flexor twitch and flexor withdrawal reflexes ipsilaterally and contralateral extensor reflexes for concomitant maintenance of posture while flexing the noxiously stimulated leg, for example.

MUSCLE SPINDLE FIBERS.   The large muscle spindle fibers (Fig. 2–10) in spinal segments project upon cells of *Clarke's nucleus* (in the thoracic segments) and of the *lateral cuneate nucleus* (comparable cells displaced rostrally into the posterior hindbrain region). Comparable fibers in the brain stem segments are still poorly identified, except for the mesencephalic trigeminal nucleus, which is the only example of a primary sensory neuron with its cell body located in the CNS, and even its association plate nucleus is still poorly identified. In addition, the large fibers send direct intrasegmental collaterals that project onto the motor plate for the monosynaptic stretch reflexes, so-called deep tendon reflexes (DTRs).

OTHER FIBERS.   The other medium-size fibers (Fig. 2–11) of spinal segments enter the posterior columns and bifurcate into primary rostral and caudal branches. From these branches secondary collaterals are given off to the neurons deep in the posterior horn, forming multisegmental association elements. In addition, many of the primary branches project upon their special association plate nuclei, the nuclei of the posterior columns (gracilis and cuneatus), which are rostrally displaced into the posterior hindbrain region. For the head, comparable trigeminal fibers project upon the main sensory trigeminal nucleus in the anterior hindbrain segment.

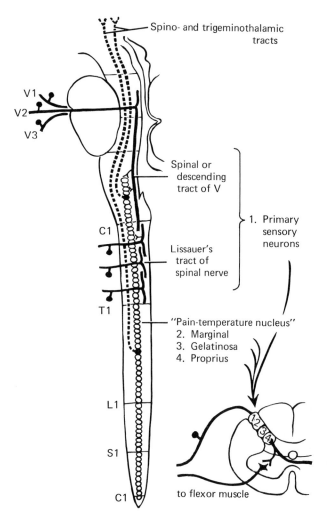

FIG. 2–9.   The small-fiber, pain–temperature system for cranial and spinal segments, with relays to the contralateral thalamus. Other primary sensory neurons in the seventh, ninth and tenth cranial nerves (not shown) join the spinal tract of the trigeminal, which thus subserves pain and temperature for the whole head.

SPECIAL SENSORY SYSTEMS.   The special sensory systems (Fig. 2–12) project upon special association plate nuclei: cochlear, vestibular and solitary in the middle and posterior hindbrain segments, and (for schematic completeness) olfactory and visual centers in the forebrain.

The Motor Plate

The motor plate is also composed of three types of cells, including voluntary motor,

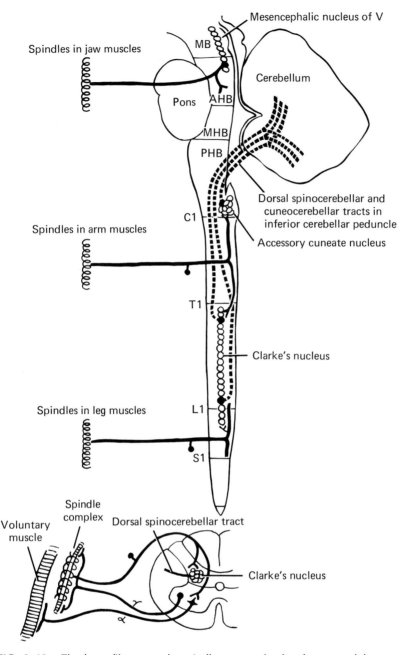

FIG. 2–10. The large-fiber, muscle–spindle system for head, arm and leg segments, with relays to the ipsilateral cerebellum.

autonomic and receptor plate regulators (Fig. 2–3).

VOLUNTARY ALPHA-MOTOR NEURONS. The voluntary alpha-motor neurons are the largest and most prominent anterior horn cells; they innervate skeletal muscles. Clus-

ters of these cells supply each muscle, but these clusters occur in two major groups: medial ones for axial muscles (paramedian, paravertebral and proximal shoulder and hip girdle muscles) and lateral ones for distal muscles (peripheral or lateral muscles, especially of the extremities). Within the brain stem segments, more or less comparable medial and lateral groups can also be easily recognized, subserving voluntary muscles in the head.

GAMMA-MOTOR NEURONS. Mingled within these clusters of large cells are small cells, gamma neurons, which send their axons out the ventral roots to supply the small muscle fibers regulating the sensitivity of the muscle spindles within the same muscle innervated by the alpha neurons. (At least one other such sensory regulator is well known in the middle hindbrain, the olivocochlear bundle, and others may exist.) It should be noted that efferent control of afferent messages is even more common centrally and is utilized almost every time one "pays attention" to some particular function, probably most often by inhibiting other messages.

AUTONOMIC NEURONS. The autonomic neurons generally have their cell bodies dorsolateral to the voluntary motor neurons and close to the primitive sulcus limitans. The small autonomic preganglionic axons leave the segments through ventral roots and end synaptically upon peripheral autonomic ganglia, whose still smaller and unmyelinated postganglionic axons project synaptically upon specific autonomic effector end organs: smooth muscles and glands. The autonomic nervous system (Fig. 2–13) is traditionally divided into thoracolumbar *sympathetic* and craniosacral *parasympathetic* components (this anatomic subdivision has other important histologic, functional and pharmacologic correlates that will be discussed later).

Although some texts include afferent neurons within the autonomic nervous system, everyone agrees that their cell bodies lie in dorsal root ganglia. It is, therefore, much simpler to regard these as more or less ordinary receptor plate elements that happen to utilize peripheral autonomic nerves (also carrying autonomic effector nerves) as the most economic way to carry afferent messages from the viscera and other autonomic end organs to the CNS. Thus the autonomic nervous system is considered as purely motor, subject to segmental and intersegmental reflex and suprasegmental controls just like the other components of the motor plate.

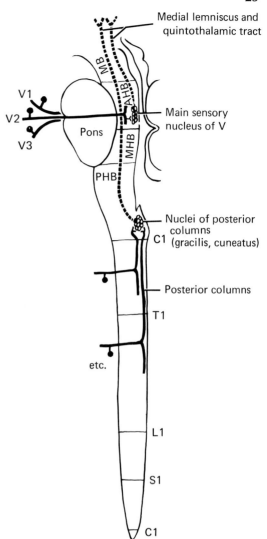

FIG. 2–11. The intermediate-size fiber, posterior column system for spinal (and corresponding cranial) segments with relays to the contralateral thalamus.

THE INTER- AND SUPRASEGMENTAL NERVOUS SYSTEM

The inter- and suprasegmental connections are quite complex, but can be divided into three parts: 1) major ascending suprasegmental *sensory* systems, 2) major descending suprasegmental *motor* systems and 3) miscellaneous intersegmental systems.

MAJOR ASCENDING SUPRASEGMENTAL SENSORY SYSTEMS

Three sizes of primary sensory (afferent) fibers end specifically upon their association

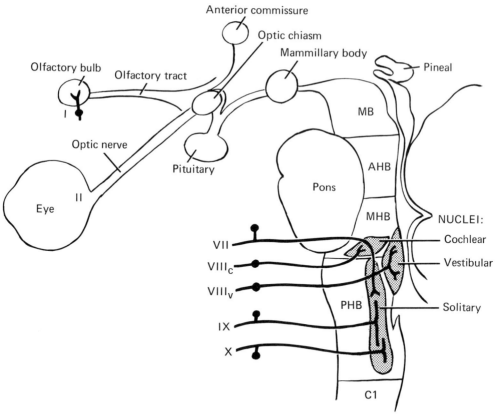

FIG. 2–12. Special sensory and association systems for olfactory, visual, auditory, vestibular and gustatory sensations and for certain medullary functions (chemo- and pressure receptors, respiratory stretch, gastric irritation) involving the solitary tract and nucleus.

plate nuclei. We can anticipate their major ascending suprasegmental tracts as follows.

THE SMALL FIBER SYSTEM. The small fiber system (Fig. 2–9) begins with the free nerve net and lightly encapsulated end organs responsive to painful (noxious, tissue-damaging) stimuli and to changes in temperature between the skin and subcutaneous blood vessels. Their centrally directed axons enter Lissauer's tract, then bifurcate into rostral and caudal primary branches running for a segment or two and giving secondary collaterals to the laminated nucleus of the posterior horn (or the equivalent spinal tract of the trigeminal nerve and its similarly laminated caudal nucleus). The deep cells of this nucleus (the nucleus proprius) not only give rise to axons that project to flexor motor neurons of the same and adjacent segments but also give rise to axons that cross the midline within a segment or two and ascend

in the ventrolateral quadrant of the spinal cord, through the brain stem to the forebrain. This spinothalamic tract (and the comparable crossed trigeminothalamic tract) is classically divided into lateral and ventral components, the former for pain and temperature and the latter for touch, but evidence obtained from cordotomies tends not to support this degree of segregation.

After synapsing on cells of the ventral posterior nucleus of the thalmus, the spinothalamic tract messages for pain and temperature may be relayed onto the sensory strip of the cerebral cortex (the postcentral gyrus, the anteriormost part of the parietal lobe), but opinions differ, and some investigators maintain that pain "reaches consciousness" at the thalamic level and does not project to the sensory cortex. It should be noted that secondary collaterals are given off the spinothalamic tract to the reticular formation in the brain stem and to the superior colliculus; indeed, perhaps only 10% of the spinothalamic tract fibers actually make it all the way to the thalamus. These secondary collaterals are important in establishing another route (the "extra lemniscal path") via the hypothalamus and medial thalamus to the frontal cortex.

THE LARGE FIBER SYSTEM. The large sensory fibers (Fig. 2–10) from the muscle spindles do not connect with association plate elements that project to the thalamus or cortex for conscious appreciation of muscle spindle stretch. Instead, in addition to the monosynaptic segmental reflex connection to alpha anterior horn cells innervating the same muscle and responsible for the DTR's, these large fibers end on cells of Clarke's nucleus in the thoracic spinal cord and on comparable cells of the lateral cuneate nucleus in the region of the medulla (posterior hindbrain). This pattern gives a single representation of leg segments in the caudal part of Clarke's nucleus and a double representation of arm segments in the rostral part of Clarke's nucleus and in the lateral cuneate nucleus. Clarke's nucleus gives rise to the large fibers of the dorsal spinocerebellar tract, which runs past the lateral cuneate nucleus, picks up comparable cuneocerebellar fibers and runs ipsilaterally into the cerebellum.

THE MEDIUM-SIZE FIBER SYSTEM. The medium-size primary sensory neurons (Fig. 2–11) have peripheral dendrites that innervate a variety of sensory end organs. Their centrally directed axons enter the spinal segments in the posterior columns. After entering, they branch into rostral and caudal primary branches, which extend at least several segments. From these secondary intersegmental systems, which probably function in various postural reflexes for standing and walking, fibers project onto segmental association cells that in turn project to the cerebellum as the ventral spinocerebellar tract (a bilateral primitive system that relays all types of sensory messages to the cerebellum).

A large part, if not the majority, of the posterior column fibers runs rostrally to end synaptically on the nuclei of the posterior columns (gracilis and cuneatus), which may be regarded as rostrally displaced segmental

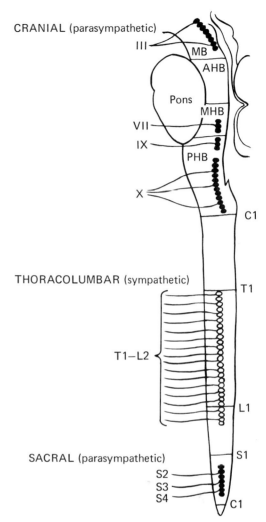

FIG. 2–13. Autonomic nervous system with thoracolumbar sympathetic and craniosacral parasympathetic preganglionic components. For simplicity, the autonomic ganglia, postganglionic axons and effector end-organs (blood vessels, other smooth muscles and glands) have been omitted.

association plate elements. The nuclei of the posterior columns give rise to fibers that cross almost immediately and ascend through the brain stem as the medial lemniscus. These fibers reach the thalamus, where they end synaptically on cells of the same ventral posterior nucleus (perhaps even on the same cells of this nucleus) as those of the spino- and trigeminothalamic tracts. Posterior column and medial lemniscus messages are then relayed onto the sensory cortex (postcentral gyrus).

lemniscus - a ribbon attached to a victor's wreath.

TABLE 2–1. SUMMARY OF PERIPHERAL NERVE FIBER SIZES

Afferents from muscle	Diameter (microns)	Afferents from skin
	20 20	
Spindle–IA		
	16 16	
Tendon–IB		
	12 12	Alpha–light punctate touch, hair movement
Flower spray, Vibration, Paccini–II		
	6 6	36 m/sec Delta-hair movement, pain, temperature
Pain, Joint movement, ligaments–III		
	1 1	
Pain–C = IV		C = 1m/sec (unmyelinated) touch, pain, temperature

It should be added that the comparable trigeminal system utilizes the main sensory trigeminal nucleus in the anterior hindbrain segment and the crossed quintothalamic tract to the ventral posterior nucleus of the thalamus. At the thalamic level, the face is represented medially, the arm and leg progressively laterally. At the cortical level, the face is represented laterally and inferiorly, the arm and leg progressively more superiorly and medially. Collaterals are given off the medial lemniscus and quintothalamic tract to the reticular formation and superior colliculus for the "extra lemniscal path" to the frontal pole via the hypothalamus and medial thalamus, as also described for the small fiber systems.

A summary of peripheral nerve fiber sizes correlated with their sources and probable functions is given in Table 2–1.

MAJOR DESCENDING SUPRASEGMENTAL MOTOR SYSTEMS

The alpha anterior horn cell is the final common path to the muscle fibers supplied by it (Fig. 2–10), and both neuron and fibers are known as the motor unit, since the neuromyal junction is generally sucessfully crossed by each nerve impulse. Repetitive stimulation of the alpha neuron leads to a fusion of single twitches into a relatively smooth tetanus and greater intensity of muscle contraction.

A wide variety of nerve fibers impinge synaptically on the alpha-motor neurons. Some of these derive from distant sources (e.g., suprasegmental organs) via long tracts (e.g., corticospinal, tectospinal, rubrospinal), some from shorter tracts (intersegmental connections of varying lengths—the longest being from the brain stem reticular formation and vestibular nucleus, shorter ones being from adjacent segments), but most from intrasegmental fibers derived from the association plate (plus some direct sensory plate fibers from the muscle spindles). Since most of the inter- and suprasegmental neurons end upon segmental association plate elements, it would appear that the anterior horn cell is most directly modulated (facilitated or inhibited) at the segmental level.

The Upper Motor Neurons

All of the descending fibers affecting the activity of the lower motor neuron are sometimes known as the *upper motor neurons,* and these are generally divided into *pyramidal* and *extrapyramidal* tracts.

THE PYRAMIDAL TRACT. The pyramidal tract specifically includes the 1,000,000 fibers passing through each pyramid of the medulla (posterior hindbrain). All of these fibers come from the cerebral cortex, most of them from the precentral (motor) cortex (only about 3% come from the Betz cells), but large numbers also come from the adjacent postcentral (sensory) cortex and premotor frontal and postsensory parietal cortex. Most of these pyramidal tract fibers cross at the caudal limit of the medulla (posterior hindbrain) and descend in the lateral white matter of the spinal cord near the posterior horn. The fibers from the sensory cortex end on cells in the posterior horn (nucleus proprius), and fibers from the motor cortex end both on cells of the association plate (intermediate between posterior and anterior horns) and on the anterior horn cells of the motor plate (this last type occurs only in primates and derives mostly from the largest fibers, probably originating from Betz cells).

Transection of the pyramidal tract in man produces an immediate hemiplegia that begins to improve in about ten days and progressively improves for about six months, after which very little detectable abnormality remains, perhaps only a Babinski sign and slight impairment of finger movements. It would appear that the pyramidal tract provides a small number of very large fibers as a relatively fast, direct connection to lower motor neurons, especially those responsible for individual, fast agile movements; in addition, a very large number of small fibers subserve other functions, probably modulation of afferent connections onto association neurons, for which adequate clinical tests have not yet been devised.

THE EXTRAPYRAMIDAL TRACTS. All of the other inter- and suprasegmental descending tracts pass through the medulla dorsal to the pyramids and can be called extrapyramidal. Probably the greatest number come from the brain stem reticular formation, upon which much of the cerebral cortex, deep cerebral nuclei (including the "basal ganglia" of telencephalic and diencephalic origin), colliculi and cerebellum project. Other long tracts include rubrospinal, tectospinal and vestibulospinal tracts. The rubrospinal tract runs laterally with the pyramidal tract but ends on the intermediate (association) gray; the vestibulospinal tract and other ventromedial tracts end upon both intermediate and anterior gray (i.e., upon both association and motor plates), but the detailed analysis is still far from complete.

The functions of these extrapyramidal tracts must be quite varied, but in general they appear to provide a variety of circuits which modulate the activity of the whole motor apparatus. Various degrees of increased muscle tone (i.e., rigidity, spasticity, dystonia) and of involuntary movements (e.g., tremors, tics, chorea, athetosis) characterize diseases of these various extrapyramidal systems.

The Gamma-Motor System

No consideration of the motor systems would be complete without discussing the gamma-motor fibers, which are known to receive descending suprasegmental and intersegmental impulses, especially from the vestibular nuclei, and which modulate the sensitivity of the muscle spindle. Since the large sensory fibers from the spindle are important sources of facilitation of voluntary alpha-motor neurons, one can easily see that stimulation of the gamma-system may reflexly excite the alpha-system (thus increasing the muscle contraction) and that transection of the dorsal roots decreases the excitability of the alpha-neurons by eliminating the potent spindle afferents.

MISCELLANEOUS INTERSEGMENTAL SYSTEMS

The reticular formation is the largest of the intersegmental systems (Fig. 2–8). Embryologically it may be considered a diffuse nerve net from which more-specialized segmental and suprasegmental structures develop. It has indistinct boundaries extending from the spinal cord to the thalamus. It includes most of the midbrain, pontine and medullary tegmentum, as well as the septal region, hypothalamus and those portions of the thalamus that do not project directly to the cortex (the nuclei of the midline, the intralaminar nuclei and the center median nucleus). It has been subdivided into a large number of nuclei but may be most simply described as those areas not recognized as major motor, sensory and association nuclei and tracts.

There are rich interconnections within the reticular formation. The dendrites of individual neurons encompass large areas with the axons covering either short or long distances. The fiber connections are extensive and complicated. In addition to the intrinsic connections, efferent fibers pass to the spinal cord, cerebellum and forebrain, including the substantia nigra, subthalamus, hypothalamus, septal region, pallidum and striatum. Afferents come from all these areas as well as from the cerebral cortex and all major sensory input systems. Reciprocal pathways relate the limbic system to the reticular formation.

The functions of the reticular formation may be subdivided into those related to 1) consciousness and affect and 2) motor and vegetative functions. Collaterals from all the ascending sensory systems (especially the trigeminal) contribute to the continuous background activity of the diffuse multisyn-

chorea - a dance

aptic system of reticular neurons projecting via the thalamus diffusely to all parts of the cortex and essential for that spectrum of behavior including various degrees of consciousness, wakefulness and alertness. Specific portions of the reticular formation play active roles in the induction and maintenance of *slow-wave* and *rapid eye movement* (REM) sleep. The oppositely directed, descending motor influences contribute highly organized patterns to relatively simple segmental and intersegmental reflexes, including postural tone, righting reflexes, gait and other alternating movements, respiration and vasomotor control and regulation of neuroendocrine functions. Particular areas of the hypothalamus relate to those visceral regulatory mechanisms that maintain the constancy of the internal environment (*e.g.*, water, electrolytes, temperature).

Certain diseases may transect the nervous system at various levels, thereby permitting the clinicophysiologic study of the separated rostral and caudal neural elements. In general, the rostral segments and suprasegmental organs will function more or less normally, consciously and voluntarily, considering the restriction of sensory inputs and motor outputs. When the transection involves the upper brain stem, one of the major difficulties is devising means of communicating with the severely restricted rostral CNS; *e.g.*, an electroencephalogram (EEG) with photic stimulation may be necessary to establish the intactness of the isolated forebrain. A pontomesencephalic transection allows wakefulness with eye movements (not laterally since the abducens cannot be innervated from the forebrain) and pupillary responses to light and near vision. Maintenance of consciousness, however, appears to require input from the trigeminal system (and pontine reticular formation). In general, the segments caudal to a transection will be severely restricted in their abilities; indeed, only reflexes will be observed, the complexity of which will depend directly upon the amount of reticular (intersegmental) formation available and functioning. Acute lesions produce *neural shock,* which frequently confuses the physician who then thinks the lesion is lower or more diffuse.

The reflexes commonly examined, in increasing order of complexity, include the following:

A. *Spinal*
   1. Segmental reflexes to muscle spindle stretch: the *Deep Tendon Reflexes* (DTR) of flexors and extensors.
   2. Segmental reflexes to pain: the flexor twitch reflex.
   3. Intersegmental reflexes to pain: the flexor withdrawal (and concomitant crossed extensor) reflexes.
   4. Intersegmental reflexes for maintenance of extensor posture: (anoxic necrosis may destroy the association interneurons that generally favor flexor reflexes, thus leading to spinal extensor tone).

B. *Brain stem*
   1. Intersegmental reflexes for vasomotor and respiratory control
      a. *Apneustic* respirations of medullary preparations (following transection near the pontomedullary junction) are so markedly ataxic that long pauses of a minute or so may occur during either inspiration or expiration, death usually occurring in one of the longer pauses.
      b. *Ataxic* respirations, with less dramatic pauses, occur with a little more pontine reticular formation functioning.
      c. *Cheyne Stokes* respirations are rhythmic but partially ataxic in their regularly varying amplitude. They appear to require still more pontomesencephalic reticular formation. Bilateral lesions in the lateral brain stem or basal ganglia commonly produce Cheyne Stokes respirations.
      d. *Central pontine hyperventilation* is not at all ataxic, and appears with bilateral lesions high in the medial reticular formation.
   2. Intersegmental reflexes for postural control
      a. Generalized flaccidity appears at pontomedullary transections but is also confusingly prominent in man even when a lot of the brain stem appears to be anatomically available (*cf.*, neural shock).

b. Extensor tone, *decerebrate* extensor posturing and tonic neck reflexes require the vestibular system plus a lot of the lateral reticular formation and are best seen in low mesencephalic transections.

c. *Decorticate* posturing (flexed upper extremities and extended lower extremities) is usually seen in man with lesions well below the cerebral cortex (since such extensive but also restricted lesions are rare), usually at or just above the midbrain.

THE SUPRASEGMENTAL NERVOUS SYSTEM

The three suprasegmental organs (cerebellum, colliculi and forebrain) are connected with each of the segments by long ascending (afferent, or sensory) and descending (efferent, or motor) fibers and are connected with each other in overlapping patterns that allow for simultaneous correlations between many systems, both at conscious and at subconscious levels.

THE CEREBELLUM

The embryologic development of the cerebellum, considered in detail in Chapter 10, can be seen as a relatively clear example of the amplification of a suprasegmental organ primarily in relation to the development of certain segmental association plate structures (Figs. 2–14 and 2–15). These segmental structures are the vestibular nuclei in the middle hindbrain (characteristic of stage I) and the trigeminal nuclei in the anterior hindbrain together with ascending spinocerebellar influences (comprising stage II). To these is added stage III, in which a third influence (the other suprasegmental organs, especially the forebrain) develops over these and other segmental association plate functions.

Since one of the major functions of the cerebellum is to coordinate smoothly all sensory and motor functions, it is pertinent to emphasize that there are important overlappings of these three stages of cerebellar development.

The cerebellum consists of cortex (molecular, Purkinje cell and granule cell layers), white matter and deep cerebellar nuclei. Except for olivocerebellar fibers, which are thought to end as climbing fibers around Purkinje cell dendrites, all cerebellar afferents (*i.e.*, fibers ascending to the cerebellar cortex) end synaptically as mossy fibers on granular cell dendrites. All cerebellar efferents (*i.e.*, fibers from the cerebellar cortex) are axons of Purkinje cells and (except for a few which pass directly to the vestibular nucleus) project to the deep cerebellar nuclei, which then project out of the cerebellum. The simplest path from the mossy endings of the ascending suprasegmental afferents involves excitatory synapses on the granule cell dendrites, thence granule cell excitatory axonal synapses on the dendrites of Purkinje cells or on the dendrites of basket cells, the axons of which then surround the soma of Purkinje cells and end as inhibitory synapses. Since the granule cell axon runs for several millimeters and excites several hundred Purkinje cells and many basket cells (each of which in turn inhibits a small central patch of about 50 Purkinje cells), the pattern of synaptic activity in the cerebellar cortex is in general a field of facilitation with a central focus of inhibition of Purkinje cells. Since the Purkinje axons end as inhibitory synapses on the deep cerebellar nuclei, this pattern is reversed with a central facilitatory and a peripheral zone of inhibition of a part of a deep cerebellar nucleus. Such a series of inhibitory synapses explains the reversal of effects observed on excising cerebellar cortex as compared to excising the deep cerebellar nucleus related to that cortex.

In general, these corticonuclear relationships occur in three parasagittal zones (Fig. 2–15a): *i.e.*, the vermis, paravermis and lateral cortex project respectively upon medial nuclei (roof or fastigial), intermediate nuclei (interpositus or globus and emboliform) and lateral (dentate) nuclei respectively. Most diagrams of the cerebellar cortex (including those of Figs. 2–14 and 2–15a) are grossly distorted since they represent only the cortex visible on the surface and ignore about seven times as much cortex which lies buried in the sulci. Braitenberg and Atwood[1] have provided an undistorted representation in Figure 2–15b, but it is obviously not useful for normal-sized texts. The total sur-

fastigial (fastigium) n. the gable end, pediment of a roof.

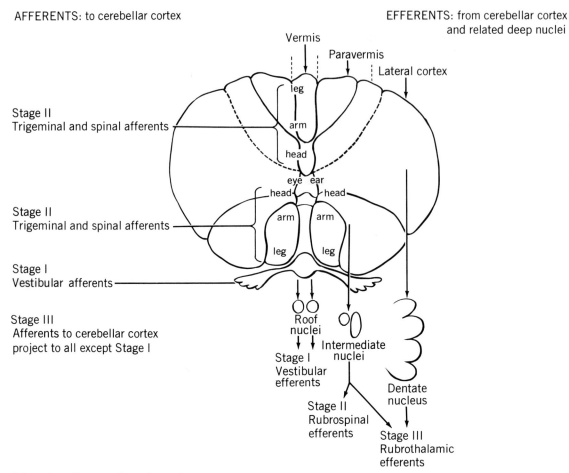

FIG. 2–14. Topographic relationships of the cerebellum. The three major stages of development have characteristic afferent and efferent neuronal systems involving predominantly horizontal and vertical cerebellar cortical areas, respectively.

face area of the cerebellar cortex is about 500 sq cm, which is one-fourth that of the cerebral cortex. There are so many cerebellar granule cells (10^{10}–10^{11}), however, that the total number of cerebellar and cerebral neurons is about the same.

At right angles to this parasagittal lamination of the efferents from the cerebellar cortex is the horizontal division into anterior, middle and posterior lobes and an approximately parallel horizontal lamination of the afferents to the cerebellar cortex. The anterior and posterior extremes of the cerebellar cortex touch each other (but are not otherwise connected) in the roof of the fourth ventricle, where the lingula and nodulus form the rostral and caudal edges of the roof.

The cerebellum is connected with the brain stem by four cerebellar peduncles (Fig. 2–16): 1) inner, 2) inferior, 3) middle and 4) superior. These are also known in most texts as the juxtarestiform body, restiform body, brachium pontis and brachium conjunctivum, respectively, but this is a needless polysyllabic terminology and only the last name serves any useful purpose in reminding one that the superior cerebellar peduncles cross in the midbrain like two conjoined arms.

THE COLLICULI (TECTUM)

The right and left superior and inferior colliculi are four small masses (corpora quadrigemina) forming a tectum (roof) over the

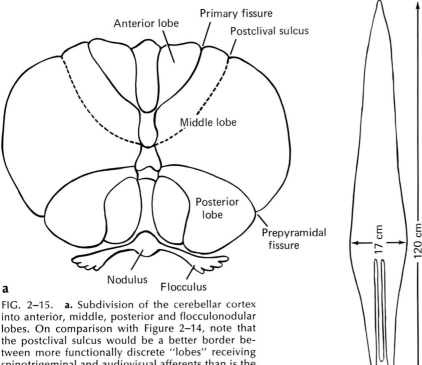

FIG. 2–15. **a.** Subdivision of the cerebellar cortex into anterior, middle, posterior and flocculonodular lobes. On comparison with Figure 2–14, note that the postclival sulcus would be a better border between more functionally discrete "lobes" receiving spinotrigeminal and audiovisual afferents than is the primary fissure between the anterior and middle lobes. **b.** Plane representation of the human cerebellar cortex with the width (17 cm) and the rostrocaudal length (120 cm) indicated in their true proportions of about 7:1. The difference between **a** and **b** is due to the large amount of cortex buried in the sulci. (Adapted from Braitenberg and Atwood, 1958)

aqueduct of Sylvius and overlying the third and fourth cranial nerve nuclei in the midbrain segment (Fig. 2–1). Each colliculus is connected with the forebrain by an arm (brachium). Although of great importance in lower animals, the colliculi are of relatively little clinical significance in man. They are discussed in detail in Chapter 11.

The inferior colliculus is a globular nucleus that receives ascending auditory fibers running in the lateral lemniscus from the cochlear nuclei (segmental association plate of the middle hindbrain) and from various other auditory nuclei in the course of these fibers: superior olive, nucleus of the trapezoid body and nuclei of the lateral lemniscus. The inferior colliculus projects to the thalamus (medial geniculate body), from which projections go to the auditory cortex in the temporal lobe (area 41, transverse gyrus of Heschl). Just what the inferior colliculus (and other nuclei) contribute to auditory messages is not clear, since at each nucleus units respond to a particular frequency of vibration at threshold and to an increasingly broad spectrum of frequencies on increasing the intensity of auditory stimulation. Presumably some of these nuclei participate in various auditory reflexes (*e.g.*, eyeblink to sound and the startle flexor reflex to sound) by establishing connections with the reticular formation and motor nuclei (*e.g.*, facial).

Parallel to the ascending fibers are descending fibers that end on a part of the superior olive. This part of the superior olive does not contribute to the ascending fibers of the lateral lemniscus but gives rise to the crossed olivocochlear bundle, which ends on the hair cells of the organ of Corti, the primary transducer converting mechanical vibrations to neural impulses. Stimulation of the olivocochlear bundle markedly inhibits the sensitivity of the hair cells and may be an important negative feedback mechanism.

The superior colliculus is a laminated

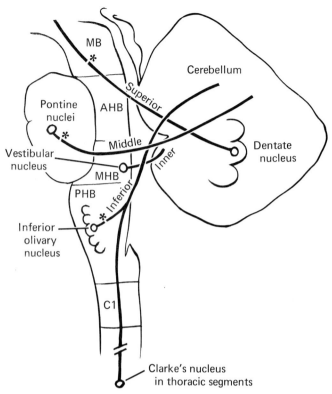

FIG. 2–16. Cerebellar peduncles: Inner (juxtarestiform body) for stage I; inferior and middle for most of the afferents for stages II and III, respectively; and superior for the efferents of stages II and III. Asterisks indicate crossings of tracts.

structure that receives visual and somato-sensory inputs (as well as related cerebral cortical inputs from sensory-motor and visual areas) and that projects both to the forebrain (hypothalamus) and to the segments (tectospinal and tectobulbar tracts). This pattern mimics the cerebellar pattern of reciprocal accessory connections between the segments and the forebrain and provides certain redundancies in the circuitry of the CNS.

Although classically regarded as a visual reflex center, current evidence indicates that the superior colliculus does not participate in conjugate gaze mechanisms. Rather, it appears to register the intensity of light: "cortically blind" people can discriminate between various intensities of light even though they cannot see them. In addition, it appears to function with the reticular formation in the rostral extralemniscal projection (via the hypothalamus, medial thalamus and frontal polar cortex) of emotionally charged components of pain (e.g., pain aggravated by worry and fear of cancer).

THE FOREBRAIN

The forebrain consists of two major embryologic expansions about the lateral ventricles (the telencephalon, see Chapters 15 and 16) and the third ventricle (the diencephalon, see Chapter 12; Figs. 2–1 and 2–2). Hollow protrusions from each of these contribute to the olfactory (telencephalic) and visual (diencephalic) systems, described in detail in Chapters 13 and 14. As the telencephalon expands laterally and posteriorly from the foramen of Monro, the floor of the telencephalic vesicle becomes fixed (as the lamina affixa) to the top of the diencephalon, so that this part of the diencephalon (the thalamus) acquires a secondary relationship also to the lateral ventricle. Just lateral to this lamina affixa, a deep nuclear mass (striatum) develops from the telencephalon and is split into two nuclei (caudate and putamen) by fibers of the internal capsule going to and from the telencephalic cortex. Argument persists concerning whether another deep nuclear mass (pallidum) originates in the diencephalon or telencephalon, but in either event it appears lateral to the internal capsule and adjacent to part of the striatum (putamen), forming the lenticular nucleus. Just medial to the lamina affixa, choroid plexus develops in the lateral ventricle; thus, the subarachnoid space of the great transverse fissure extends between the medial floors of the two lateral ventricles and above the roof of the third ventricle.

Perhaps the simplest approach to the forebrain would be to consider an analogy with the cerebellum, *i.e.,* to recognize the cerebral cortex, the cerebral white matter and the *deep cerebral nuclei.* The connections of the forebrain are more complex than those of the cerebellum, however; in addition to cerebral cortico-deep nuclear connections (similar to those of the cerebellum), there are long cerebral cortical efferent tracts bypassing the deep nuclei (corticopontine, corticoreticular, corticobulbar and corticospinal tracts) and extensive corticocortical connections between adjacent and distant, even contralateral, areas of cerebral cortex. Another major difference is that practically all of the cerebral cortical afferents (excepting only the olfactory) come from the deep nuclei (especially the thalamus, to which we have already noted that spinal and trigeminal somatosensory and cerebellar tracts project).

The Diencephalon

The diencephalon develops in four dorsoventral nuclear masses separated by sulci visible in the wall of the third ventricle. These are the epithalamus, dorsal thalamus, ventral thalamus and hypothalamus. The ventral thalamus migrates laterally to form parts of other thalamic nuclei and possibly the pallidum and subthalamic nucleus, thus leaving only three masses and two sulci visible from the third ventricle.

THE EPITHALAMUS. The epithalamus consists of the epithalamic striae (striae medullares thalami, serving as the attachment of the roof of the third ventricle), habenular ganglion and pineal body.

THE THALAMUS. The dorsal thalamus (or "thalamus" in most everyday usage) consists of three major mediolateral nuclear masses: medial, intralaminar and lateral. The geographic terminology of each is generally referred to the center median nucleus within the intralaminar complex, such that anterior, posterior, dorsal, ventral, medial and lateral are understandable in this three-dimensional frame of reference.

THE HYPOTHALAMUS. The hypothalamus may give rise to the pallidum and subthalamic nucleus, but in its mature pattern it is divided into medial and lateral portions in reference to the fornix that plunges into the hypothalamus just below the foramen of Monro on its way to the mammillary body.

fornix— an arch, a vault.

Diencephalic Systems

Within the diencephalon there develop several small areas (predominantly within the hypothalamus; Fig. 2–17) containing neurons that are sensitive to changes in humoral factors (water, sodium, blood volume, various hormones and blood temperature). These neurons respond either by the release of specific humoral factors from their axon terminals locally or by the activation of descending suprasegmental neural impulses directed at the segmental autonomic preganglionic neurons.

WATER BALANCE. The supraoptic and part of the paraventricular nucleus in the hypothalamus are rich in capillaries that are more permeable than most CNS blood vessels. The large neurons in these areas manufacture a protein carrier and vasopressin (an octapeptide with antidiuretic hormonal—ADH—effects). These travel down the axons to be stored at the axon terminals in the posterior pituitary (pars nervosa of the hypophysis). In response to decreasing water concentration of the blood (or to nonspecific stress) electrical impulses in these neurons stimulate the release of vasopressin into the capillaries of the posterior pituitary for circulation to the kidney, where cells in the distal part of the tubule are stimulated to reabsorb

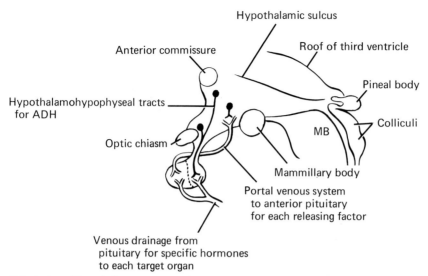

FIG. 2–17. Hypothalamus in sagittal section emphasizing neurosecretory functions related to anterior and posterior portions of the pituitary gland. *luteum - saffron yellow*

more water from the urine into the blood. This circuit restores water to the blood, thus maintaining water balance. (Oxytocin is also made by the cells of the supraoptic and paraventricular nuclei and similarly participates in uterine contraction during delivery of the baby and in "milk let down" during lactation.)

SODIUM BALANCE. The subcommissural organ, although anatomically a midbrain structure in the roof of the aqueduct of Sylvius, consists of modified ependymal cells that are said to secrete aldosterone-stimulating hormone in response to decreasing sodium concentration in the blood (or to decreasing blood volume). The hormone is carried to the adrenal medulla, where the cells of the zona glomerulosa secrete aldosterone. This is then carried to the kidney, where cells in the proximal part of the tubule are stimulated to reabsorb more sodium from the urine into the blood. This circuit restores sodium to the blood, thus maintaining sodium balance and blood volume by the concomitant osmotic drawing of water with the sodium.

ENDOCRINE BALANCE. Cells in the ventral region of the hypothalamus are responsive to various specific hormones (or nonspecific stress) and secrete specific releasing factors, which enter the adjacent capillaries and are carried by a short portal system of veins to capillaries in the anterior pituitary (adenohypophysis). From specific cells of the anterior pituitary specific tropic or stimulating hormones are secreted to be carried to the specific endocrine target glands: thyroid (TH), adrenal cortex (ACTH), ovarian corpus luteum (LH), ovarian follicle (FSH), gonads (GTH), growing tissues (GH), melanophores (MSH). From each of these target cells other specific hormones, steroids or other biologically active compounds may be secreted to influence still more distal cells and to feed back onto the hypothalamus and anterior pituitary in complex neuroendocrine circuits that maintain most of the endocrines in balance.

THE PINEAL BODY. The pineal body also contains capillaries that are more permeable than most CNS vessels. It stores serotonin and melatonin, but just how these potent chemicals are released for normal body functions is not known. The pineal cells, at least in animals such as the rat, show a diurnal pattern of activity controlled by postganglionic sympathetic and parasympathetic nerves that enter the pineal from the adjacent tentorium (via conary nerves) and are affected indirectly by light via the hypothalamus, descending central suprasegmental autonomic tracts and ascending peripheral sympathetic fibers (whose postganglionic cells lie in the superior cervical ganglion). No comparable information is available in man.

TEMPERATURE CONTROL. Cells within the anterior hypothalamus are sensitive to increasing blood temperature and respond by sending neural impulses down suprasegmental autonomic tracts to activate segmental preganglionic autonomic neurons for sweating (evaporation of fluid cools the surface of the skin), vasodilation (inhibition of vasoconstriction) at the surface (bringing more blood to the surface for cooling), and in hairy animals panting and inhibition of pilo-erection. When these cells are destroyed (as in subarachnoid hemorrhage, trauma, tumor), heat-loss mechanisms are impaired and body temperature rises to levels that may be fatal by coagulation of proteins (107° F, 42° C).

Cells within the posterior hypothalamus are sensitive to decreasing blood temperature and respond with opposite effects: peripheral vasoconstriction, pilo-erection (to increase the immediate environmental insulation), increased muscular activity, inhibition of sweating—all designed to conserve or increase body heat. Infections by many bacteria, viruses and other microorganisms stimulate the release of endogenous pyrogen from leucocytes, and the pyrogen affects the cells of the hypothalamus to conserve body heat, the body temperature rising to produce fever. Such fever of most infections tends not to exceed 103° F (40° C).

Thalamic Relay Systems

Also within the diencephalon are groups of cells that make up the various nuclei of the thalamus. In general, cells of the thalamus are in two-way connections related to particular parts of the cerebral cortex. In addition, many of the thalamic nuclei relay onto the cerebral cortex neural messages arriving over particular long tracts: cerebellar (dentatorubrothalamic tract) to the nucleus ventralis lateralis (VL) and thence to precentral motor and premotor cortex (areas 4 and 6); somatosensory (spino-, trigemino- and quintothalamic tracts and medial lemniscus) to the nucleus ventralis posteriorus

(VP) and thence to postcentral somatosensory cortex (areas 3, 1 and 2); auditory (brachium of inferior colliculus) to the medial geniculate nucleus (MG) and thence to temporal auditory cortex (area 41); and visual (optic nerve, chiasm and tract from retina) to the lateral geniculate nucleus (LG) and thence to occipital visual cortex (area 17). Another similar relay already mentioned, the extralemniscal pain pathway, involves a chain of neurons from the reticular formation and superior colliculus to the hypothalamus, medial thalamus and anterior frontal lobe cortex (areas 8, 10 and 12).

Another relay is peculiar to the forebrain and completes the circuit of the limbic lobe: afferents from paralimbic cortex (primary olfactory and medial parts of frontal, parietal, occipital and temporal lobes) converge on the cingulate gyrus and hippocampal gyrus (parahippocampus), the two major gyri of the limbic lobe. Cingulate gyrus efferents form the cingulum, a bundle of fibers sweeping in a posterior descending loop deep to the cingulate gyrus and hippocampal gyrus, which also contributes fibers to the cingulum. The cingulum ends on cells of the parahippocampus, which then projects to the dentate gyrus and hippocampus, whose large pyramidal cells give rise to the fibers of the fornix. The fornix spirals successively posteriorly, superiorly, anteriorly and finally inferiorly, forming the roof and anterior edge of the foramen of Monro before it penetrates the hypothalamus and ends in the mammillary body. The mammillothalamic tract then projects to the anterior nucleus of the thalamus, from which fibers then project back to the cingulate gyrus, thus completing the limbic loop. In addition, the two sides are connected together by fibers of the fornix that cross in the hippocampal commissure (psalterium) to join the right and left hippocampi.

Ways out of this limbic circuit, which has been implicated in memory and emotions, are not so numerous as ways into it, but include fornix connections to other hypothalamic nuclei and mammillotegmental fibers to the reticular formation. Because of the paucity of ways out, reverberating circuits can occur within the limbic system, as in cases of psychomotor epilepsy. In such cases relatively little effect may be seen on immediate conscious sensations or behavior

psalterium - a stringed instrument.

or even on the ordinary EEG's of electrical activity of most of the cerebral cortex, but recent memories fail to be recorded and high voltage electrical activity can be recorded rather selectively from the limbic system for peroids lasting anywhere from minutes to hours.

Other relays from other deep cerebral nuclei via the thalamus to the cortex or to other deep nuclei are favorites of the diagram-makers, but when all is said and done almost everything is connected to almost everything else and back to itself! In general, one can find short and long neural loops that could through extrapyramidal tracts modulate motor (and sensory) activity initiated and maintained through pyramidal (and extrapyramidal) tracts. Emphasis has traditionally been upon modulation of motor activity, and especially upon abnormalities of such modulation as are seen in "diseases of the basal ganglia and extrapyramidal system." These diseases include Parkinsonism (regular rhythmic tremor at rest, lead pipe or cogwheel rigidity depending on how much the increased tone is interrupted by the tremor, and bradykinesia or slowness in initiating movements) and a spectrum of nonrhythmic movements and increased tone ranging from ballism and chorea through athetosis to dystonic movements and dystonic postures. In most of these disorders a more normal balance of power can be obtained by the destruction of one or another of the deep cerebral nuclei, especially the ventralis lateralis (VL) in the thalamus. Since the VL plays back most immediately upon the motor and premotor cortex, from which a large part of the pyramidal and extrapyramidal systems originate, one can visualize the surgical destruction of an important cortical afferent in terms of removing a disease-induced hyperactivity of the VL— and one can speculate that various diseases themselves destroy other components that tend to inhibit the VL.

Among the larger extrapyramidal loops are the corticopontocerebellar and deep nuclear–central tegmental tract–inferior olivary circuits described with stage III of the cerebellum and feeding back directly upon the VL by way of the dentatorubrothalamic fibers. Another major system involves cerebral cortex, striatum and pallidum with the VL and other deep nuclei (*e.g.,* hypo-thalamus, subthalamus, substantia nigra). But pretty soon we will be falling into the trap of making more and more diagrams! The commonly observed lesions (in the striatum in chorea, in the subthalamus in ballism, in the substantia nigra in Parkinsonism and in the thalamus in athetosis) probably only represent the tip of the iceberg, with more diffuse lesions being overlooked, especially in the cerebellum and cerebral cortex.

It seems quite likely that the destruction of at least some of the extrapyramidal systems along with the pyramidal tract accounts for the spasticity and relative permanence of *capsular hemiplegia.* Although little has been done experimentally, it seems possible that an additional lesion in an appropriate part of the extrapyramidal systems might restore a more normal balance to the almost completely reversible *pure pyramidal hemiplegia.*

The Telencephalon

Within the telencephalon the deep nuclei (striatum) and the limbic lobe have been briefly considered above. We should now consider some of the features of the rest of the telencephalon, *i.e.,* the cerebral cortex (pallium) and white matter.

DEVELOPMENT. In contrast to some organs, such as the heart and the liver, which tend to enlarge parallel to general bodily development, the brain (especially its telencephalon) grows most rapidly just before and after birth (see Chapter 3). From 350 g at birth it increases to 1000 g by 18 months of age and practically reaches the adult's 1300 g by 3 years. A gradual decrease occurs after age 25. The gray matter constitutes about 40% of the forebrain and the white matter 60%. The gray matter contains more water and less lipid than the white. The area of the cerebral cortex is approximately 2.5 sq ft (1111 sq cm) on each side, only one-third of which is visible on the surface. There are about 2.6×10^9 cortical neurons.[5]

THE CEREBRAL CORTEX. There is considerable histologic variation in the neuronal components of the layers of the cerebral cortex from one region to another. In general, however, there is activation of a vertical column of neurons by afferent fibers that end synaptically on small neurons (granule cells) in the middle of the cortex (layer 4). From here vertical association elements, especially the superficial granule and small pyramidal cells of layers 2 and 3, provide synaptic connections onto the deep layers of large pyramidal and other neurons of layers 5 and 6, which provide efferent fibers out of the cortex. In general, there are only two ways into the cerebral cortex (from the thalamus and from other cortex) and only two ways out of the cerebral cortex ("pyramidal" via corticosegmental, corticobulbar, corticospinal tracts and "extrapyramidal" via many tracts from the deep cerebral nuclei, other cerebral cortex and the reticular formation).

Characteristic areas that can be relatively easily identified grossly and microscopically include basal olfactory cortex, hippocampal formation, precental motor cortex (with Betz cells) and visual cortex (with the line of Gennari). Some of Brodmann's numerical areas recur in neurologic conversations: the precentral motor strip (area 4) and premotor cortex (area 6), the postcentral sensory gyrus (areas 3, 1 and 2), the frontal eye field (area 8), the pericalcarine primary visual cortex (area 17) and the temporal primary auditory cortex (area 41). The sensory-motor representation of the body in the *central lobe* (comprising adjacent parts of the more classic frontal and parietal lobes) can be recalled by imagining a person hanging upside down with his leg superiormedially and his face inferior-laterally. The localization of focal epileptic seizures or of focal neurologic deficits takes advantage of the relatively wide separation of these areas in the cerebral cortex as contrasted with their concentration in the internal capsule, brain stem and spinal cord.

DISEASES LOCALIZING IN THE TELENCEPHALON. Since the telencephalon makes up so much of the CNS, it is to be expected that its diseases are the most numerous. It is subject to all the bacterial infections (abscesses, tuberculoma), demyelinating diseases (multiple sclerosis, diffuse sclerosis), vascular diseases (infarcts, hemorrhages), trauma (laceration, contusion) and gliomas (astrocytoma, glioblastoma multiforme) that affect parts of the CNS approximately in proportion to the mass (number of neurons, glia, vessels). In addition, its specialized and complex development subject it to many other diseases that localize more or less specifically in the cerebral cortex and white matter: many infections due to viruses (herpes simplex, rabies, kuru, subacute sclerosing panencephalitis, progressive multifocal leucoencephalopathy and Jakob–Creutzfeldt) or spirochetes (general paresis), many metabolic and toxic diseases (anoxia, hypoglycemia, lipidoses) and many degenerative diseases (the senile and presenile dementias of Alzheimer and Pick). Although most of these diseases occur rather rarely in the immature brain, they must at least be mentioned to provide a frame of reference for the common neurologic entities. Reactions characteristically occurring in the immature brain will be the subject of the rest of this book.

REFERENCES

1. Braitenberg V, Atwood RP: Morphological observations on the cerebellar cortex. J Comp Neurol 109:1–33, 1958
2. Hausman L: Atlas III, Illustrations of the Nervous System. Springfield, CC Thomas, 1961
3. Meyer A, Hausman L: A reconstruction course in the functional anatomy of the nervous system. Arch Neurol Psychiatr 7:287–310, 1922
4. Meyer A, Hausman L. The forebrain: A study and reconstruction based on the method outlined by the authors. Arch Neurol Psychiatr 19:573–593, 1928
5. Pakkenberg H: The number of nerve cells in the cerebral cortex of man. J Comp Neurol 128: 17–20, 1967
6. Streeter GL: Developmental horizons in human embryos. Description of age groups XV, XVI, XVII and XVIII, being the third issue of a survey of the Carnegie collection. Contrib Embryol 32: 133–203, 1948

chapter 3

CELLULAR KINETICS, MYELINATION AND PATTERNS OF GROWTH OF THE NERVOUS SYSTEM

As described in Chapter 2 in general terms, the nervous system starts as a single layer of neuroepithelial germinal cells on the dorsal surface of the developing embryo. More specific information concerning the mechanisms involved in their further differentiation has become available over the past twenty years as new techniques have been developed and refined. Although most of this information has been derived from experimental work on animals, it seems quite likely that fundamentally similar mechanisms of embryonic cellular kinetics exist in the early stages of the development of the human nervous system. These will be described first. Since the later stages of embryonic and fetal growth become increasingly species-specific, we will conclude this chapter by reviewing the rates of myelination of different tracts and certain patterns of growth of the human nervous system, including the weights of various parts.

EMBRYONIC CELLULAR KINETICS

The classic division of the early neural tube into ependymal, mantle and marginal layers was until recently considered of fundamental importance in the cellular kinetics of differentiation of neurons and glia. However, since practically all cell division occurs in the ependymal layer, it is more accurate to refer to the ependymal layer as the germinal layer. Furthermore, since the daughter cells migrate radially, first as neurons and later as glia, it is now apparent that the mantle and marginal layers must be relegated to grosser regions of the developing neural tube.

THE EPENDYMAL, OR GERMINAL, LAYER

It had long been known that cells undergoing mitosis were only found adjacent to the lumen of the neural tube, and it was suspected that one daughter cell remained there to further divide while the other migrated out to differentiate into a neuroblast in the mantle layer. Sauer[25, 26, 27, 28] accurately described, on the basis of purely morphologic observations, that the wall of the early neural tube was composed entirely of germinal cells arranged in a pseudostratified epithelium whose nuclei were moving through the cytoplasm radially, peripherally and then centrally, repeating this to-and-fro cycle many times. Near the lumen of the neural tube, the nucleus underwent mitosis, and the nuclei of the resultant daughter cells then migrated back toward the periphery. Later, both nuclei returned toward the lumen to divide again, the to-and-fro cycle repeating many times.

The concept of interkinetic germinal cell migration was generally disregarded until studies in the 1950s and 1960s both confirmed and extended it. Recent reviews by Watterston,[35] Sidman[31] and Jacobson[14] provide readable, well-documented summaries on the kinetics of these germinal cells. Two types of experiments provided the proof.

1. *Mitotic inhibition:* Watterston *et al.*[35, 36] applied colchicine (which blocks mitosis at metaphase) to early neural tubes in chick embryos. Initially, a single layer of arrested mitotic figures was seen at the surface of the lumen and none in the periphery. With time, additional layers of cells which were arrested at metaphase began to accumulate near the lumen, thus indicating that more than just the germinal cells along the lumen were involved in the mitotic process.
2. *Radioautographs of labeled DNA:* Beginning with the studies of Sauer and Walker[29] and Sidman *et al.*[32] numerous experiments[1, 10, 14, 19, 21, 23, 35] have clearly documented the interkinetic germinal cell migration. The basic technique used in these studies was pulse-labeling of the neuroepithelial germinal cells with tritiated thymidine (thymidine-H[3]) at varying stages of development. Initially, the labeled nuclei (which incorporate the thymidine for DNA synthesis) are found only in the peripheral layer. With time, they are seen to move toward the lumen and divide, and with more time, the resultant daughter cell nuclei move back to the periphery of the neural tube. From these observations, specific phases of the cell cycle have been defined.

PHASES OF THE CELL CYCLE

Sidman[31] has designated the various phases of the interkinetic germinal cell cycle as follows:

M phase: The period of mitosis of a given population of nuclei located on the luminal surface of the neural tube. No incorporation of thymidine occurs.

G1 phase: The first gap phase, when the daughter nuclei of a given population are moving back to the periphery of the neural tube. Some early incorporation of thymidine takes place.

S phase: The period when the most synthesis of DNA and the most incorporation of thymidine occur in nuclei located in the peripheral layer.

G2 phase: The second gap phase, when nuclei are moving from the periphery toward the lumen. Some thymidine is incorporated and some DNA synthesized during this period.

Depending on the species, the region of the neural tube and the gestational age when the cells are labeled, there are varying *generation times*, defined as the time required for one complete cycle.[14] In general, the earlier in gestation, the shorter the generation time. For example, the neural tube of the mouse at 10 days has an 8-1/2 hour cycle, and at 11 days, its cycle is from 10-1/2 to 11 hours. The subependymal glioblasts of the neonatal mouse have a generation time of 65 hours, whereas the cerebellar glioblasts of the mouse at from 1 to 3 days postnatally have a generation time of 120 hours.

THE MANTLE LAYER

The mantle layer is formed shortly after closure of the neural tube, just after some of the germinal cells differentiate into neuroblasts. These neuroblasts have a large round nucleus, a dark nucleolus and a pale cytoplasm. Their inability to synthesize DNA also distinguishes them from germinal cells.[19] In order to understand the possible mechanisms by which these cells detach from the lumen, one must first recognize that the original pseudostratified germinal cells are attached to each other by terminal bars affixed as a protein frame around each cell at its luminal end. At the time of mitosis, providing that the cleavage furrow during metaphase is perpendicular to the lumen, each daughter cell receives one-half of the maternal terminal bar, and the two daughter cells remain attached to each other. Although there are conflicting observations, it seems that prior to closure of the neural tube all such cleavage furrows are perpendicular to the lumen, whereas after closure of the tube some are parallel, thus leaving the outermost daughter cell unattached to the luminal surface.[19-21] In this manner, the outermost daughter cell is free to migrate out of the ependymal zone and become a neuroblast in the formation of the mantle zone.

Not only neuroblasts are derived from the germinal cells, glioblasts also develop by a similar mechanism. It is not yet clear whether the original germinal cell can give rise to both neuroblasts and glioblasts, whether the original glioblast can subsequently differentiate into both astrocytes and oligodendrocytes, or whether all three cell types have separate cell lines.[14] It is generally agreed that microglia are derived from the mesoderm, predominantly from leucocytes in the bone marrow, and that they migrate into the CNS by way of blood vessels. There is still disagreement about the length of time that the microglia persist in the normal nervous system, but there is general agreement that about two-thirds of the phagocytic cells that react in various inflammatory or traumatic states enter promptly from the circulating blood. Recent studies by Vaughn and Pease[34] indicate that adventitial cells or multipotential neuroglial cells derived from neuroectoderm may account for the other one-third of these phagocytic cells; indeed, in situations such as Wallerian degeneration, without inflammation or vascular injury these multipotential neuroglia may predominate.

Around the ventricular cavities, a zone of proliferating cells, termed the subependymal zone, is found to exist between the germinal (ependymal) layer and the mantle layer. The cells within the subependymal zone have the capacity to divide, but they do not seem to have the same interkinetic migrations seen in the original germinal cells. Although the fate of the cells derived from the subependymal zone is not entirely clear, at least some of them give rise to small neurons.

Jacobson[14] believes that the many studies of interkinetic cell migrations have shown several features to be common to all regions of the brain: 1) There is a spatial gradient such that the cells originate in an inside-out sequence. 2) There is a temporal gradient such that the rostral portion develops before the caudal. 3) There are differences in the time of origin of the different types of neurons such that the large ones are produced before the small ones. For example, the large neurons are formed first in the spinal cord; the Purkinje cells are formed before the basket and stellate cells in the cerebellum; and the pyramidal cells are formed first and the granule cells later in the cerebral cortex.

Nearly all of the radioautographic studies have been carried out in subhuman species, but Rakic and Sidman,[23] utilizing thymidine-H[3], showed that an 18-1/2-week-old human fetus was similar to the mouse (17th gestational day) with respect to the germinal cells and cells derived from them. Their study included descriptions of these cells in the lateral ventricles, cerebral cortex, olfactory bulb, third ventricle, cerebral aqueduct and cerebellum.

MYELINATION

THE MARGINAL LAYER

One large component of the developing CNS is the marginal layer, which consists of axons and glial cells that eventually make up the white matter of the CNS. Most axons become myelinated. The myelin in the CNS is formed from oligodendrocytes, and that in the peripheral nervous system from Schwann cells.[14]

The Schwann cells are generally considered to be derived from neural crest cells that migrate out along the axons of the peripheral nerves. The Schwann cells attach to the axons in a proximal-distal manner, and after attachment are capable of mitotic division. The proliferation of these Schwann cells continues as long as the axon grows in length, but proliferation ceases once a Schwann cell begins to form myelin by wrapping its cytoplasm in jelly roll fashion around the axon. Although the earliest wrappings are visible by electron microscopy, myelin is not recognized by light microscopy until about seven lamellae have formed. Whether or not a Schwann cell forms myelin is apparently determined by the size of the axon. All axons become surrounded by Schwann cell cytoplasm, but the smallest peripheral nerve fibers never become myelinated; i.e., they are embedded in Schwann cell cytoplasm visible by electron microscopy, but not repetitively wrapped by Schwann cell membrane.

The CNS myelin is formed by oligodendrocytes. In contrast to the Schwann cell, only one of which wraps one segment of a peripheral axon, a single oligodendrocyte myelinates more than one central axon. Thus, in this feature, an oligodendrocyte is similar to a peripheral non-myelin-forming Schwann cell, which is related to many unmyelinated peripheral axons; but in actual electron microscopic observations this feature is extremely difficult to prove since the attachments of the lamellae of myelin to the perinuclear cytoplasm of the oligodendrocyte are very delicate and generally not in the plane of section. In contrast to peripheral nerves, the mature central white matter has no unmyelinated axons. Prior to the formation of myelin in a particular region of the CNS, there is an intense proliferation of oligodendrocytes (this process has been termed myelination gliosis, which is a poor designation, since gliosis usually implies a pathologic rather than a normal process, and since the normal myelination gliosis has been confused with the abnormal glial fatty metamorphosis, one of the reactions of the premyelin glia to metabolic stress and other injuries, as discussed in Chapter 16). Myelination is also preceded by an increase in vascularization in that area.[14]

The formation of the marginal layer is a relatively late event. Malínský and Malínská[19] identified the earliest myelin in the human spinal cord between 75- and 105-mm CR length by electron microscopy and between 105- and 145-mm CR length by light microscopy. Not only does myelination begin later than many other aspects of neural differentiation, it also continues for a longer period of time, in many cases into the second decade of life and in some cases even longer.[37] It is obviously difficult to define when a process such as myelination actually ends; the CNS tracts are generally not homogeneous, and the best criterion would be the number of lamellae in each myelin sheath defined electron microscopically. Since the human in particular is not available for adequate fixation for electron microscopy, it will probably be some time before we have adequate human data. Figures 3-1 and 3-2 provide examples of the timing of myelination of some tracts in the human CNS as defined by light microscopy. Figure 3-3 provides data more closely approximating the actual onset of myelination as defined by electron microscopy.[3, 4, 5, 8, 9, 11, 12, 16, 22] The considerable differences in time between Figures 3-1 and 3-3 relate to the fact that 7-10 lamellae are required for resolution by light microscopy.[24, 30] Some of the variability in the results reported may relate to the level actually studied, since Friede and Hu[9] noted a striking proximodistal

difference in development of myelin in the human optic nerves and tracts.

PATTERNS OF GROWTH AND DEGENERATION OF THE NERVOUS SYSTEM

The original germinal cellular differentiation and the later myelination of the CNS eventually result in a large increase in overall size. The weight of the brain and its major components is easily measured and can provide preliminary information about underlying diseases. Table 3-1 and Figures 3-4 to 3-6 provide data correlating brain weight with prenatal[7, 13, 15, 17, 33] and postnatal[2, 6, 17] ages.

Considerable information is available concerning the pyramidal (corticospinal) tract. It originates from a large area of cerebral cortex, both frontal and parietal (including all of areas 1-8 of Brodmann) and continues to enlarge in cross-sectional area until about 30 years of age (Fig. 3-7). Following destruction of its cells or fibers at any level rostral to the medulla, a major part of its Wallerian degeneration can be followed as sudanophilic lipids (cholesterol esters) appear and are subsequently absorbed. The rates of appearance and disappearance of these lipids are much more rapid in the immature CNS (Fig. 3-8) than in the adult (Fig. 3-9), indeed approaching the rates observed in peripheral nerves.

TABLE 3-1. WEIGHTS OF CEREBRUM AND BRAIN STEM (INCLUDING CEREBELLUM, MIDBRAIN, PONS AND MEDULLA) DURING THE FETAL PERIOD*

CH length (mm)	Weights (g)	
	Cerebrum	Brain stem
100-150	5.7	.82
150-200	12.4	1.22
200-250	29.7	2.34
250-300	44.9	2.95
300-350	80.0	5.07
350-400	132.8	9.4
400-450	191.5	14.2
450-500	287.2	25.7
500-550	345.8	29.9

* Modified from Table 41, Dunn.[7]

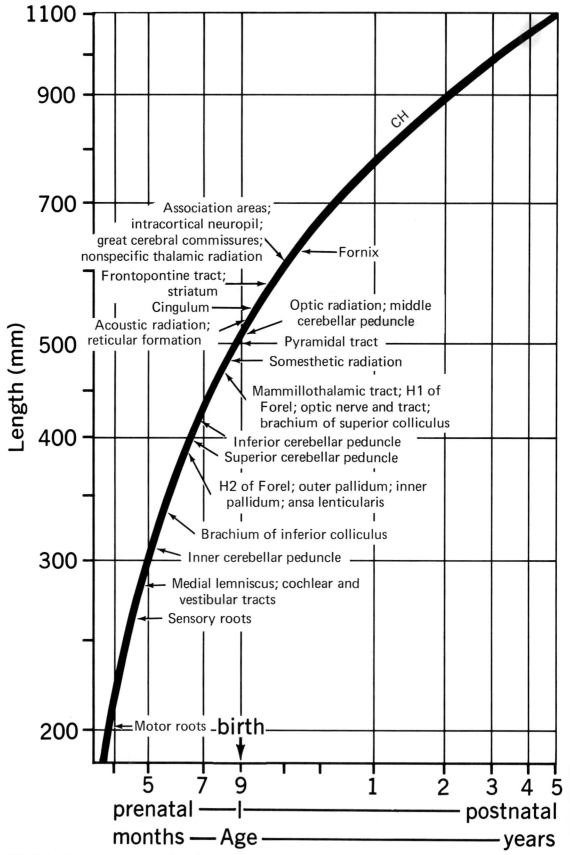

FIG. 3–1. Approximate onset of myelination in various parts of the nervous system as observed by light microscopy. The ordinate depicts CH length and the abscissa approximate ages. (Adapted from Yakovlev and LeCours, 1967)

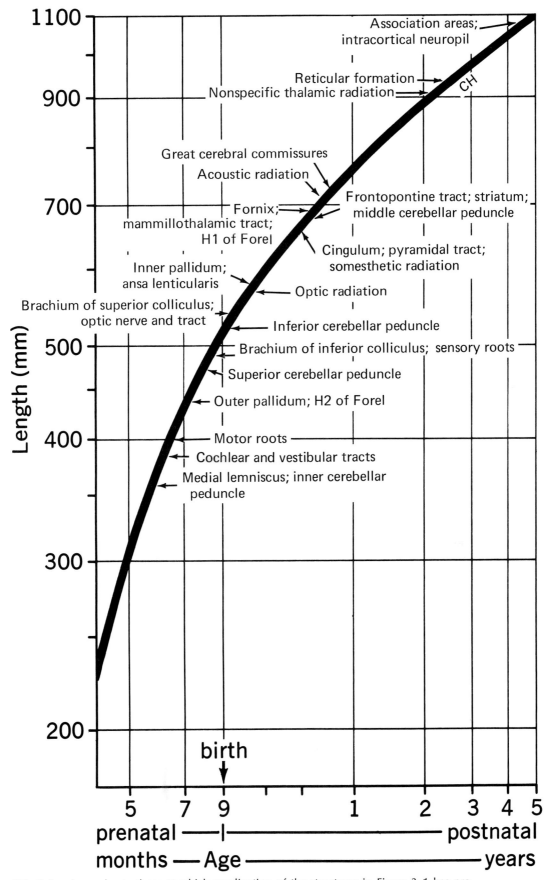

FIG. 3–2. Approximate times at which myelination of the structures in Figure 3–1 has progressed to 50% completion as observed by light microscopy. The ordinate depicts CH length and the abscissa approximate ages. (Adapted from Yakovlev and LeCours, 1967)

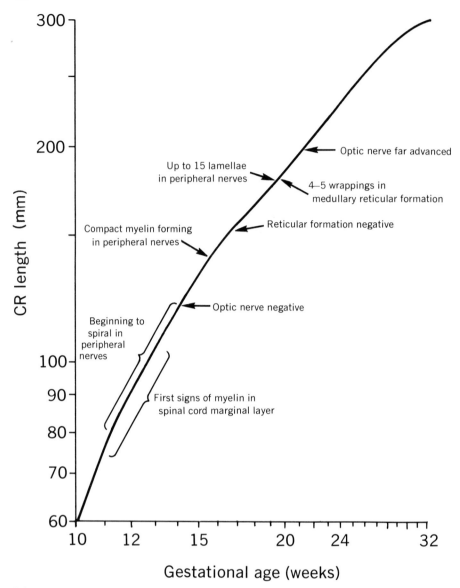

FIG. 3–3.   Approximate onset of myelination in various parts of the nervous system as observed by electron microscopy. The ordinate depicts CR length, and the abscissa the approximate ages. (Adapted from Cravioto, 1965; Dunn, 1970; Gamble, 1966, 1968; Ochoa, 1971; Davidson et al., 1973 and Kogon, unpublished data)

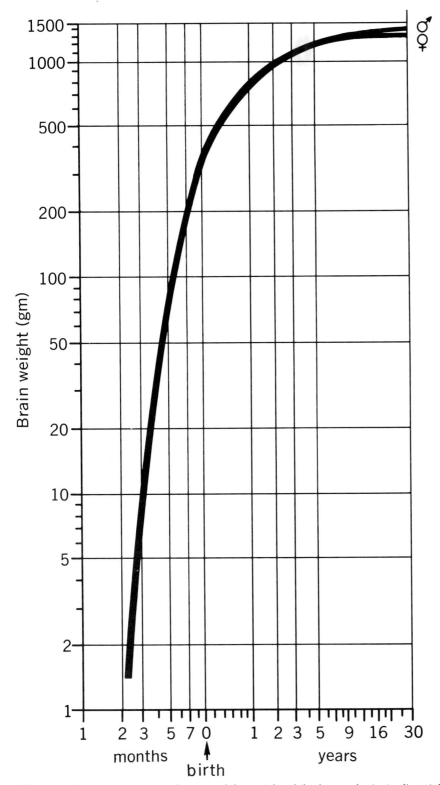

FIG. 3–4. Representative growth curve of the weight of the human brain (ordinate) from the tenth gestational week into adult life.

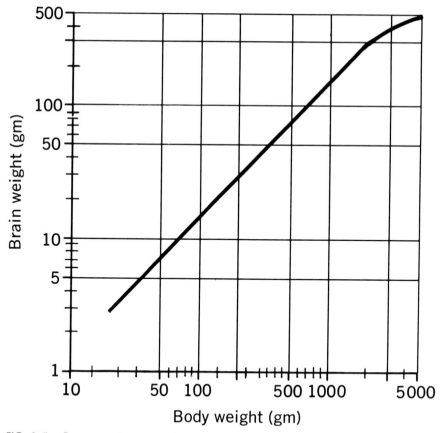

FIG. 3–5.   Representative curve depicting the weight of the brain as compared with body weight in prenatal and early postnatal periods.

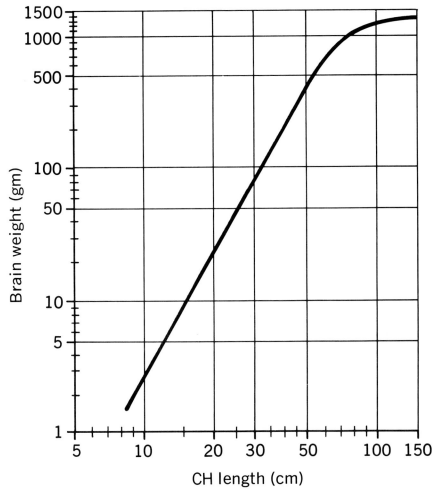

FIG. 3–6. Representative curve depicting the weight of the brain as compared with body length prenatally and postnatally.

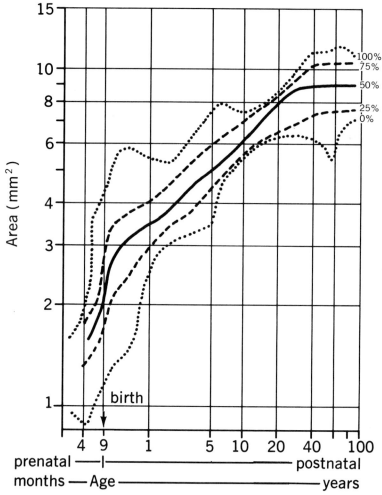

FIG. 3–7. Cross sectional area of one pyramidal tract at the midolivary level as a function of age. The areas were measured on frozen sections of gelatin-embedded tissue (without significant shrinkage) or on sections from paraffin-embedded tissue (corrected for an average shrinkage to about 83% of the actual area as determined on paired specimens).

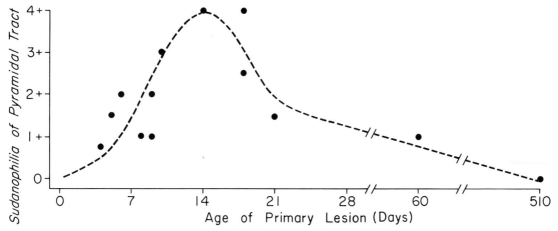

FIG. 3–8. Wallerian degeneration (as indicated by accumulation of sudanophilic lipids) in the pyramidal tract of infants at various times after massive cerebral lesions. (From Leech and Alvord, 1974)

FIG. 3–9. Wallerian degeneration in the pyramidal tract of adults as compared to infants. Note the variance in time scale from Figure 3–8 due to the marked difference in age-related rates of degeneration. (From Leech and Alvord, 1974)

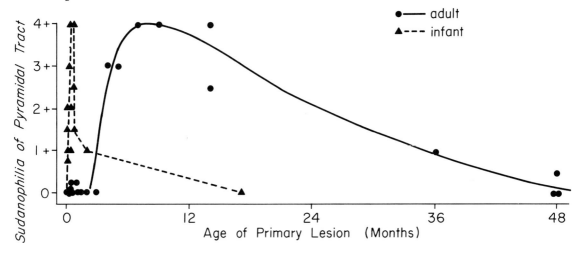

REFERENCES

1. Adrian EK Jr, Walker BE: Incorporation of thymidine-H^3 by cells in the normal and injured mouse spinal cord. J Neuropathol Exp Neurol 21:597–609, 1962

2. Coppoletta JM, Wolbach SB: Body length and organ weights of infants and children. A study of the body length and normal weights of the more important vital organs of the body between birth and twelve years of age. Am J Pathol 9: 55–70, 1933

3. Cravioto H: Electron microscopic studies on the developing human nervous system. II. The optic nerves. J Neuropathol Exp Neurol 24:166–167, 1965

4. Cravioto H: The role of Schwann cells in the development of human peripheral nerves. An electron microscopic study. J Ultrastruct Res 12:634–651, 1965

5. Davison AN, Duckett S, Oxberry JM: Correlative morphological and biochemical studies of the human fetal sciatic nerve. Brain Res 58: 327–342, 1973

6. Dobbing J, Sands J: Quantitative growth and development of human brain. Arch Dis Child 48:757–767, 1973

7. Dunn HL: The growth of the central nervous system in the human fetus as expressed by

graphic analysis and empirical formulae. J Comp Neurol 33:405–491, 1921

8. Dunn JS: Developing myelin in human peripheral nerve. Scott Med J 15:108–117, 1970

9. Friede RL, Hu KH: Proximo-distal differences in myelin development in human optic fibers. Z Zellforsch Mikrosk Anat 79:259–264, 1967

10. Fugita S: Kinetics of cellular proliferation. Exp Cell Res 28:52–60, 1962

11. Gamble HJ: Further electron microscopic studies of human foetal peripheral nerves. J Anat 100:487–502, 1966

12. Gamble HJ: Axon ensheathing by ependymal cells in the human embryonic and foetal spinal cord. Nature 218:182–183, 1968

13. Gruenwald P, Minh HN: Evaluation of body and organ weights in perinatal pathology: 1. Normal standards derived from autopsies. J Clin Pathol 34:247–253, 1960

14. Jacobson M: Developmental Neurobiology. New York, Holt, Rinehart and Winston, 1970

15. Jenkins GB: Relative weight and volume of the component parts of the brain of the human embryo at different stages of development. Contrib Embryol 13:43–59, 1921

16. Kogon M: Electron microscopic observations on the development of myelin in the human central nervous system. (in prep)

17. Krogman WM: Growth of man. Tabulae Biol 20:1–963, 1941

18. Leech RW, Alvord EC Jr: Wallerian degeneration in the premature human. J Neuropathol Exp Neurol 34:92, 1975

19. Malínský J, Malínská J: Developmental stages of prenatal spinal cord in man. Folia Morphol (Praha) 18:228–235, 1970

20. Martin AH: Significance of mitotic spindle fiber orientation in the neural tube. Nature 216:1133–1134, 1967

21. Martin A, Langman J: The development of the spinal cord examined by autoradiography. J Embryol Exp Morphol 14:25–35, 1965

22. Ochoa J: The sural nerve of the human foetus: electron microscopic observations and counts of axons. J Anat 108:231–245, 1971

23. Rakic P, Sidman RL: Supravital DNA synthesis in the developing human and mouse brain. J Neuropathol Exp Neurol 27:246–276, 1968

24. Samorajski T, Friede RL: A quantitative electron microscopic study of myelination in the pyramidal tract of rat. J Comp Neurol 134:323–338, 1968

25. Sauer FC: Mitosis in the neural tube. J Comp Neurol 62:377–405, 1935a

26. Sauer FC: The cellular structure of the neural tube. J Comp Neurol 63:13–23, 1935b

27. Sauer FC: The interkinetic migration of embryonic epithelial nuclei. J Morphol 60:1–11, 1936

28. Sauer FC: Some factors in the morphogenesis of vertebrate embryonic epithelium. J Morphol 61:563–579, 1937

29. Sauer ME, Walker BE: Radioautographic study of interkinetic nuclear migration in the neural tube. Proc Soc Exp Biol Med 101:557–560, 1959

30. Schonbach J, Hu KH, Friede RL: Cellular and chemical changes during myelination. Histologic, autoradiographic, histochemical and biochemical data on myelination in the pyramidal tract and corpus callosum of rat. J Comp Neurol 134:21–38, 1968

31. Sidman RL: Cellular proliferation and migration in the developing brain. Drugs and Poisons in Relation to the Developing Nervous System. Public Health Serv Publ #1791, 1967, pp. 5–11

32. Sidman RL, Miale IL, Feder N: Cell proliferation and migration in the primitive ependymal zone; an autoradiographic study of histogenesis in the nervous system. Exp Neurol 1:322–333, 1959

33. Tanimura T, Nelson T, Hollingworth RR, Shepard TH: Weight standards for organs from early human fetuses. Anat Rec 171:227–236, 1971

34. Vaughn JE, Pease DC: Electron microscopic studies of Wallerian degeneration in rat optic nerves. II. Astrocytes, oligodendrocytes and adventitial cells. J Comp Neurol 140:207–226, 1970

35. Watterston RL: Structure and mitotic behavior of the early neural tube. Organogenesis. Edited by RL DeHaan and H Ursprung. New York, Holt, Rinehart and Winston, 1965, pp. 129–159

36. Watterston RL, Veneziano P, Bartha A: Absence of a true germinal zone in neural tubes of young chick embryos as demonstrated by the colchicine technique. (abstracted) Anat Rec 124:379, 1956

37. Yakovlev PI, LeCours AR: The myelogenetic cycles of regional maturation of the brain. Regional Development of the Brain in Early Life. Edited by A Minkowski. Oxford, Blackwell, 1967, pp. 3–70

NEURAL TUBE CLOSURE AND DIFFERENTIATION

chapter 4

NEURULATION

The early development of the human neural tube is complex, and not all of the classical concepts that apply to its rostral portion are applicable to caudal structures. However, in discussing the initial formation of the tube and the malformations detectable in the early embryo, it is convenient to divide the overall development into three phases that can be defined on a morphologic basis. During the first phase of neural tube closure and differentiation (neurulation) the neuroectoderm is in contact with the amniotic cavity. The second (canalization) and third (retrogressive differentiation) phases apply only to the caudal neural tube and are discussed in Chapter 5. During these later periods, the neural tube has a complete covering of ectoderm. Therefore, the separation of the nervous system from the amniotic space is an essential feature of neurulation. Figures 4–1 and 4–2 show some of the major morphologic events associated with neurulation.

NORMAL DEVELOPMENT OF THE NEURAL TUBE*

NEURAL PLATE

Following implantation in stage V (see Chapter 1), the first defined rostrocaudal axis arises in stage VI when the primitive streak appears and in stage VII (0.4-mm) when the notochordal process is found. Rostral to the primitive streak is the primitive node (Hensen's node) which separates the streak from the notochord. During stage

* See Chapter 1 for background information on embryologic development and staging system.

VIII (1- to 1.5-mm) the primitive pit and neurenteric canal are present. At this time the notochord contains a canal that extends rostrally from the primitive node. The neurenteric canal is derived from a breakdown of the ventral wall of the notochordal canal at the level of the primitive pit during this same stage of development.[31] The notochord is in direct continuity with the surface layer, and some believe that the notochord plays a role in the induction of the neural plate that first becomes evident during stage VIII. Studies with the light microscope in chick embryos have demonstrated regular indentations of the overlying neural plate by the notochord at intervals of 30–50 μ.[16] These indentations are transient and are not seen in later stages.

NEURAL FOLDS AND GROOVE

During the latter part of stage VIII or early in stage IX (1.5-mm CR), the first differentiation toward a tubular structure takes place as the neural folds are formed and a neural groove thus created. Several theories exist describing the initiation and progression of neural fold formation, but this dynamic event has not yet been serially studied in human embryos; most of the available knowledge has been obtained from subhuman species such as avians[9] and amphibians.[35] Intra- and inter-cellular factors involved in the progressive closure of the neural tube include changes in the shape of ependymal cells and in their connections with surrounding cells. Contractile filaments have been reported, but their role in neurulation is not clearly understood. Changes in the surrounding mesoderm are also impor-

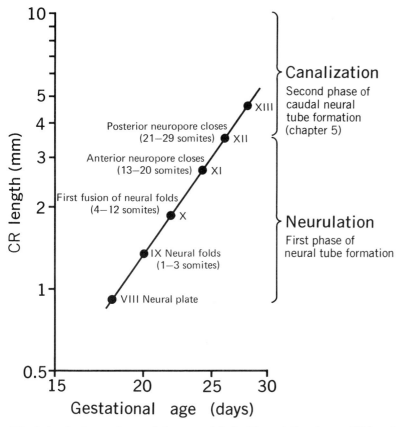

FIG. 4–1. Features of neurulation correlated with gestational age, CR length and developmental stage.

tant in the overall closure mechanism. However, one cannot presume that neurulation in humans is identical to that in amphibians since the number of cells differs and their interaction with surrounding tissues is more complex in humans.

FUSION OF NEURAL FOLDS

Stage X (2- to 3.5-mm CR) encompasses development between 4 and 12 somites when the first fusion of neural folds occurs. This takes place at the 6- to 7-somite stage and the site of initial fusion is at the level of the 3rd or 4th somite.[15] Although there is some variation in this site, the process proceeds caudally in such a manner that the level of fusion is at the most recently formed somite. In the older embryos of this stage, the tube is fused from the otic plate level of the rhombencephalon down to the 12th somite.

CLOSURE OF THE ANTERIOR NEUROPORE

Approximately three days after the neural tube begins to fuse, the cephalic portion undergoes a marked differentiation to form the forebrain (see Chapters 12–16). It is important to recognize that the more precocious development of the tectum with respect to the tegmentum is largely responsible for the production of the cephalic flexure, which is further accentuated by the downward growth of the hypothalamic region. During stage XI (2.5- to 4.5-mm CR) the embryo has between 13 and 20 somites. The younger embryos show fusion of the neural folds to the level of the colliculi, and this fusion progresses to complete closure rostrally in the older ones. The site of final closure, called the anterior neuropore, is located at the most rostral portion of the neural groove, which corresponds to the region of the lamina terminalis in older

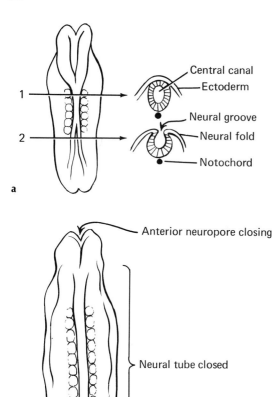

FIG. 4–2. **a.** Neurulation. Dorsal view of a stage X embryo during initial fusion of neural folds. On the right side are cross sections taken at the levels of arrows *1* and *2*. **b.** Dorsal view of a stage XI embryo. A large part of the neural tube has closed. The anterior neuropore, while still open in this drawing, closes during this stage. The posterior neuropore closes in stage XII.

specimens. The development of the primordia of the thalamus and corpus striatum and the optic evaginations markedly distort the configuration of the anterior neuropore. Its appearance, initially oval, becomes slit-like as the lateral lips advance toward the midline.[39] As with the entire neural tube, the opposing neuroectoderm fuses, as does the surface ectoderm. The central canal is thereafter in continuity with the amniotic cavity only through the posterior neuropore.

CLOSURE OF THE POSTERIOR NEUROPORE

Precisely where and when the posterior neuropore closes during stage XII (21–29 somites) have not been determined. Whether there are any unusual morphogenetic cellular movements is not known.

Simple calculations indicate that the site of the posterior neuropore must be at one of the lumbar segments: the first 3 or 4 somites contribute to the formation of the occipital bone and the next 20 to the cervical and thoracic segments, thus accounting for 23 or 24 of the 21–29 somites present during stage XII when the posterior neuropore closes. Since the posterior neuropore is open in the younger specimens and closed in the older specimens of this stage, closure probably occurs during the middle of this period, when the embryo has about 25 somites. This would locate the site of closure about the first or second lumbar segment (L1 to L2) with a probable variation of not more than two segments rostral or caudal (*i.e.*, T11 to L4).

When the posterior neuropore closes, the first phase of neural tube formation is completed. The internal cavities of the nervous system are completely sealed, and there is no longer a connection between the central canal and the amniotic fluid. This factor becomes important with respect to the discussion of certain theories of pathologic conditions, especially meningomyelocele.

ABNORMAL DEVELOPMENT

The malformations generally attributed to faulty neurulation are among the most severe anomalies found in humans. With the exception of meningomyelocele, all are incompatible with prolonged extrauterine life. If the developmental sequence is arrested prior to closure of the posterior neuropore, differing types of defects occur. In general, the earlier the defect arises, the more severe it is.

THEORIES OF OPEN NEURAL TUBE LESIONS

Theories regarding the development of open lesions of the neural tube fall into two basic groups: 1) those postulating that the tube

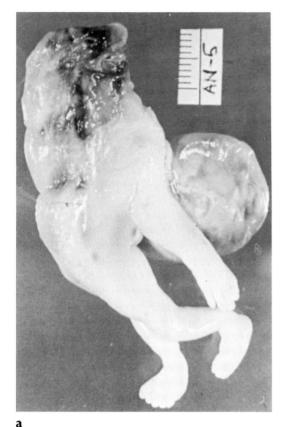

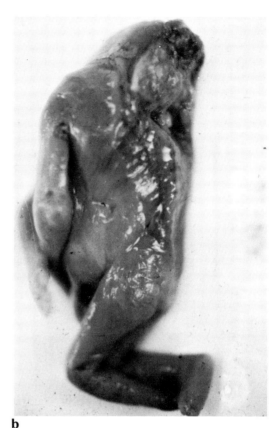

a

b

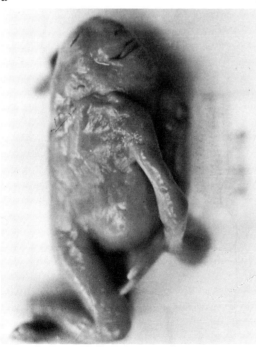

c

FIG. 4–3. **a.** Dorsolateral view of a human fetus with total dysraphism (complete craniorachischisis). The specimen measured 42-mm CR length and had an estimated gestational age of 109 days. On the right side, a large omphalocele that contains bowel, liver and lung can be seen. There were numerous other anomalies. Note the rotational deformities of the legs. (#H-587) **b.** Dorsolateral view of a human fetus (52-mm CR length) with complete craniorachischisis. The specimen has extreme spinal retroflexion and anterior cervical spina bifida in addition to numerous other anomalies. (#H-800) **c.** Ventrolateral view of the specimen shown in Figure 4–3**b** with craniorachischisis and spinal retroflexion.

never undergoes a normal closure, either totally or at a given site and 2) those postulating that it closes normally but then reopens. It is important that this controversy be resolved, as the period of development during which teratogenic agents could produce the defects is entirely different in the two cases.

The theory of a normal closure followed by reopening has most recently been popularized by Gardner,[12, 13, 14] who credits

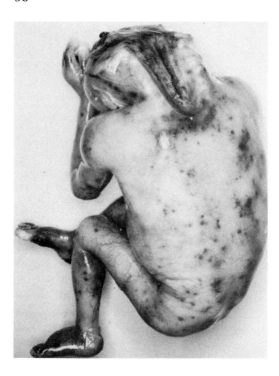

FIG. 4–4. Dorsal view of an 84-mm CR length human fetus with craniorachischisis (holoacrania and cervical rachischisis). (#H-1537)

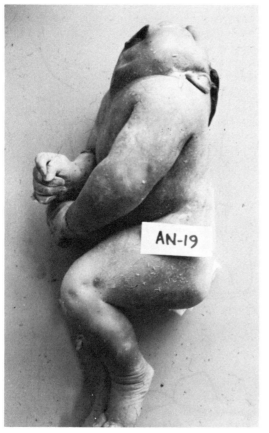

FIG. 4–5. **a.** Lateral view of a 213-mm CR length, 2180-g human fetus with extreme spinal retroflexion and craniorachischisis. Note absence of the neck. There were several visceral anomalies. (#H-865) **b.** Dorsal view of the head and upper spine of the fetus shown in Figure 4–5a.

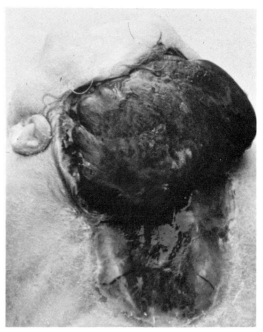

a

b

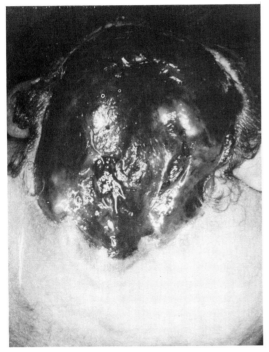

FIG. 4–6. Dorsal view of a human anencephalic with holoacrania and cervical rachischisis. The neural lesion is similar to that in the specimen shown in Figure 4–5a and **b** except for the absence of spinal retroflexion. (#H-1057)

Morgagni[23] with the original hypothesis. Although there are several variations of the theory, the basic premise is that the embryo undergoes a normal phase of neurulation followed by an abnormal process in which a reopening, or rupture, occurs. Gardner believes this is due to abnormal distention and pressure within the central canal (hydrocephalomyelia) secondary to the thin roof of the fourth ventricle becoming impermeable to the passage of cerebral spinal fluid (CSF) and cites the studies of Weed[44] as supporting this viewpoint. Weed followed the development of the cerebrospinal spaces in pig and human embryos by injecting dye. Although Weed's excellent morphologic studies did show a normal phase in which the roof of the fourth ventricle is seemingly impermeable to the egress of fluid, the interpretation that this supports Gardner's hypothesis is open to question.

More recently, Padget[32, 33] has proposed that the neural tube closes normally and then undergoes a process of "neuroschisis," in which a cleft in the dorsal neuroectoderm

allows the escape of CSF into the subectodermal space. Depending upon a varied sequence of events thereafter, the ectoderm can be secondarily ruptured and the neuroectoderm exposed to the amniotic cavity. Her evidence is based upon a survey of this process in many human embryos in the collection of the Carnegie Institute. At present, this hypothesis, while attractive, must await confirmation by other investigators before the more traditional theory of nonclosure is discarded.

A less popular hypothesis has been advanced by Vogel,[42] who believed that the changes in anencephaly are secondary to malformations in the pattern of the cerebral vasculature. Evidence for this is based in part on dye injections in older specimens and has not been studied in the earlier, more crucial stages. It is also based in part on experimental occlusion of the internal carotid artery with arrest of subsequent development of the cerebrum, but as yet without the production of anencephaly. Whether the hypothesis should be presented under those proposing a reopening mechanism is open to question, since any hypothesis concerning the internal carotid does not explain

FIG. 4–7. Dorsal view of the head of an anencephalic fetus of the holoacrania type, i.e., the defect is through the level of the foramen magnum. Compare the external appearance of the brain remnants in this case with that in Figure 4–5**b** which appears as an undifferentiated hemorrhagic mass. (#H-1302)

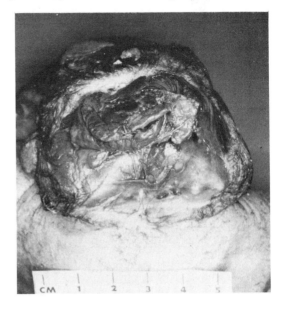

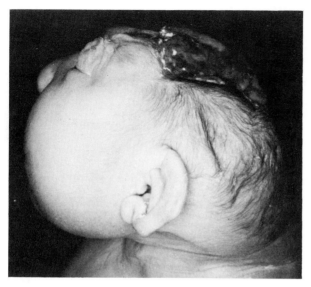

FIG. 4–8.   Lateral view of an anencephalic fetus of the meroacrania type, *i.e.*, the defect does not extend to the level of the foramen magnum. (#H-1264)

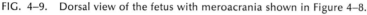

FIG. 4–9.   Dorsal view of the fetus with meroacrania shown in Figure 4–8.

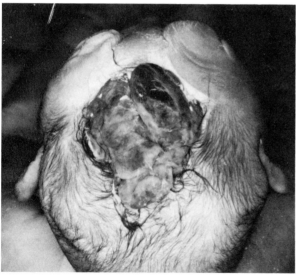

the lack of skin covering the typical anencephalic lesion, the skin being supplied by the external carotid artery. Thus, while the preservation of the ophthalmic artery may be important for the preservation of the eyes in the typical anencephalic specimen, the more distal occlusion of the internal carotid artery is not sufficient. But at least Vogel's hypothesis falls into the encephaloclastic group.

Experimental studies in animals lend only a little support for the reopening theories. Murakami *et al.*[24] have produced midbrain deformities in rat fetuses whose mothers were injected with vincristine. Histologic examination revealed a variety of abnormalities that were consistent with the concept of reopening in that the midbrain was exposed to the surface but the rest of the neural tube was closed. Fowler[11] has shown that chick embryo neural tubes can be reopened

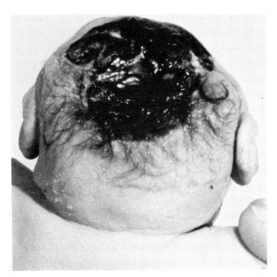

FIG. 4–10. Dorsal view of another human fetus with meroacrania, in which the exposed tissue is hemorrhagic. Compare with the nonhemorrhagic tissue in Fig. 4–9 (#H-319).

mechanically. However, this is accomplished only by external manipulation of the embryo with a sharp instrument and cannot be considered direct substantiation of the internal mechanisms proposed by either Gardner or Padget. Bonnevie[5] advanced further evidence on the basis of a strain of mice having myelencephalic blebs that supposedly arose secondary to the escape of CSF from a closed neural tube. These observations have been questioned.[17] There are undoubtedly selected specimens that support the reopening hypothesis, but most neuroembryologists favor the hypothesis that the neural tube never closes.

Several studies support the view that dysraphia can arise from neural tubes that never closed properly,[17,43] and human specimens recovered from both spontaneous and therapeutic abortions provide additional evidence favoring this theory. Dekaban and Bartelmez[8] report a 14-somite embryo with complete dysraphia and review previous similar specimens in the literature. Several stage XIV human embryos with caudal myeloschisis have been reported.[21,29,30,41] In addition to unfused neural folds, some specimens contain portions of primitive neural plate that had apparently not even begun the folding process.

Patten's[34] observation that an overgrowth

of nervous tissue is found in some cases of dysraphia provides one explanation of how neural folds could be prohibited from fusing properly. The growth of neuroectoderm over surface ectoderm has been observed experimentally[43] in rodents and human embryos with myeloschisis,[30,40] but the question of whether this overgrowth of neuroectoderm is primary or secondary has not been determined. The observations of Dekaban and Bartelmez[8] and of Lemire et al.[21] support the concept that cellular orientation of the neuroectoderm is disturbed, but it is still unclear as to whether the primary defects are in the ectoderm or mesoderm.[22]

TYPES OF DYSRAPHIA

Abnormal development during neurulation expresses itself in varying types of dysraphia in humans. In the normal process of fusion of the neural folds, small areas are occasionally skipped. These may close in soon afterward or may persist as defects of partial dysraphia or partial craniorachischisis. This defect most commonly occurs at either end and is associated with a failure of closure of the normal anterior or posterior neuropores, but it may occur at any point in between, associated with failure of closure of these "skipped areas." Thus, any portion of the neural tube can be involved. The most common anomalies include craniorachischisis (complete dysraphia), anencephaly (acrania

FIG. 4–11. Another human fetus with meroacrania showing distortion of the cranium as viewed from above. (#Np 366)

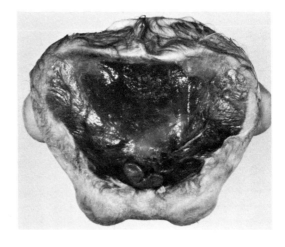

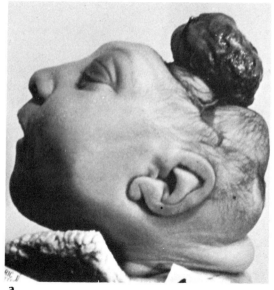

a

FIG. 4–12.   **a.** Lateral view of an infant with meroacrania who lived for several weeks. Since there is
no skin covering, the basic lesion is that of anencephaly rather than of encephalocele (which is skin
covered). **b.** Dorsal view of the patient shown in
Figure 4–12a. Note that occipital bone and foramen
magnum are intact. Because there is a significant
protrusion of dysplastic cerebral cortex, it can also
be classified as exencephaly. (COHMC #A67-119)

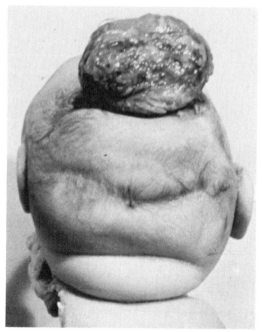

b

or cranioschisis), exencephaly and meningomyelocele (myelocele, caudal myeloschisis).

These malformations are recognized as
failures of neurulation since CNS tissue is
directly exposed to the outside of the body.
Although many similar lesions to be discussed in Chapter 5 also involve the caudal
spine, they have an intact skin covering.

Craniorachischisis

The incidence of complete dysraphia is not
known as most embryos so severely malformed are spontaneously aborted early in
pregnancy. The onset of this malformation
would not be later than stages IX or X (1.5-
to 3.5-mm CR) during the formation of the
neural folds. The earliest case recovered is
the 14-somite embryo of Dekaban and
Bartelmez.[8] Some human specimens with
complete craniorachischisis do undergo
further development into the young fetal
stages (Fig. 4–3a, 4–3b, 4–3c) but rarely beyond.[20] This condition represents the most
severe malformation associated with defec-

tive neurulation. The term craniorachischisis
is also applied to cases in which the brain and
a part of the spinal cord (Figs. 4–4 to 4–6) are
exposed to the surface, and it is not therefore
synonymous with complete dysraphism.

Anencephaly

The characteristic appearance of the anencephalic newborn is well known to most
physicians. The incidence of this anomaly
ranges from 1/1000 live births in the United
States to 5/1000 in areas of Ireland and
Wales. The true incidence is not known because many anencephalic embryos are spontaneously aborted early in pregnancy.
Anencephaly has been reported in twins and
triplets.[36] Epidemiologic studies have implicated race, social class, season of conception
and viruses as possible causes.[18, 26] Whether
underlying genetic mechanisms are involved
is not known,[45] but an interaction between
genetic, immediate and intergenerational
effects has been recently postulated.[10]
Nakano[27] has reviewed studies relating to
the above factors and others.

There are several varieties of anencephaly.
The most common is called holoacrania or
holoanencephaly, in which case the open
defect extends through the level of the fora-

men magnum (Fig. 4–7). If there is an accompanying rachischisis of the cervical spine, the defect is termed holoacrania with cervical rachischisis (sometimes craniorachischisis is used, as discussed above). If the defect in the skull does not extend to the foramen magnum, it is classified as mero-acrania or meroanencephaly (Figs. 4–8 to 4–12b).

Some cases of anencephaly have extreme retroflexion of the upper spine and other anomalies that are similar to a different condition called iniencephaly. The presence of the membranous neurocranium in inienceph-

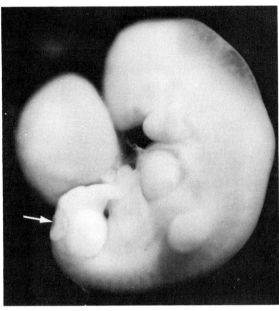

FIG. 4–13. Lateral view of a stage XIV (5.5-mm CR) human embryo with caudal myeloschisis (*arrow*), the forerunner of myelocele (or meningomyelocele). (#H-22)

FIG. 4–14. Cross section through area of myeloschisis in embryo shown in Figure 4–13. Note overgrowth of neural tissue (*arrow*).

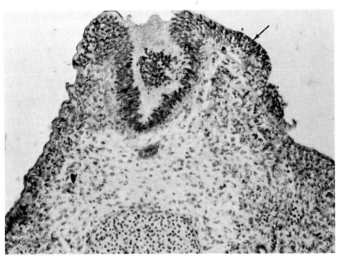

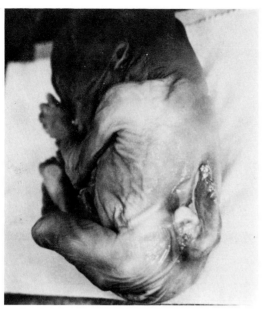

FIG. 4–15. Laterodorsal view of 173-mm CR length human fetus with a thoracolumbar myelocele. (#H-1302)

aly provides the major distinction between the two entities. Otherwise they have enough similarities to be considered within one spectrum of morphologic anomalies.[19]

Anencephaly probably arises no later than stage XI (2.5- to 4.5-mm CR) at which time the cephalic portion of the neural folds is undergoing closure. The extent of the lesion varies, as described above, but all cases show varying degrees of absence of the membranous neurocranium and skin. The exposed neural tissue is represented by a hemorrhagic, fibrotic, degenerated mass of neurons and glia without any well-defined cortex. This lesion always involves practically all of the forebrain and may involve other structures of the base of the brain from the level of the lamina terminalis to the foramen magnum. The optic chiasm is usually present, as are the distal optic nerves, but some specimens show a marked hypoplasia of the nerves just distal to the chiasm. Although there has been some controversy about whether the entire pituitary gland is present, careful studies have documented that it is usually present but malformed.[1,2,7] The hypothalamus is usually absent. Naeye and Blanc[25] separated anencephalics into two groups: 1) normal (or prolonged) ges-

tation, normal body weight (corrected for absence of the brain) and presence of pituitary and 2) premature birth, subnormal body weight and absent (or markedly hypoplastic) pituitary. They suggest that the second group may be so affected because of decreased growth hormone.

Associated malformations of every organ system have been found. One such malformation, adrenal hypoplasia, has interesting implications with respect to the pituitary-adrenal axis. Virtually all anencephalics of term gestation have markedly hypoplastic adrenal glands that are nearly all medulla. The interest in the functional significance of tropic hormones from the pituitary gland involves the fact that the fetal adrenal cortex apparently undergoes normal development[2,4] until about midway through gestation, after which time it progressively deteriorates and is lost at birth. Experimental evidence suggests that the adrenal hypoplasia is secondary to pituitary dysfunction.[3]

Another unique feature of term anencephalics is the frequent overgrowth of the upper extremities relative to the lower extremities.[28] This is expressed in a proximal-distal relation, with the upper arms showing the most and the hands the least excessive growth. The studies by Nañagas[28] include only older specimens, and the time of onset of this condition is not known. The lower extremities show normal growth when correction for total body length is made. Other structures that show overgrowth are the thymus (frequent) and the mandible (infrequent).

Exencephaly

Exencephaly is a condition in which the brain is outside of the skull. In humans this is most commonly found in embryos as an early stage of anencephaly. As gestation progresses, the neural tissue gradually degenerates; it is unusual to find a term infant with this entity (see Figs. 4–11 and 4–12).

Meningomyelocele

Meningomyelocele probably develops no later than stage XII (3- to 5-mm CR), but opposing viewpoints exist (see previous discussion under "Theories of Open Neural Tube Lesions"). Of all neural tube lesions

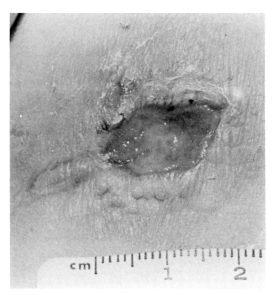

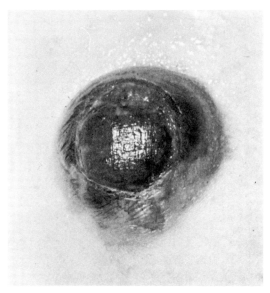

FIG. 4–16.   Dorsal view of a small (1.5-cm) myelocele in a neonate. The lesion is flat with the surface
of the back.

FIG. 4–17.   Dorsal view of a small meningomyelocele with dysplastic spinal cord in the center. An
enlarged subarachnoid space ventral to the cord
accounts for the protrusion above the level of the
back as compared with the case illustrated in
Figure 4–16.

FIG. 4–18.   Lateral view of the meningomyelocele
shown in Figure 4–17.

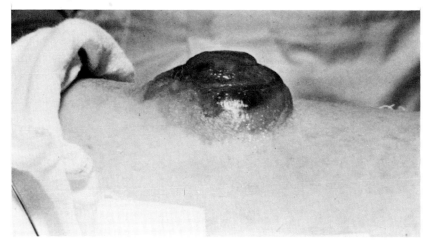

associated with faulty neurulation, this is the
most important since most infants with the
defect survive for many years. Like anencephaly, the incidence varies from 1/1000 to
5/1000 live births and is highest in certain
areas in Ireland, Scotland and Wales. Although the incidence in spontaneous abortions is not known, it is surprisingly high in
therapeutic abortions.[29, 30, 40] There is presently a controversy over the role of environmental versus genetic factors. Through the
experimental production of this malformation in animals, some insight has been
gained into the mechanisms of pathogenesis.[17]

Numerous human embryos and fetuses

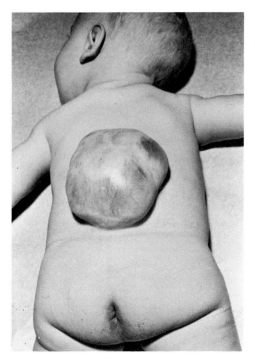

FIG. 4–19. Dorsal view of a large thoracolumbar meningomyelocele which has completely epithelialized. The patient was nine months old and had a functioning ventriculoatrial shunt for hydrocephalus. (UWH#10-25-49)

FIG. 4–20. Closeup lateral view of an epithelialized meningomyelocele.

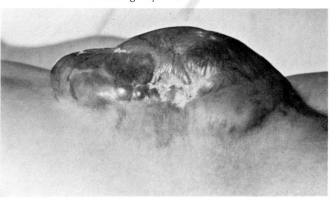

with meningomyelocele have been described (Figs. 4–13 to 4–15). Most show an open neural groove and/or neural plate, and many have an overgrowth of neural tissue. The early embryos and fetuses do not have the enlarged subarachnoid cystic cavity ventral to the dysraphic cord that is frequently found in newborns. When and how this space arises are not known. Virtually all patients born with meningomyelocele have an Arnold–Chiari malformation involving the cerebellum and medulla at the foramen magnum, but the etiopathogenetic interrelation is unclear (see Chapter 10).

The several varieties of meningomyeloceles can be separated on the basis of the level of the vertebral, motor or sensory deficits; the size of the superficial lesion; and whether it appears as a flat open lesion or as a bulging membranous sac. The flat lesion usually shows a recognizable spinal cord on the surface with CSF frequently leaking onto the exposed area. This type is usually referred to as a myelocele (Fig. 4–16). Meningomyeloceles are myeloceles in which an enlarged subarachnoid space ventral to the cord is associated with dorsal displacement of the cord creating a sac on the back

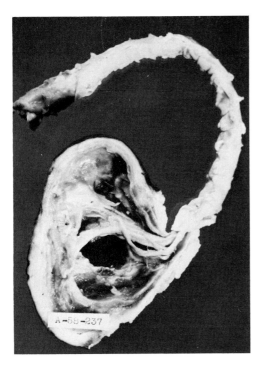

FIG. 4–21. Midsagittal view of the sac of a meningomyelocele from a 15-month-old infant. Above is the spinal cord (artificially curved) which enters the sac and projects to the roof of the sac at the left. Most of the sac is formed by a large subarachnoid space ventral to the cord. (JDH #A58-237)

FIG. 4–22. Coronal section of the sac of a meningomyelocele from a 45-day-old infant. The duplicated spinal cord is incorporated in the epithelialized lesion, and spinal nerves can be seen coursing ventrally through the sac. (JDH #A-56-375)

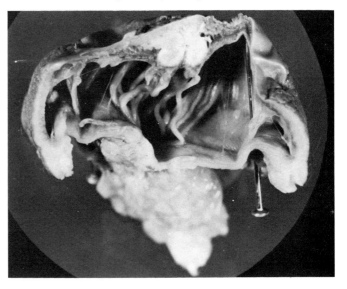

(Figs. 4–17 and 4–18). The center of the lesion is called the zona medullovasculosa (the dorsally reflected spinal cord plus a vascular network around it), while the remainder is referred to as the zona epitheliosa. The latter term refers to the fact that the covering of these lesions occurs by a gradual growth of epithelial tissue toward the center,[6] the entire process of epithelialization requiring many weeks (Figs. 4–19 to 4–22). Only the extreme lateral borders have normal skin with skin appendages.

At the time of birth, most meningomyeloceles have an opening in the epithelial covering through which there is a continual escape of CSF. If the sac is not resected, it usually undergoes gradual spontaneous closure over several weeks or months. Many infants with meningomyelocele develop hydrocephalus during the first few weeks. Some disagreement exists about whether the neurologic prognosis is better if the sac is resected during the first day of life[37] or is left to close spontaneously and later resected as an elective procedure,[38] but immediate closure has the distinct advantage of de-creasing the likelihood of infection. In either case, it is important that serial neurologic examinations be made of lower extremity and bladder functions, as either can deterio-rate over short periods of time. Continuous comprehensive medical and surgical man-agement can enhance the prognosis for better physical and mental development even though the neurologic deficits remain fixed.

REFERENCES

1. Anderson ABM, Laurence KM, Turnbull AC: The relationship in anencephaly between the size of the adrenal cortex and the length of gestation. J Obstet Gynaecol Br Commonw 76: 196–199, 1969

2. Angevine DM: Pathologic anatomy of hypophy-sis and adrenals in anencephaly. Arch Pathol 26:507–518, 1938

3. Bearn JG: The thymus and pituitary-adrenal axis in anencephaly. Br J Exp Pathol 49:136–144, 1968

4. Benirschke K: Adrenals in anencephaly and hydrocephaly. Obstet Gynecol 8:412–425, 1956

5. Bonnevie K: Embryological analysis of gene manifestation in Little and Bagg's abnormal mouse tribe. J Exp Zool 67:443–520, 1934

6. Cameron AH: The spinal cord lesion in spina bifida cystica. Lancet 271:171–174, 1956

7. Covell WP: A quantitative study of the hy-pophysis of the human anencephalic fetus. Am J Pathol 3:17–28, 1927

8. Dekaban AS, Bartelmez GW: Complete dys-raphism in 14 somite human embryo. Am J Anat 115:27–42, 1964

9. diVirgilio G, Lavenda N, Worden JL: Sequence of events in neural tube closure and the forma-tion of neural crest in the chick embryo. Acta Anat (Basel) 68:127–146, 1967

10. Emanuel I, Sever LE: Questions concerning the possible association of potatoes and neural-tube defects, and an alternate hypothesis re-lating to maternal growth and development. Teratology 8:325–332, 1973

11. Fowler I: Responses of the chick neural tube in mechanically produced spina bifida. J Exp Zool 123:115–151, 1953

12. Gardner WJ: Myelomeningocele, the result of rupture of the embryonic neural tube. Cleve Clin Q 27:88–100, 1960

13. Gardner WJ: Rupture of neural tube: Cause of myelomeningocele. Arch Neurol 4:1–7, 1961

14. Gardner WJ: The Dysraphic States: From Syr-ingomyelia to Anencephaly. Amsterdam, Ex-cerpta Medica, 1973

15. Heuser CH, Corner GW: Developmental hori-zons in human embryos. Description of age group X, 4 to 12 somites. Contrib Embryol 36: 29–39, 1957

16. Jurand A: The development of the notochord in chick embryos. J Embryol Exp Morphol 10: 602–621, 1962

17. Kalter H: Teratology of the Central Nervous System. Chicago, Univ Chicago Press, 1968

18. Laurence KM, Carter CO, David PA: Major central nervous system malformations in South Wales. II. Pregnancy factors, seasonal variation and social class effects. Br J Prev Soc Med 22: 212–222, 1968

19. Lemire RJ, Beckwith JB, Shepard TH: Inien-cephaly and anencephaly with spinal retroflex-ion. A comparative study of eight human speci-mens. Teratology 6:27–36, 1972

20. Lemire RJ, Beckwith JB, Warkany J: Unpub-lished data, 1975

21. Lemire RJ, Shepard TH, Alvord EC Jr: Caudal myeloschisis (lumbo-sacral spina bifida cystica) in a five millimeter (Horizon XIV) human em-bryo. Anat Rec 152:9–16, 1965

22. Marin-Padilla M, Ferm VH: Somite necrosis and developmental malformations induced by vita-min A in the golden hamster. J Embryol Exp Morphol 13:1–8, 1965

23. Morgagni JB: 1769 (quoted by WJ Gardner, 1960)

24. Murakami U, Hoshino K, Inoye M: An experi-mental observation on the morphogenesis of reopening of the cranium. Proc Congen Anom Res Assoc Japan 12:157–171, 1972

25. Naeye RL, Blanc WA: Organ and body growth in anencephaly. Arch Pathol 91:140–147, 1971

26. Naggan L, MacMahon B: Ethnic differences in the prevalence of anencephaly and spina bifida in Boston, Massachusetts. N Engl J Med 277: 1119–1123, 1967

27. Nakano KK: Anencephaly: A review. Dev Med Child Neurol 15:383–400, 1973

28. Nañagas JC: A comparison of the growth of the body dimensions of anencephalic human fetuses with normal fetal growth as determined by graphic analysis and empirical formulae. Am J Anat 35:455–494, 1925

29. Nishimura H, Takano K, Tanimura T, Yasuda M,

Uchida T: High incidence of several malformations in the early human embryos as compared with infants. Biol Neonate 10:93–107, 1966

30. Nishimura H, Tanimura T, Swinyard CA: A study of 26 human embryos (Horizon 11–22 Streeter) with central nervous system defects (abstracted). Teratology 2:267, 1969

31. O'Rahilly R: Developmental Stages in Human Embryos, Part A: Embryos of the First Three Weeks (Stages 1 to 9). Washington DC, Carnegie Inst Wash, 1973

32. Padget DH: Spina bifida and embryonic neuroschisis: A causal relationship. Johns Hopkins Med J 123:233–252, 1968

33. Padget DH: Neuroschisis and human embryonic maldevelopment. J Neuropathol Exp Neurol 29:192–216, 1970

34. Patten BM: Embryological stages in the establishing of myeloschisis with spina bifida. Am J Anat 93:365–395, 1953

35. Schroeder TE: Neurulation in Xenopus laevis. An analysis and model based upon light and electron microscopy. J Embryol Exp Morphol 23:427–462, 1970

36. Scott JM, Paterson L: Monozygous anencephalic triplets—a case report. J Obstet Gynaecol Br Commonw 73:147–151, 1966

37. Sharrard WJW, Zachary RB, Lorber J, Bruce AM: A controlled trial of immediate and delayed closure of spina bifida cystica. Arch Dis Child 38:18–22, 1963

38. Shurtleff DB, Foltz EL: Comparative study of meningomyelocele repair of cerebrospinal fluid shunt as primary treatment in spina bifida. Dev Med Child Neurol [Suppl] 13:57–64, 1967

39. Streeter GL: Developmental horizons in human embryos. Description of age group XI, 13 to 20 somites, and age group XII, 21 to 29 somites. Contrib Embryol 30:211–245, 1942

40. Swinyard CA, Chaube S, Nishimura H: Embryogenetic aspects of human meningomyelocele. Pediatr Ann 2:26–43, 1973

41. Tanimura T, Takano K, Nishimura H: Congenital anomalies found in the central nervous system of 450 human embryos (abstracted). Proc Congen Anom Res Assoc Japan 4:44, 1964

42. Vogel FS: The anatomic character of the vascular anomalies associated with anencephaly. Am J Pathol 39:163–174, 1961

43. Warkany J, Wilson JG, Geiger JF: Myeloschisis and myelomeningocele produced experimentally in the rat. J Comp Neurol 109:35–64, 1958

44. Weed LH: Development of cerebro-spinal spaces in pig and in man. Contrib Embryol 5:1–116, 1917

45. Yen S, MacMahon B: Genetics of anencephaly and spina bifida. Lancet 2:623–626, 1968

chapter 5

SECONDARY CAUDAL
NEURAL TUBE FORMATION

After the posterior neuropore closes in stage XII (3- to 5-mm CR) the second phase of caudal neural tube formation begins. The neural tube is now completely covered with ectoderm, and since the low lumbar, sacral and coccygeal segments have not yet developed, further development of these segments has to come about by a process entirely different from neurulation. How this is done in human embryos is poorly understood, but the studies of Ikeda,[12] Bolli[4] and Lemire[20] suggest a process similar to that occurring in avians.[17,24] An understanding of this process requires description of the *caudal cell mass* and of *retrogressive differentiation*. The temporal relationships of these developments are shown in Figure 5–1.

NORMAL DEVELOPMENT*

CAUDAL CELL MASS

The caudal end of the neural tube and the notochord, which are in contact, blend into a large aggregate of undifferentiated cells extending into the tail fold. At this point in development, the other structures in this region are mesonephros and hindgut. Although the caudal cell mass initially contains only undifferentiated cells, some cells near the end of the neural tube orient themselves around small vacuoles. At this time, probably in stages XIII or XIV (4- to 7-mm CR), the cells undergo a transformation and

* See Chapter 1 for background information on embryologic development and staging system.

begin to attain the appearance of ependymal cells. This change initially involves only the cells immediately surrounding the vacuoles, but as the vacuoles coalesce, two or three layers of cells take on the appearance of neural cells. The coalescing vacuoles enlarge and make contact with the central canal of that portion of the neural tube previously formed by the process of neurulation. This new process, referred to as canalization (Figs. 5–2 to 5–5), is one way the caudal neural tube might elongate during this second phase of formation. The role of the tail in this elongation has been studied by Gaertner,[8] Kunitomo,[18] Seichert and Jelínek,[25] Jelínek *et al.*[15] and Klika and Jelínek.[17]

From stages XIII to XX a variety of morphologic patterns are found in the caudal neural tube.[20] Accessory lumens are sometimes seen in either a dorsoventral or a lateral plane with neural cells being oriented in layers around each lumen (Figs. 5–6 to 5–9). In most cases the main central canal is usually easily distinguished from the accessory one. Some embryos show partial obliteration of the lumen by either folds of tissue or actual ependymal masses projecting into it (Fig. 5–10). Both the accessory lumens and the cellular proliferations into the lumen are possibly formed by the canalization process that is still taking place distal to the point where they are found. Bollí[4] found accessory lumens in 35% of embryos between 4- and 31-mm CR length and subdivided them on a morphologic basis. One type originated within a thickened ventral portion of the neural tube, and the second type showed

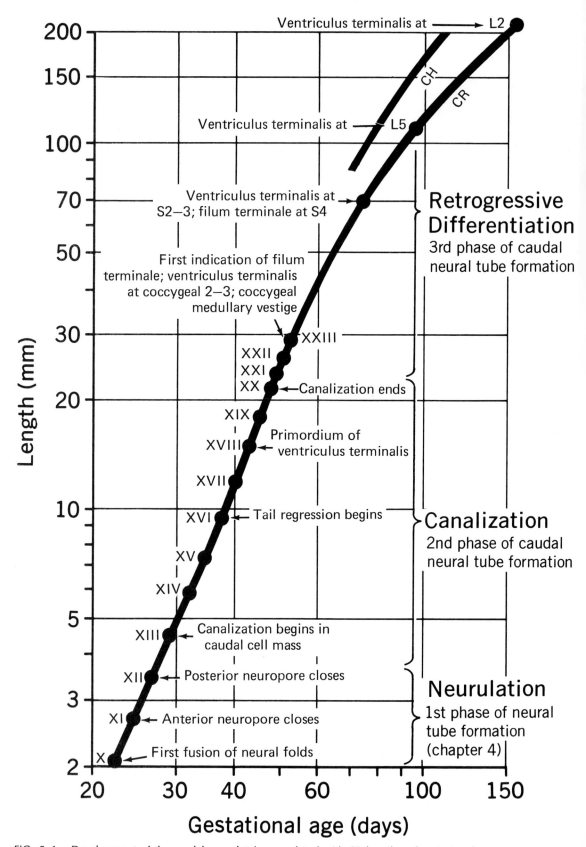

FIG. 5–1. Development of the caudal neural tube correlated with CR length and gestational age.

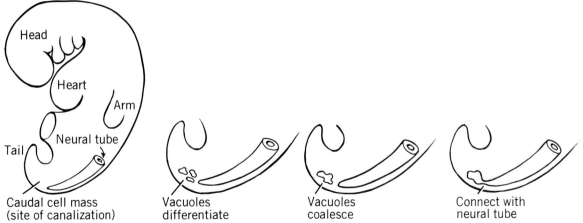

FIG. 5–2. Canalization as a possible factor in the elongation of the neural tube after closure of the posterior neuropore.

complete separation of the canals. In the former type he noted that the notochordal sheath was either absent or poorly differentiated. While the relationship of these findings is still unclear, it is worth noting that development of the neural tube in this area seems to lack the precision of neurulation.

RETROGRESSIVE DIFFERENTIATION

The third phase in the formation of the caudal neural tube involves the regression of those structures derived during the canalization phase. Since this takes place in a remarkably precise manner, Streeter[27] believed that it was not a degenerative process and referred to it as "retrogressive differentiation." Even more-severe degenerative changes, including necrosis, are now recognized in various stages of normal development, so that there is no longer serious argument about the concept that degeneration ("necrobiosis") occurs normally. The following descriptions are taken from Streeter's study as well as from those of Kunitomo[18] and Kernohan.[16]

At about stage XVI (8- to 11-mm CR), when the process of canalization is still continuing, the tail structures show the first sign of a regression that will ultimately result in the complete disappearance of the embryonic tail, a subject of considerable evolutionary controversy. Indication of regression of the neural tube itself probably starts no sooner than stage XVIII or XX. From this point, the third phase of neural tube forma-

tion continues until some time after birth. Although the development of the caudal vertebral structures is intimately involved, these structures will here be used only as landmarks; they are described more completely in Chapter 19.

The relations of three derivatives of the embryonic neural tube (the ventriculus terminalis, filum terminale and coccygeal medullary vestige) are important to an understanding of retrogressive differentiation (Fig. 5–11). As the lumen of the central canal begins to decrease in size, one portion (the ventriculus terminalis) will remain throughout life as an identifiable space. This space is found in most cases within that portion of the caudal spinal cord known as the conus medullaris; in other cases it is found in the upper filum terminale. There is some question about when the ventriculus terminalis first becomes an identifiable structure in the embryo and fetus. Kernohan[16] was not able to locate it in embryos of 15-, 18-and 20-mm CR length (corresponding to stages XVIII and XIX) but could measure it in an embryo of 22-mm CR length (corresponding to stage XX). Thereafter, he was able to identify it in all larger specimens. On the other hand, Kunitomo[18] noted that the "primordium" of the ventriculus terminalis could be seen in a 15.5-mm CR length embryo (corresponding to stage XVIII). By this stage the embryonic neural tube can be divided into a rostral portion, which has ependymal, mantle and marginal zones, and a caudal portion, which has only ependyma.

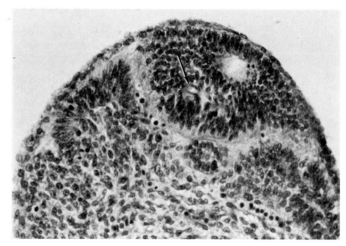

FIG. 5–3

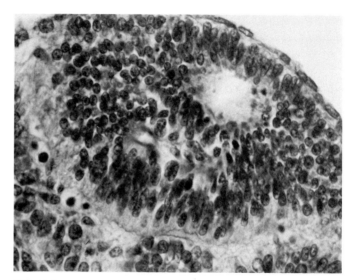

FIG. 5–4

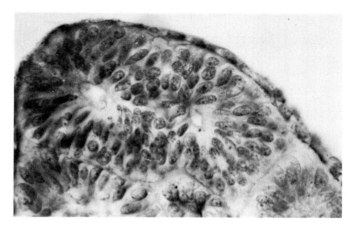

FIG. 5–5

◀ FIG. 5–3. Photomicrograph of a cross section of the caudal neural tube of a stage XIV (7-mm CR) human embryo showing a small lumen ventral and slightly to the left of the main lumen (*arrow*). These lumina connect at another level. (#H-254)

◀ FIG. 5–4. This higher power view of Figure 5–3 shows the lumina in greater detail.

◀ FIG. 5–5. Photomicrograph of a cross section of the caudal neural tube in a stage XIV (6-mm CR) embryo showing two lateral lumina, each with two to three layers of cells (#H-783).

The primordium of the ventriculus terminalis can be defined at this point as a small dilation of the central canal just caudal to this morphologic junction, which corresponds to the level of the developing 32nd vertebra (coccygeal 2). Its presence has been confirmed in our own series of embryos at this stage.[21] Streeter[27] has further defined its level at coccygeal vertebrae 2 and 3 by stage XXIII, sacral 2 at 67-mm CR length, lumbar 5 at 111-mm CR length and lumbar 2 at 221-mm CR length. At this last fetal stage it is approximately 1.5 mm in both the anteroposterior and lateral dimensions.[16]

The first indication of the filum terminale is shown by Streeter[27] in a 30-mm CR embryo (stage XXIII). As the caudal neural tube atrophies, a small ependymal rest known as the coccygeal medullary vestige remains at the tip of the coccygeal segments. Between this and the ventriculus terminalis,

the spinal cord (neural tube) atrophies into a fibrous band, the filum terminale. Ependymal rests are found within the filum during early fetal development, and many persist into postnatal life. The time at which the coccygeal medullary vestige disappears is not known. The filum terminale, of course, persists throughout life and is divided into a rostral intradural and subarachnoid part and a caudal part fused with the dura.

ABNORMAL DEVELOPMENT

The following distinctions characterize malformations that arise during each of the three phases of caudal neural tube development discussed in Chapters 4 and 5.

1. Malformations dating back to the first phase (neurulation) are those in which nervous tissue is found externally, *i.e.*, not covered with intact ectoderm or skin. This phase begins by stage VIII when the neural plate appears and ends during stage XII when the posterior neuropore closes.
2. Malformations arising during the second phase are covered by intact skin. This phase begins in stage XIII and ends about stage XX, during which the caudal neural tube undergoes further elongation by the process of canalization.
3. Malformations arising during the third

FIG. 5–6. Photomicrograph of the caudal neural tube in a stage XVIII (16-mm CR) human embryo in which a small lumen can be seen ventral to the main canal. (This is not the notochord, which is more ventral and not included here.) The accessory lumen connects with the main central canal at another level. (#H-134)

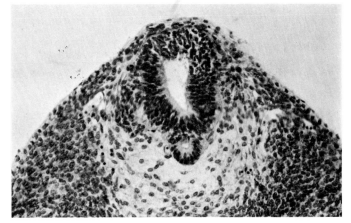

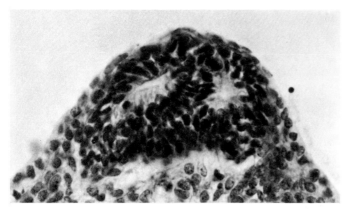

FIG. 5–7. Photomicrograph of a section taken more caudally in the embryo shown in Figure 5–6. At this level are two laterally placed lumina, and there is less differentiation of the surounding cells.

FIG. 5–8. Photomicrograph of a cross section through the caudal neural tube of a stage XVIII (14-mm CR) embryo with an accessory ventral lumen that connects with the main canal at another level. (#H-50)

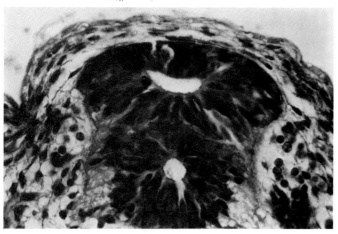

FIG. 5–9. Photomicrograph of a cross section of a stage XIX (18-mm CR) human embryo with a lateral division of the caudal neural tube. The notochord, which is ventral in this section, passes between the two neural tubes in caudal sections. (#H-203)

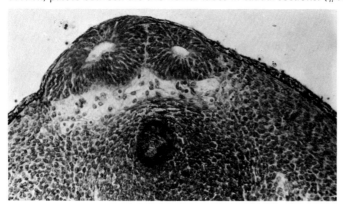

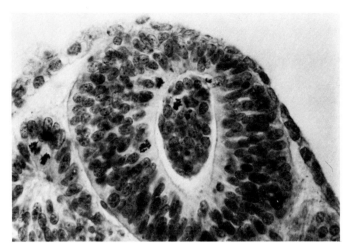

FIG. 5–10. Photomicrograph of a cellular mass projecting into the central canal of the caudal neural tube of a stage XV (9-mm CR) human embryo. (#H-443)

period are also covered with intact skin and involve the structures formed during normal regression. This phase of retrogressive differentiation or regression and atrophy of neural tissue within the tail of the embryo overlaps the second phase in time and continues into childhood. During this period the ventriculus terminalis and filum terminale are formed.

Most malformations of the caudal neural tube that arise during the second and third phases of development are difficult to separate with respect to time of onset and will be discussed together. Similarly, some vertebral malformations found in conjunction with neural defects arise during this period and are part of more generalized complexes of anomalies involving many structures. The malformations associated with canalization and retrogressive differentiation of the caudal neural tube and spine include myelocystocele, disastematomyelia (diplomyelia or split cord syndrome), lumbosacral lipoma and lumbosacral meningocele.

MYELOCYSTOCELE

The incidence and pathogenesis of this unusual anomaly is unknown. First described by Recklinghausen,[23] it consists of a localized cystic dilatation of the central canal.

The typical patient is born with a cystic mass over the lower spine that is covered with intact skin. There is frequently cloacal exstrophy and other malformations (Figs. 5–12 and 5–13). Vertebral defects are common and consist of lordosis, scoliosis and agenesis of sacral parts. Ballantyne[2] stated that myelocystocele can be found in association with a meningocele (dorsal or ventral), in which case it is termed a myelocystomeningocele. A variety of sensory and motor deficits of the lower extremities are also associated. Myelocystocele, with the accompanying cloacal exstrophy, represents one of the most severe malformations of a newborn compatible with life.

Examination reveals the sac to be covered with fat and skin. The wall is lined by ependyma and ill-defined membranes. No nerves are present within the cavity, and those exiting from the area can pass through vertebral foramina or between bony clefts.

It is difficult to date the onset of this malformation as there are presently no good clues to its pathogenesis. Since the defect is covered with intact skin, it should arise from the neural tube that is formed after closure of the posterior neuropore in stage XII (3- to 5-mm CR). The only point where there is any physiologic dilatation of the central canal in that region is the ventriculus terminalis, but there is no evidence that this site is actually involved. The sacral vertebrae are usually deformed or absent. Since the segments that will form the sacral vertebrae are formed during stage XIII (4- to 6-mm CR), it is possible that an arrest in development at this stage might account for those cases with

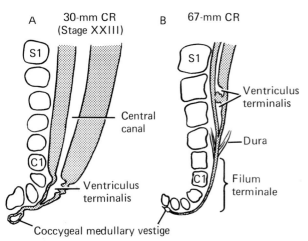

FIG. 5–11. Relationship of selected structures involved in retrogressive differentiation. (Adapted from Streeter, 1919)

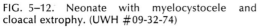

FIG. 5–12. Neonate with myelocystocele and cloacal extrophy. (UWH #09-32-74)

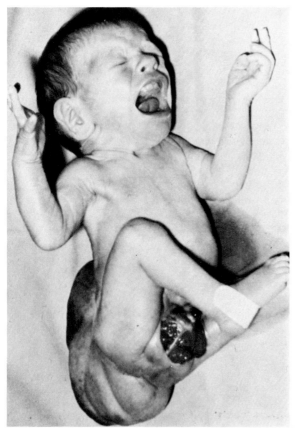

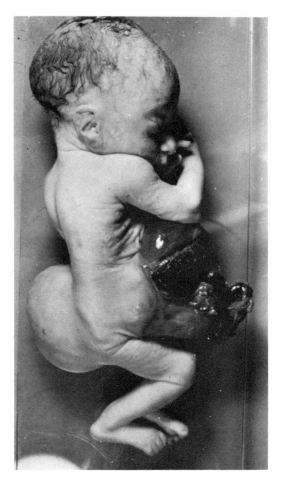

FIG. 5–13. Human fetus of 220-mm CR length with a myelocystocele and gastropleuralschisis. (#H-78)

agenesis of the sacrum. Myelocystoceles have been experimentally produced in the offspring of golden hamsters treated with retinoic acid.[26] Dr. Shenefelt (personal communication) has produced myelocystoceles with such treatments both before and after closure of the posterior neuropore. His findings were "consistent with changes secondary to necrotizing damage in a limited zone of the spinal cord and adjacent mesoderm, with the size and location of the zone varying systematically according to both dosage and time of treatment."

DIASTEMATOMYELIA

Diastematomyelia (Fig. 5–14) implies a spinal cord that is bifid at some portion. In

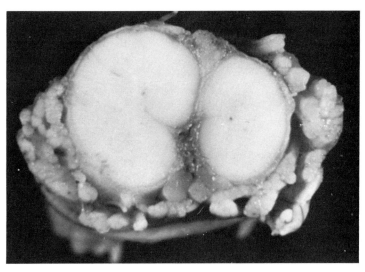

FIG. 5–14. Diastematomyelia shown in cross section of a human spinal cord. The ventral aspects of each cord are directed toward the center. Another example of diastematomyelia (but associated with syringomyelia) is shown in Figure 9–8.

some cases the cord has a normal singular rostral component, then splits into two parts for the remainder of its caudal length; in other cases it is singular, then divides, and later becomes singular again in a rostro-caudal dimension. These anatomic variations have led to confusion regarding pathogenesis and clinical importance.

James and Lassman[13] helped to clarify these problems by separating cases on the basis of whether 1) each cord was invested with a separate sheath of dura mater or 2) both cords were within one dural tube. In their 13 cases with separate dural tubes, either a bone, cartilage or fibrous septum was always present and occupied most of the space between the two dural tubes. By contrast, in 11 cases having both cords within a single dural tube, no septum was present. In the latter group, the bifid cords always rejoined caudally to form an "apparently normal" single spinal cord. James and Lassman[14] later extended their observations to 41 cases, 19 of which had a septum, 21 of which did not and 1 was mixed with 3 areas of diastematomyelia. In 15 of the cases without a septum they noted anomalous "bands" consisting of dense fibrous tissue or aberrant dorsal nerve roots. These bands were located between the spinal cord and neural arch in 11 cases, and between the spinal cord and dura mater in 3 cases; in 1 case the band was

attached to the filum terminale (its other attachment was not mentioned).

The above anatomic division seems clearer than that of Cohen and Sledge,[5] who attempted to distinguish between diastematomyelia and diplomyelia. They defined the former as a congenital splitting of the spinal cord with each portion having a separate arachnoid but sharing a common dura and the latter as a duplication of part or all of the cord, in which all eight segmental nerve roots are present (four for each segment of the two cords). Cohen and Sledge[5] believed that the available descriptive evidence favored persistence of the neurenteric canal as the underlying defect, whereas Gardner[9] implicated nonpermeability of the rhombencephalic roof causing hydrocephalomyelia and subsequent rupture of the distal neural tube as the major pathogenetic factor.

Diastematomyelia and/or diplomyelia have been described as occurring spontaneously in dogs, swine and cattle. They have also been reported in the offspring of rodents subjected to trypan blue, irradiation or insulin injections during pregnancy. In humans the malformation can exist without associated neurologic deficits, but in most patients with separate dural tubes, compression of the spinal cords occurs with subsequent neurologic impairment.

The previous discussion regarding the

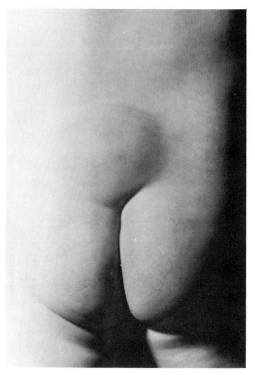

FIG. 5–15. Dorsal view of a lumbosacral lipoma in an infant. While the neurologic examination was normal, the subcutaneous component traversed the dura and connected to a deep lipoma enmeshed with the conus medullaris and cauda equina. (UWH #15-23-49)

normal development of the caudal neural tube suggests that many types of duplications may arise during canalization. Persistence of these might well account for some cases of diplomyelia without such mechanisms as splitting by a neurenteric canal. The role of the notochord in this process is not known, but it may be the key to the pathogenesis. The notochordal cells arise in continuity with Hensen's node, and although the latter continues to assume a more caudal position as growth continues, an arrest in the development of the tail fold might leave it in a position of influence. In chick embryos, Grabowski[10] has shown the excision of Hensen's node to be associated with duplications of the neural tube in which there is a complete separation of spinal cord, notochord and developing vertebrae. This merely indicates that a midline process can create this condition experimentally; it is not evidence that either the node or the notochord is involved in the malformation.

LUMBOSACRAL LIPOMA

Several varieties of lipomas involving the caudal neural tube appear to be formed during the second and third phases of development. Some are associated with diastematomyelia or meningocele, and they are difficult to classify in a way that provides both pathogenetic and clinical information. Two general subdivisions within the category of lumbosacral lipoma are lipoma and lipomeningocele. In the former there is a subcutaneous fatty mass that may or may not have associated spina bifida occulta, but does not have any attachment to the dura mater and has no intradural component. By contrast, in the latter (lipomeningocele) the subcutaneous fatty mass is attached to or pentrates the dura mater by way of a fibrous stalk and may be associated with an intradural fatty component. The cystic component of the lesions may be apparent superficially or be hidden beneath the lipoma.[22] Lassman and James[19] and Anderson[1] have given detailed accounts of the varying connections that the overlying fatty tumor can have with different portions of the caudal neural tube structures.

From the outside the lesion usually appears as a soft mass with intact skin (Figs. 5–15 to 5–18). There can be associated hair, sinuses or nevi. Radiographs frequently reveal a widened spinal canal of the lower lumbar vertebrae. In addition, various degrees of agenesis or deformity of the sacrum have been reported. The superficial aspect of the mass is fairly typical of subcutaneous fat, and this part is not usually encapsulated. The fat may be lobulated, and, as deeper structures are approached, it becomes more fibrous. A stalk of fibrous fatty tissue can be found to traverse the dura and be associated with an intradural lipomatous component in a large percentage of patients with a subcutaneous midline lipoma. The mass within the spinal canal may involve several sites (conus medullaris, cauda equina or filum terminale) and, depending upon its size, can compress the cord or nerves. Neurologic deficits obviously depend upon these underlying neural involvements. While the incidence of symptomatic lumbosacral lipomas is unclear, Emery and Lendon[7] have found a high frequency of such lesions in patients

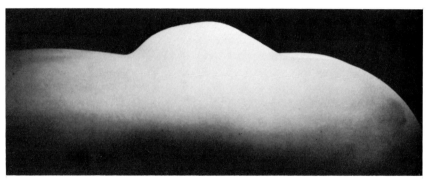

FIG. 5–16.   Lateral view of the lumbosacral lipoma shown in Figure 5–15.

FIG. 5–17.   Small subcutaneous lumbosacral lipoma in a teen-age male. This was associated with diastematomyelia and neurologic deficits. (UWH #11-17-54)

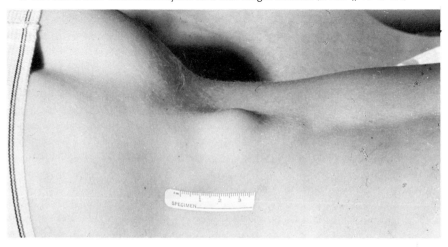

with meningomyelocele. These were most commonly associated with the filum terminale (intra- and extrathecal), but they also involved the dura, leptomeninges and area of a diastematomyelia. Barson[3] found four symptomless intradural lipomas in 300 spinal cords, an incidence of 1.3%.

The pathogenesis varies with the type of lesion. Most lesions probably originate early in the fetal period during the development of the structures that form the distal spinal cord (the fetal phase of retrogressive differentiation). The caudal cell mass seems to have totipotent characteristics, and a small clone of lipomatous cells developing in that region would not necessarily inhibit the growth of surrounding structures but could form the basis of the lesion seen at birth. The associated vertebral maldevelopment would also favor this later period since the dorsal components of the spinal canal are the last to form, thus permitting connections between the dorsal subcutaneous tissues and the spinal cord.

It is important for clinicians dealing with lumbosacral lipoma to realize that progressive neurologic impairment can develop in patients who initially seem to be normal. It is frequently impossible to determine the extent of the involvement on clinical examination alone if results of radiographic and neurologic examinations are normal. Dubowitz et al.[6] have stressed the importance of considering intradural connections of the superficial mass in all cases. However, surgical therapy seems to be effective even if some of the lipomatous mass is left within the conus.

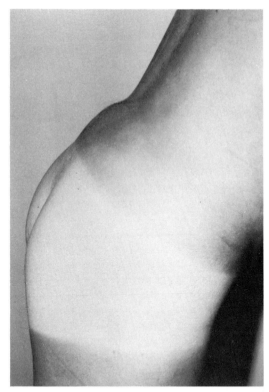

FIG. 5–18. Lumbosacral lipoma in a 34-year-old male.

MENINGOCELE

Meningocele over the lower spine is a rare lesion that does not directly involve the neural tube but it must be considered in the differential diagnosis of skin-covered cystic masses in this region. In a typical case the posterior spinous processes of some lower lumbar vertebrae are not fused, and there is a dorsal prolapse of arachnoid and dura mater. An abnormal subarachnoid space is formed over the spinal cord, which itself is intact and normal. No neurologic deficits are associated with true meningoceles, and most do not require resection if small. If a meningocele is large enough to hinder daily activities, an elective operation may be performed to reduce the size. Meningocele is generally not associated with hydrocephaly or other anomalies, and the prognosis is excellent.

There is no predilection for one sex over the other, and the exact incidence is not known, probably not more often than about 1/10 meningomyeloceles and therefore about 1/10,000 live births. Since the development of the dura mater begins ventral and lateral to the neural tube in stage XIX (16- to 18-mm CR), it is unlikely that the dorsal prolapse could arise until near the end of the embryonic period. Since the caudal neural tube remains close to the overlying skin until the vertebral laminae fuse even in early fetal life (see Chapter 19), it is more likely that such a prolapse of the dura would occur between the 50th and 70th gestational days.

Meningoceles that present ventrally through a sacral defect are very rare and are termed "anterior sacral meningoceles" (see Chapter 19).

MISCELLANEOUS SKIN-COVERED LESIONS[22, 28]

The differential diagnosis of lesions found over the caudal spine that are covered by intact skin and probably arise at varying times during the fetal period includes the following:

Myelocystocele
Meningocele
Lumbosacral lipoma
Teratoma
Duplication of rectum
Abscess
Hemangioma
Bone malformation
Bone tumor
Epidermoid (Dermoid) cyst
Pilonidal cyst
Chondroma
Neuroblastoma
Glioma
Chordoma

While not all are associated with the development of the nervous system, it is important that they be correctly diagnosed to provide the distinction.

Congenital dermal sinuses and cysts are probably derived as a result of an invagination of ectoderm that is carried by the neural tube as it separates from the surface.[11] They may occur at any level but are especially common in the posterior fossa and lumbosacral regions. They are of clinical importance in that they are associated with an increased risk for meningitis and should therefore be resected.

REFERENCES

1. Anderson FM: Occult spinal dysraphism: Diagnosis and management. J Pediatr 73:163–177, 1968

2. Ballantyne JW: Manual of Antenatal Pathology and Hygiene II. The Embryo. New York, William Wood, 1905

3. Barson AJ: Symptomless intradural spinal lipomas in infancy. J Pathol 104:141–144, 1971

4. Bolli P: Sekundäre Lumenbildungen im Neuralrohr und Rückenmark menschlicher Embryonen. Acta Anat (Basel) 64:48–81, 1966

5. Cohen J, Sledge CG: Diastematomyelia. Am J Dis Child 100: 257–263, 1960

6. Dubowitz V, Lorber J, Zachary RB: Lipoma of the cauda equina. Arch Dis Child 40:207–213, 1965

7. Emery JL, Lendon RG: Lipomas of the cauda equina and other fatty tumors related to neurospinal dysraphism. Dev Med Child Neurol [Suppl] 20:62–70, 1969

8. Gaertner RA: Development of the posterior trunk and tail of the chick embryo. J Exp Zool 111:157–174, 1949

9. Gardner WJ: Diastematomyelia and Klippel–Feil syndrome. Cleve Clin Q 31:19–44, 1964

10. Grabowski CT: The effects of the excision of Hensen's node on the early development of the chick embryo. J Exp Zool 133:301–344, 1956

11. Haworth JC, Zachary RB: Congenital dermal sinuses in children: Their relation to pilonidal sinuses. Lancet 2:10–14, 1955

12. Ikeda Y: Beiträge zur normalen und abnormalen Entwicklungsgeschichte des caudalen Abschnittes des Rückenmarks bei menschlichen Embryonen. Z Anat Entwicklungsgesch 92:380–490, 1930. (Quoted by Klika and Jelínek, 1969)

13. James CCM, Lassman LP: Diastematomyelia: a critical survey of 24 cases submitted to laminectomy. Arch Dis Child 39:125–130, 1964

14. James CCM, Lassman LP: Spinal Dysraphism: Spina Bifida Occulta. New York, Appleton-Century-Crofts, 1972

15. Jelínek R, Seichert V, Klika E: Mechanism of morphogenesis of caudal neural tube in the chick embryo. Folia Morphol (Praha) 17:355–367, 1969

16. Kernohan JW: The ventriculus terminalis: its growth and development. J Comp Neurol 38:107–125, 1925

17. Klika E, Jelínek R: The structure of the end and tail bud of the chick embryo. Folia Morphol (Praha) 17:29–40, 1969

18. Kunitomo K: The development and reduction of the tail and of the caudal end of the spinal cord. Contrib Embryol 8:161–198, 1918

19. Lassman LP, James CCM: Lumbosacral lipomas: critical survey of 26 cases submitted to laminectomy. J Neurol Neurosurg Psychiatry 30:174–181, 1967

20. Lemire RJ: Variations in development of the caudal neural tube in human embryos (Horizons XIV–XXI). Teratology 2:361–370, 1969

21. Lemire RJ: Development of the caudal neural tube in human embryos (Horizons XIII–XXI) (abstracted). Teratology 2:264, 1969

22. Lemire RJ, Graham CB, Beckwith JB: Skin-covered sacrococcygeal masses in infants and children. J Pediatr 79:948–954, 1971

23. Recklinghausen F: Untersuchungen über die Spina bifida. Berlin, Georg Reimer, 1886

24. Romanoff AL: The Avian Embryo. New York, Macmillan, 1960

25. Seichert V, Jelínek R: Tissue shifts in the end and tail bud of the chick embryo. Folia Morphol (Praha) 16:436–446, 1968

26. Shenefelt RE: Morphogenesis of malformations in hamsters caused by retinoic acid: Relation to dose and stage at treatment. Teratology 5:103–118, 1972

27. Streeter GL: Factors involved in the formation of the filum terminale. Am J Anat 25:1–11, 1919

28. Werner JL, Taybi H: Presacral masses in childhood. Am J Roentgenol Radium Ther Nucl Med 109:403–410, 1970

chapter 6

EPENDYMA AND DERIVATIVES

Ependyma, the postnatal lining of the ventricles, is originally comprised of neuroectodermal cells, most of which are actively dividing germinal cells destined to migrate radially and form the neurons and glia of the CNS. A few form several small but highly specialized organs, including the paraphysis, epiphysis, neurohypophysis, subcommissural organ and area postrema. A relatively inactive layer of these cells remains to line the ventricles, cover the choroid plexus and line the central canal of the spinal cord, including the portion that atrophies to form the filum terminale with the ventriculus terminalis and coccygeal medullary vestige (as described in Chapter 5). The major features of the development of the choroid plexus and other ependymal derivatives are summarized in Fig. 6–1.

NORMAL DEVELOPMENT*

CHOROID PLEXUS

Collectively, the choroid plexuses in the adult constitute approximately 100 million cells with a total surface area of 200 sq cm.[6, 30] They have been extensively studied both morphologically and functionally.[6, 7, 18, 35] Although they have long been regarded as a primary source for the production of CSF, recent data suggest that this may not be completely true.[17] The embryology of the choroid plexuses has been studied by Bailey,[1] Kappers,[14] Bartelmez and Dekaban[2] and Shuangshoti and Netsky.[25]

* See Chapter 1 for background information on embryologic development and staging system.

Choroid plexus first appears in the roof of the fourth ventricle at 16-mm CR (stage XVIII), in the lateral ventricles at 18-mm CR (stage XIX) and in the third ventricle at 23-mm CR (stage XXI). Kappers[14] quotes earlier studies suggesting that the anlage of choroid plexus may be present in some embryos of from 13- to 14-mm CR (stage XVII). The primordia appear as simple or club-shaped folds protruding into the ventricles. The ependymal lining is composed of pseudostratified columnar cells, 50–70 μ thick, with nuclei that are hyperchromatic, centrally placed and oval or fusiform. A brush border is seen in some areas. Very quickly (in the same stages), a central stalk is defined with ependymal cells containing few mitoses as opposed to the distal portion where numerous mitotic figures are found.

The first major changes in the choroid plexuses of the lateral ventricles are seen at from 22- to 23-mm CR (stage XXI), when they become lobulated as early vascularization of the stroma begins. At this time, the distal ependyma cells commence to change into a single columnar layer and become shorter (20–30 μ). Small vacuoles appear in their bases at this stage according to Kappers,[14] although Shuangshoti and Netsky[25] did not find them until later.

Progressive lobulation occurs, and at from 29- to 30-mm CR (stage XXIII) the distal ependyma is characterized as low columnar (20–25 μ) with apically placed nuclei, the base of each cell being occupied by PAS-positive vacuoles. The proximal ependyma remains pseudostratified, as do some cells at the depths of the interlobular clefts; both groups are devoid of vacuoles.

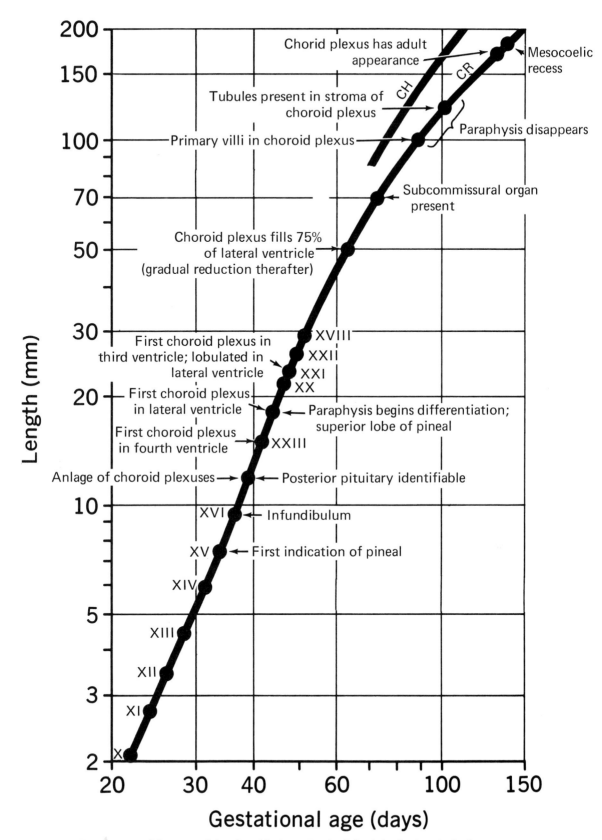

FIG. 6–1. Developmental features of the choroid plexus (to the left of the line) and of other ependymal derivatives (to the right of the line) are correlated with CR length and gestational age.

Increased amounts of PAS-positive material and generalized growth occur between 30- and 50-mm CR length, when the choroid plexus fills 75% of the lateral ventricle. At this time, portions of the interlobular clefts are pinched off, resulting in ependymal cells being entrapped in the stroma, which, previously more "gelatinous," now contains a few fibroblasts.

Between 85- and 120-mm CR length, the apically placed ependymal nuclei move centrally as the PAS-positive vacuoles decrease in size. At 100-mm CR length, primary villi begin to appear and the stroma is characterized by large numbers of fibroblasts. "Tubules" (thought to arise from the pinched-off interlobular clefts) become prominent in the stroma after 120-mm CR length. The stroma gains more collagen by 140-mm CR length. Beyond this time, there is a continued reduction in ependymal cell size with most cells ending as simple cuboidal epithelium, about 10 μ. Throughout the entire period there are changes in the vascular pattern and nature of other stromal elements. After 50-mm CR length, the choroid plexus undergoes a progressive reduction in size relative to the ventricular volume.

In comparing the development of the choroid plexuses of the third and fourth ventricles with that of the lateral ventricles, Shuangshoti and Netsky[25] state that those in the third and fourth ventricles complete their differentiation sooner, having the adult appearance by approximately 170-mm CR. Different amounts of glycogen occur in different sites, being greatest in lateral ventricle, next in the fourth ventricle and least in the third ventricle choroid plexuses.

PARAPHYSIS

Probably no single derivative of ependyma has been the subject of as much controversy as the transitory paraphysis, the most rostral of the dorsal recesses of the telencephalic part of the third ventricle. It arises just rostral to the velum transversum, which separates the telencephalon from the diencephalon. Earlier studies[15] found the paraphysis absent in embryos between 4- and 17-mm CR (stages XIII–XIX), present between 21- and 25.5-mm CR (stages XX–XXII) and absent thereafter. Kappers,[13] with excellent documentation, found it present in 30 speci-

mens between 17-mm CR (stage XIX) and 100-mm CR length, but he was unable to locate it in an additional fetus of 145-mm CR length. Kappers[13] showed that the paraphysis starts as a thickening of the ependyma, followed by the formation of a vacuole that is at first not in continuity with the ventricle. Eventually the vacuole and ventricle communicate, and the gland acquires several lobules before it regresses into obscurity.

PINEAL GLAND (EPIPHYSIS)

The pineal gland develops from a recess located between the habenular commissure rostrally and the posterior commissure caudally; the apex of its body is in the midline above the superior colliculi. Recent reviews of its function,[22] of its phylogeny[36] and of its postnatal histology[23] in humans have been published. The two lobes (superior and inferior) of the pineal are comprised of lobules, the parenchyma of which is divided by connective tissue septa. Around the entire body is a capsule of large astrocytes that are interconnected with astroglia within the lobules. Pinealocytes, blood vessels, myelineated and unmyelineated nerve fibers and oligodendrocytes fill the gland. The adult pineal weighs 100–180 g and is 5–9 mm wide.[36] It is innervated by sympathetic nerves from the superior cervical ganglia and has a propensity to undergo calcification and cystic degeneration. Although microscopic calcification may be seen in infants,[36] roentgenographically demonstrable amounts do not accumulate until puberty in most cases, and only then in approximately 25% of people.

Hochstetter,[12] Streeter[28] and Bartelmez and Dekaban[2] provide landmarks in the development of the pineal. The primordium of the pineal starts as a slight thickening of the midline ependyma early in stage XV (7- to 8-mm CR) followed by a small evagination (recess). Its site is further demarcated in stage XVI (8- to 11-mm CR), when fibers can be identified in the posterior commissure. During stage XVII (14- to 16-mm CR), the neuroblasts of the mantle zone acquire a follicular pattern, creating vacuoles that are not connected with the lumen. In older embryos of stage XIX (17-mm CR), the superior lobe begins to differentiate.

SUBCOMMISSURAL ORGAN AND MESOCOELIC RECESS

The posterior commissure forms the caudal boundary of the pineal and the rostral boundary of the subcommissural organ, an ependymal derivative located dorsally at the junction of the third ventricle and cerebral aqueduct. The subcommissural organ is better defined in lower vertebrates as its secretory activity produces Reissner's fiber, which is said to extend from the subcommissural organ down the length of the central canal of the spinal cord. It is also considered to be the source of aldosterone-stimulating hormone. In humans it is composed of two parts: 1) the organ proper, an area of tall columnar ciliated epithelium which faces the third ventricle and secretes a PAS-positive substance and 2) the mesocoelic recess, an evagination of the cerebral aqueduct lined by smaller ependymal cells with basally located nuclei. Although there is some disagreement as to whether or not the organ atrophies in adult life,[11] it has been identified as being present with secretory activity as early as 70-mm CR in the human fetus.[34] In a study of human specimens from 20 weeks gestational age (about 180-mm CR, according to our estimate) through adulthood, Rakic[21] found the mesocoelic recess in all cases until 11 months postnatally and sporadically thereafter.

POSTERIOR PITUITARY

Tilney,[29] Streeter[28] and Bartelmez and Dekaban[2] have studied this region carefully. In stage XV (7- to 9-mm CR) the position of the oral hypophysis marks the site of the future infundibulum (posterior pituitary, neurohypophysis, neural lobe or pars neuralis). The first evagination of the infundibulum on the floor of the diencephalon is found in stage XVI (8- to 11-mm CR). During stage XVII (11- to 14-mm CR) this evagination takes on the appearance of a "wrinkled sac" that can be termed the posterior pituitary. Between stages XVIII and XXIII, the main changes in the posterior pituitary are an increase in size and a deepening of the foldings. In stage XXI the infundibulum still has a narrow canal that communicates with the ventricle and expands distally into a small pouch within the infundibular process.

During the fetal period there are several changes in the posterior pituitary.[24, 29] Between 55- and 100-mm CR length, it is triangular, and the outer zone is relatively acellular. The canal contains many densely packed nuclei with little cytoplasm. At 120-mm CR length the stem elongates downward and backward to form an angle of 20° with the ventricular floor. Glandular tissue is present, and cellular processes appear about this time. When the fetus reaches 170-mm CR length, the infundibular angle is 45°, and thereafter it gradually increases until birth, when it is nearly perpendicular. Cellular changes between 170- and 200-mm CR length further define the posterior pituitary gland. Proximally the cells, called pituicytes, and their processes are arranged in whorls around connective tissue trabeculae. Their nuclei are oval, but the entire cell is stellate with from three to six processes. Inter- and intracellular granules are present. The distal portion of the posterior pituitary has oval or fusiform cells with either one or two processes. In contrast to the proximal cells, there are no intracellular granules, but some intercellular granules exist.

At the time of birth the proximal portion of the posterior pituitary exhibits an increase in connective tissue trabeculae, whereas the distal portion does not have this increase. The pituicytes enlarge and many of their processes form an anastomotic network.

ABNORMAL DEVELOPMENT

EXPERIMENTAL CONSIDERATIONS

Before considering human anomalies, we should consider the reactions of the ependyma (and neural tube) in several experimental situations. Many of the following remarks are taken from the article by Watterston.[32]

Irradiation

If the early ependyma is x-irradiated, many of the cells have a propensity to form *rosettes, i.e.,* vacuoles surrounded by several layers of germinal cells. These rosettes are somewhat similar to the vacuoles normally found in the differentiating caudal cell mass during the canalization phase after closure of the posterior neuropore. Irradiation also has an effect on the cell cycle by temporarily blocking cells in the G2 phase just prior to mitosis[9] without affecting either DNA synthesis (S phase) or cells in mitosis (M phase).

Mechanical Injury

Mechanical injury can be applied to the neural tube in a variety of situations, such as by direct puncture with a needle or extirpation of a segment. Studies utilizing this general approach have provided information with respect to the importance of several structures in normal differentiation. If one lateral half of a recently closed neural tube is removed, the remaining three-fourths differentiate normally, and only cell groups derived from the extirpated segment are missing. This type of experiment is helpful in determining which portions of the early ependyma contribute cells to specific cell groups.

Inductive Influence of the Notochord

The inductive influence of both notochord and mesoderm on ependymal differentiation has also been studied experimentally. That the ependyma in the recently closed neural tube is normally thinnest ventrally (toward the notochord) and thickest laterally (toward the somite) suggests corresponding inhibitory and stimulatory effects on the interkinetic cell cycle. This has been further shown in experiments where duplication of the notochord produces two areas of ventral thinning.

Most of these experimental observations do not have direct human applications, but some insight may be gained in attempting to understand deficiencies arising in the migration of cells from the ependymal zone to other sites.

HETEROTOPIAS AND CELL RESTS

Neuronal and glial heterotopias are found in the CNS in a variety of clinical entities discussed throughout this book. These cells are derivatives of ependyma, but the manner in which they arrive and differentiate at these various sites is unclear.

Ependymal *rests* are normally found in the filum terminale and at other sites where the ventricular walls have collapsed upon each other (*e.g.*, occipital horn, angles of ventricles). Their presence in other areas not associated with the previous central canal must be considered anomalous.

CHOROID PLEXUS

An important lesion of the choroid plexus, the papilloma (Figures 6–2 and 6–3), is rare but most commonly occurs in the glomus of the lateral ventricle. Communicating nonobstructive hydrocephalus is caused by the overproduction of CSF, sometimes many liters per day. It may be converted to an obstructive type either by hemorrhage from the friable tumor producing a hemogenic meningitis, or by shedding of the tips of papillae and seeding throughout the leptomeningeal spaces.

In addition, there are a variety of cysts, the most common of which is the result of hemorrhage (*xanthomas*) into the stroma of the glomus of the choroid plexus in the trigone of the lateral ventricle. Occasionally, a benign cyst[26] is found incidentally in fetuses and adults. Choroid plexus is one of the elements typically found among the neural derivatives in sacrococcygeal teratomas (see Chapter 22).

PARAPHYSIS

Colloid cysts of the third ventricle are only one of a number of cysts found in the CNS that Shuangshoti and Netsky[26] believe are more appropriately called *neuroepithelial cysts.*[26]

Sjövall[27] is credited as the first person to suggest either in 1909[5] the "ependymal" origin or in 1910[26] the "paraphyseal" origin of colloid cysts in the third ventricle. Dandy[5] is frequently given credit for popularizing these lesions by collecting 31 cases from the literature and adding 5 cases of his own, the largest series reported up to that time. By 1958, over 250 cases had been reported, including a series of 54 cases reviewed by Yenermen *et al.*[37] There is no sexual pre-

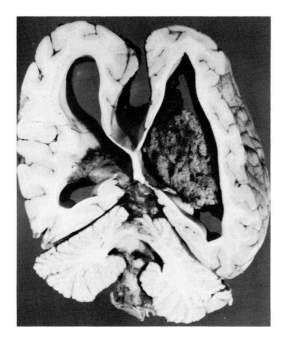

FIG. 6–2. Choroid plexus papilloma of a 4-year-old girl who had an enlarged head and retarded development of speech and motor coordination, but was not seen medically until hospitalized for an upper respiratory infection. Ventriculography demonstrated marked hydrocephalus and a mass in the left lateral ventricle, but she died with bronchopneumonia 12 days later without surgical intervention. (#D 932)

FIG. 6–3. Papilloma of the choroid plexus of the third ventricle of an 18-month-old girl with an abnormally enlarging head since age 6 months. At the terminal stage, CSF was bloody, and nests of neoplastic cells were found microscopically in the basal leptomeninges. (#Np 2254)

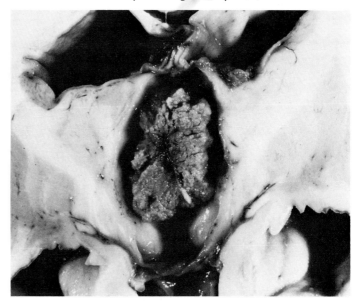

dilection. Although they can occur in infants,[10] they more often present symptomatically after the 20th postnatal year.[8] These cysts usually arise in the rostral midline roof of the third ventricle adjacent to the presumed site of the transient paraphysis (Figs. 6–4, 6–5a and 6–5b). They are attached to the choroid plexus in 50% of the cases (Figs. 6–6 and 6–7); they contain a mucinous material [19] (Fig. 6–8) which may be phagocytosed (Fig. 6–9); they cause obstructive symptoms at the foramina of Monro. If large or more caudally located, they can produce third ventricular outlet obstruction.

FIG. 6–4

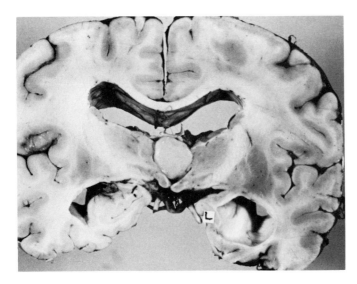

FIG. 6–5

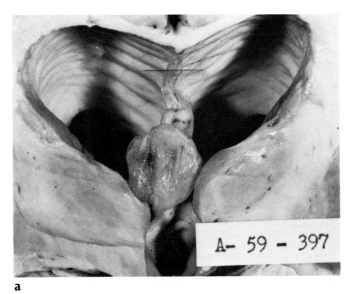

a

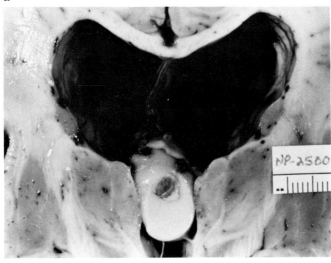

b

◀ FIG. 6–4. Coronal section of the brain of a 68-year-old man with a colloid cyst in the third ventricle (the most common location). The cyst was lined by ciliated epithelium and obstructed the flow of CSF, with resultant hydrocephalus. (#Np 380)

◀ FIG. 6–5. **a.** Coronal section of the brain of a 58-year-old woman with a colloid cyst originating from the roof of the third ventricle and obstructing the foramina of Monro. Note the ventricular dilatation. (HH#A 59-397) **b.** Coronal section of the brain of an 84-year-old woman with the plane of section passing through the colloid cyst. This cyst, lined by ciliated epithelium, acted as an obstruction and caused dilatation of the lateral ventricles. (#Np 2500)

The popularity for the paraphyseal origin of colloid cysts is indicated in the titles of many articles[3, 10] and in books,[33] but Kappers[13] accepts only the two cases of Zeitlin and Lichtenstein[38] as paraphyseal in origin on the basis that their cells are not ciliated. Shuangshoti and Netsky[26] agree that some colloid cysts of the third ventricle may arise from the paraphysis, but they disagree with Kapper's criteria. Other investigators, while providing excellent clinical[37] or histologic[4] studies, have expressed no preference for the origin of these cysts. Since these cysts only very rarely occur elsewhere,[20, 26] the argument seems academic.

PINEAL

Warkany[31] provides an excellent discussion of anomalies of the pineal body. These include primary aplasia of unknown etiology and aplasia secondary to hydrocephalus. Varying degrees of hypoplasia have been reported. In one case, there was associated micrencephaly, microgyria, porencephaly and chorioretinitis; in another the hypoplasia of the main pineal was accompanied by an accessory pineal and arachnoid cysts. Hyperplasia without neoplasia has also been

FIG. 6–6. Photomicrograph of an asymptomatic small colloid cyst of the third ventricle developing between the choroid plexus and the left fornix in an 82-year-old man. The epithelium was not ciliated. (#Np 1042)

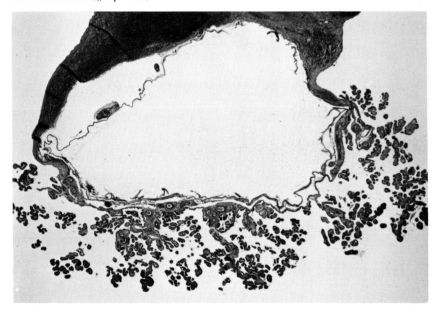

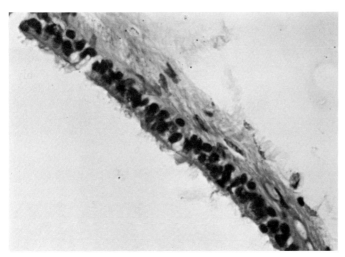

FIG. 6–7. Photomicrograph of the colloid cyst in Fig. 6–5**b** showing ciliated low columnar cells on a layer of collagen.

FIG. 6–8. Low-power photomicrograph of a colloid cyst of the third ventricle of a 13-year-old boy, stained with periodic-acid-Schiff. The mass of lipid-filled macrophages on the left arises at a site where nonciliated epithelium is absent. This cyst was attached to the fornices, but not directly to the choroid plexus. (#Np 3440)

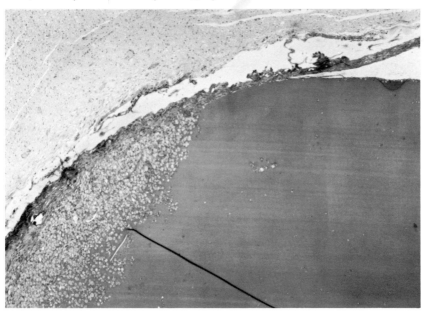

found. Pineal rests have been found in the quadrigeminal plate,[36] and neuroepithelial pineal cysts can occur independently or associated with pinealoma.[26] Neoplasms (pinealoma, pineal germinoma or teratoma) are discussed in Chapter 22.

SUBCOMMISSURAL ORGAN

We have been unable to locate any anomalies that specifically involve the subcommissural organ or mesocoelic recess. Since the latter is actually within the aqueduct of

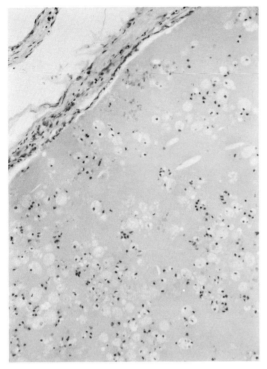

FIG. 6–9. High-power photomicrograph of the macrophages in the colloid cyst in Figure 6–8.

Sylvius, it may be the source of neuroepithelial cysts, termed mesencephalic cysts. Lu et al.[16] reported one such case in a 5-year-old child who had meningitis (*Listeria monocytogenes*) as an infant; the authors, however, concluded that the cyst was of developmental origin. The patient had obstructive hydrocephalus; neuropathologic exam revealed "broad" convolutions of the cerebral cortex, small choroid plexuses, and a trabecula dividing the opening to the aqueduct, one channel of which communicated with the cyst. Histologically, most of the cyst wall was lined with ependyma surrounded by glia. Shuangshoti and Netsky[26] reported another similar cyst (case 4) lined by simple cuboidal or columnar ependyma with numerous papillary projections resembling choroid plexus. No communication between the dorsally placed cyst and the aqueduct could be found, so that it probably represented an area of "pinched-off" ependyma.

POSTERIOR PITUITARY

Anomalies of the pituitary gland are discussed in Chapter 21.

REFERENCES

1. Bailey P: Morphology of the roof plate of the forebrain and the lateral choroid plexuses in the human embryo. J Comp Neurol 26:79–120, 1916

2. Bartelmez GW, Dekaban AS: The early development of the human brain. Contrib Embryol 37:13–32, 1962

3. Bull JWD, Sutton D: The diagnosis of paraphysial cysts. Brain 72:487–516, 1949

4. Coxe WS, Luse SA: Colloid cyst of third ventricle. J Neuropathol Exp Neurol 23:431–445, 1964

5. Dandy WE: Benign Tumors of the Third Ventricle of the Brain: Diagnosis and Treatment. Springfield, CC Thomas, 1933

6. Dohrmann GJ: The choroid plexus: a historical review. Brain Res 18:197–218, 1970

7. Dunn J Jr, Kernohan JW: Histologic changes within the choroid plexus of the lateral ventricle: their relation to age. Proc Staff Mayo Clinic 30:607–615, 1955

8. Ferry DJ, Kempe LG: Colloid cyst of the third ventricle. Milit Med 133:734–737, 1968

9. Fujita S, Horii M, Tanimura T, Nishimura H: H3-thymidine autoradiographic studies on cytokinetic responses to X-ray irradiation and to thio-TEPA in the neural tube of mouse embryos. Anat Rec 149:37–48, 1964

10. Gemperlein J: Paraphyseal cysts of the third ventricle. Report of two cases in infants. J Neuropathol Exp Neurol 19:133–134, 1960

11. Gilbert G: The subcommissural organ. Neurology (Minneap) 10:138–142, 1960

12. Hochstetter F: Beiträge zur Entwicklungsgeschichte des menschlichen Gehirns, 2, part 1. Die Entwicklung der Zirbeldruse. Vienna and Leipzig, Franz Deuticke, 1923, pp. 1–46

13. Kappers JA: The development of the paraphysis cerebri in man with comments on its relationship to the intercolumnar tubercle and its significance for the origin of cystic tumors in the third ventricle. J Comp Neurol 102:425–510, 1955

14. Kappers JA: Structural and functional changes in the telencephalic choroid plexus during human ontogenesis. The Cerebrospinal Fluid. Edited by GEW Wolstenholme and CM O'Connor. Ciba Foundation Symposium. Boston, Little, Brown and Co, 1958, pp. 3–25

15. Krabbe KH: Studies on the existence of a paraphysis in mammalian embryos. Brain 59:483–493, 1936

16. Lu AT, Yuen TGH, Bassler TJ: Mesencephalic cyst in fourth ventricle causing obstructive hydrocephalus. Bull Los Angeles Neurol Soc 27:79–86, 1962

17. Milhorat TH: Choroid plexus and cerebrospinal fluid production. Science 166:1514–1516, 1969

18. Millen JW, Woollam DHM: The Anatomy of the Cerebrospinal Fluid. New York, Oxford Univ Press, 1962

19. Mosberg WH Jr, Blackwood W: Mucus-secreting cells in colloid cysts of the third ventricle. J Neuropathol Exp Neurol 13:417–426, 1954

20. Parkinson D, Childe AE: Colloid cyst of the fourth ventricle. J. Neurosurg 9:404–409, 1952

21. Rakic P: Mesocoelic recess in the human brain. Neurology (Minneap) 15:708–715, 1965

22. Relkin R: The pineal gland. N Engl J Med 274:944–950, 1966

23. Scharenberg K, Liss L: The histologic structure of the human pineal body. Prog Brain Res 10:193–217, 1965

24. Shanklin WM: Differentiation of pituicytes in the human foetus. J Anat 74:459–463, 1940

25. Shuangshoti S, Netsky MG: Histogenesis of the choroid plexus in man. Am J Anat 118:283–316, 1966

26. Shuangshoti S, Netsky MG: Neuroepithelial (colloid) cysts of the nervous system. Neurology (Minneap) 16:887–903, 1966

27. Sjövall E: (quoted by Dandy, 1933; Shuangshoti and Netsky, 1966)

28. Streeter GL: Developmental Horizons in Human Embryos, Age Groups XI–XXIII. Embryol Reprint, vol II, Washington DC, Carnegie Inst Wash, 1951

29. Tilney F: The development and constituents of the human hypophysis. Bull Neurol Inst NY 5:387–436, 1936

30. Voetmann E: On the structure and surface area of the human choroid plexuses (a quantitative anatomical study). Acta Anat (Basel) [Suppl] 10:1–116, 1949

31. Warkany J: Congenital Malformations. Chicago, Year Book Medical Publishers, 1971

32. Watterson RL: Structure and mitotic behavior of the early neural tube, Organogenesis. Edited by RL DeHaan and H Ursprung. New York, Holt, Rinehart and Winston, 1965, pp. 129–159

33. Willis RA: The Borderland of Embryology and Pathology, ed 2. Washington, Butterworths, 1962

34. Wislocki GB, Roth WD: Selective staining of the human subcommissural organ. Anat Rec 130:125–133, 1958

35. Wolstenholme GEW, O'Connor CM (eds): The Cerebrospinal Fluid. CIBA Foundation Symposium. Boston, Little, Brown and Co, 1958

36. Wurtman R, Axelrod J, Kelly DE: The Pineal. New York, Academic Press, 1968

37. Yenermen MH, Bowerman CI, Haymaker W: Colloid cyst of the third ventricle. Acta Neurovegetativa 17:211–277, 1958

38. Zeitlin H, Lichtenstein BW: Cystic tumor of the third ventricle containing colloid material. Arch Neurol Psychiatr 38:268–287, 1947

chapter 7

VENTRICULAR SYSTEM AND CEREBROSPINAL FLUID (CSF) FLOW

The adult central nervous system is surrounded by cerebrospinal fluid (CSF), which is mainly secreted by the choroid plexuses within the lateral, third and fourth ventricles. The mechanical effects of this fluid environment are well established; the role that it plays in the physiologic functions of the brain and spinal cord is less well known. This chapter focuses upon the development of the ventricular system and CSF flow and some of the expressions of errors in morphogenesis that are visualized in extrauterine life. The works of Bartelmez and Dekaban,[5] Heuser and Corner[12] and Streeter[25-28] provided most of the data on normal development.

NORMAL DEVELOPMENT*

It is important to emphasize that the CNS from its earliest form as the neural plate is bathed by fluid, at first by the amnionic fluid and after neurulation has occurred, by CSF. Whereas amnionic circulation apparently is capable of providing essential nutrients, the CSF is not; capillary ingrowth occurs as soon as neurulation has occurred and differentiation within the neural tube results in a multilayered structure. Circulation of blood within the vascular system of the embryo is required for further cellular differentiation.

As schematized in Figure 7–1 closure of the neural tube is completed by stage XII (3- to 5-mm CR). The ventricular system at this

* See Chapter 1 for background information on embryologic development and staging system.

time is clearly demarcated into the cavities of the prosencephalon, mesencephalon, metencephalon and myelencephalon continuous with the central canal of the spinal cord. The mammillary recesses develop at the junction of the prosencephalon and mesencephalon during this stage. Caudal to the posterior neuropore, the differentiating neural tube forms small vesicles that serially coalesce by the process of canalization (see Chapter 5) to extend the central canal of the spinal cord. By stage XIII (4- to 6-mm CR) the evaginations of the optic vesicles are clearly seen. At this time the rhombencephalic ventricle rapidly enlarges, and the rhombencephalic roof protrudes from the dorsal surface of the embryo. The earliest differentiation of the primitive leptomeninx into pia can be seen at this time; the process starts in the region of the medulla. During stage XIV (5- to 7-mm CR) the rhombencephalic roof becomes attenuated and differs from the remainder of the dorsal nervous system because of the absence of neuroblasts. The ventricle of the telencephalon medianum rapidly enlarges. In stage XV (7- to 9-mm CR) the evaginations of the cerebral hemispheres develop on either side of the telencephalon medianum, and the velum transversum demarcates the diencephalic ventricle from the telencephalic anterior portion of the third ventricle. By stage XV pia can be clearly identified surrounding the brain stem.

Stage XVI (8- to 11-mm CR) is characterized by the development of the marginal ridge between the thalamus and the hypothalamus and by the evagination of the neu-

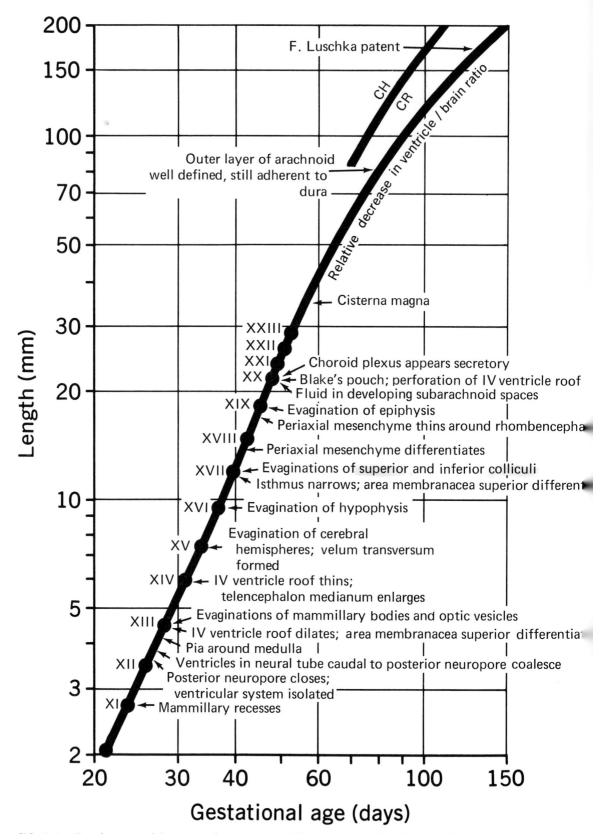

FIG. 7–1. Development of the ventricular system and CSF pathway correlated with CR length and gestational age.

rohypophysis from the floor of the hypo-thalamus. During stage XVII (11- to 14-mm CR) the evaginations of the superior and inferior colliculi become distinct, and the growth of the basal plate begins to reduce the relative size of the ventricular lumina throughout the neuraxis. In stage XIX (16- to 18-mm CR) the evagination of the epi-physis is first seen. The growth of the cere-bral evaginations is so rapid that by stage XX (18- to 22-mm CR) the cerebral hemispheres overlap the diencephalon and the lateral ven-tricles are the largest portion of the ventric-ular system.

At this stage the roof of the rhombenceph-alon becomes uniquely differentiated; the ependymal lining loses its mitotic activity and forms a single epithelial layer. Caudal to the plica choroidea of the fourth ventricle the roof of the fourth ventricle becomes per-forated and forms the foramen of Magendie. The exact time of this critical event has been debated for over a century; indeed, the mere presence of this foramen in man has been, for much of this century, a source of heated discussion and polemic, which was finally laid to rest by Barr[4] in 1948.

During stage XX major changes alter the appearance of the choroid plexus and the leptomeninx. The cellular elements of the choroid plexus become granulated and de-velop the appearance of secretory epi-thelium. The loose syncytial network of peri-axial mesenchyme rapidly differentiates as soon as CSF is found outside the fourth ventricle; this process starts in the region of the cisterna magna and spreads to other basal regions and thence over the hemi-spheres and spinal cord. The metamorphosis of the leptomeninges into thin arachnoid trabeculae that create a fluid-containing space occurs within several days of the first appearance of extraventricular CSF, al-though the arachnoid membrane itself does not delaminate from the dura mater until much later.

Stages XX–XXII are important to the de-velopment of normal ventricular and CSF flow systems. Three critical events are closely related in time: 1) perforation of the roof of the fourth ventricle, 2) development of secretory epithelium in the choroid plexus and 3) differentiation of leptomeninx into arachnoid trabeculae with the formation of subarachnoid space. Histologic studies of the roof of the fourth ventricle[9] clearly show that it is not the buildup of CSF pressure that leads to the perforation of the roof of the fourth ventricle, but rather an active process of differentiation which is initiated just prior to the development of function of the choroid plexus.

The development of the foramen of Magendie is one of the most important events in the dynamics of CSF circulation. This region of the brain has been intensively studied in man and many other species. The classic works of Weed[30] and Blake[8] are the basis of many subsequent studies.[23, 31] Blake[8] described a closed pouch that evagi-nates from the caudal fourth ventricle and persists as a pouch in some species but is lost in man. Barr[4] has measured the cross-sec-tional area of the foramen of Magendie in normal adult humans and found that it is practically always patent.

The other outlets from the fourth ventricle are the foramina of Luschka, which are found at the lateral margin of the choroidal fissure of the fourth ventricle, adjacent to cranial nerves VII and VIII. These are usu-ally patent in the term human fetus (Brock-elhurst[9] describes them as patent at 220-mm CR length and others[22, 29] at 195-mm CR length), but the size of the embryo or fetus when they first open has never been ascer-tained. In general, those animals with a large foramen of Magendie have small foramina of Luschka and vice versa. Normal man has all three foramina patent at the time of birth, although Alexander[1] showed that about 20% of otherwise normal humans have congeni-tally impatent foramina of Luschka, almost always bilaterally symmetric.

The development of the ventricular system during fetal life mirrors the growth of each segment of the CNS. The central canal of the spinal cord is usually obliterated after birth because of the growth of the neuronal and glial elements; the ventricular system then terminates at the level of the obex. Epen-dymal remnants persist into adult life in the spinal cord. The aqueduct (Fig. 7-2) nar-rows both relatively and absolutely as the mesencephalon develops until about six months gestation and then enlarges some-what. The relative size of the lateral ventri-cles is reduced by hemispheral cortical and white matter development. The volume of the ventricular system in relation to that of

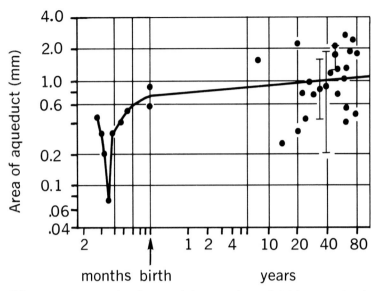

FIG. 7–2. Cross sectional area of the aqueduct of Sylvius correlated with age. (Adapted from Alvord, 1961)

the CNS steadily decreases as the neural tube differentiates into its various components; the absolute volume obviously increases until full brain growth is achieved in childhood.

ABNORMAL DEVELOPMENT

HYDROCEPHALUS

The main anomaly associated with the development of the ventricular system and CSF flow is hydrocephalus, a condition in which all or part of the ventricular system is dilated, most frequently secondary to increased intraventricular pressure due to obstruction in the flow of CSF. Actually, any abnormal collection of fluid within the ventricles can be termed hydrocephalus, those cases without increased CSF pressure usually being termed hydrocephalus *ex vacuo*, although a few may be examples of arrested hydrocephalus after some resolution of the previously increased pressure.

In recent years patients with hydrocephalus have been successfully treated by draining CSF from the brain to some other site by way of polyethylene tubes with interposed reservoirs and pressure valves, these shunts being named after the sites involved, *e.g.*, ventriculoatrial (VA), ventriculoperitoneal (VP). Because adequate therapy is now available for this condition, a problem that was previously quite devastating has a more optimistic prognosis.

The incidence of hydrocephalus (with and without meningomyelocele) is 1/1200 live births overall with marked variations throughout the world.[11,19] In addition to the fact that it commonly accompanies meningomyelocele, hydrocephalus has been found to be associated with prenatal infections (cytomegalovirus, toxoplasmosis and possibly mumps) and with some recessively inherited syndromes (*e.g.*, Hurler).

Hydrocephalus has been found to occur spontaneously and can be readily produced experimentally in several species of animals. Rodents are particularly susceptible to hydrocephalus induced by numerous teratogenic agents (*e.g.*, irradiation, drugs, dyes) as well as by dietary alterations (*e.g.*, folic acid and pantothenic acid deficiencies). Kalter[15] provides extensive discussions of the studies reported to 1968. Recent experimental studies on hydrocephalus have been published by Woodard and Newberne,[33] who found aqueductal stenosis (associated with aplasia of the subcommissural organ and other CNS malformations) in offspring of vitamin B_{12}-deficient rats; Margolis and Kilham,[18] who inoculated Reovirus type 1 in suckling hamsters; Wisniewski *et al.*,[32] who

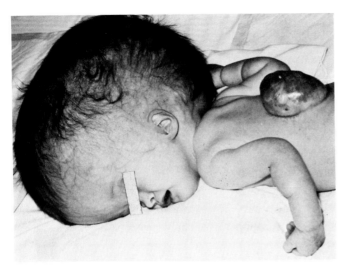

FIG. 7–3. An untreated infant with thoracic meningomyelocele and hydrocephalus. The head is large, and the scalp veins are prominently dilated. The eyes manifest the "setting-sun sign."

FIG. 7–4. Hair in fibrotic leptomeninges in a patient with a meningomyelocele and the Arnold–Chiari malformation.

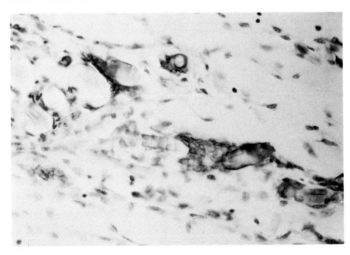

injected silicone oil into the subarachnoid space of dogs and rabbits; and Chamberlain,[10] who gave 6-aminonicotinamide to pregnant rats, the offspring of which were noted to have intracranial hemorrhage, hypoplastic choroid plexuses and hydrocephalus.

A variety of acquired pathologic processes and congenital anomalies can lead to a failure of the subarachnoid spaces to be competent and this can in turn lead to an enlarge-ment of the ventricles. Malformations of the brain and spinal cord can lead to accompanying changes in the size and contours of the ventricles, but these are probably not malformations whose pathogenesis is related to the original fluid-containing spaces. Untreated hydrocephalus of any etiology can lead to the cosmetic and neurologic sequelae shown in Figure 7–3.

Table 7–1 relates causes of hydrocephalus found in infants and children to sites at

TABLE 7–1. COMMON CAUSES OF
HYDROCEPHALUS

Site of Block	Etiology
Arachnoid Villi	Failure to develop, obstruction by infection or hemorrhage
Subarachnoid Spaces	Meningitis, pyogenic or tuberculous
	Subarachnoid hemorrhage traumatic ruptured arteriovenous malformation or neoplasm from subependymal and intraventricular hemorrhage in the premature infant
Fourth Ventricular Outlet	Meningitis, tuberculous
	Arnold–Chiari malformation
	Dandy–Walker malformation
	Neoplasm
	Cysts of posterior fossa
Fourth Ventricle	Arnold–Chiari malformation
	Neoplasm (medulloblastoma, ependymoma, choroid plexus papilloma)
Aqueduct of Sylvius	Ependymitis mumps pyogenic meningitis
	Genetic trait (X-linked)
	Arnold–Chiari malformation
	Aneurysm of the Vein of Galen
	Mesencephalic tumor or arteriovenous malformation
	Pinealoma
	"Disuse atrophy" or collapse after shunt
Third Ventricle	Pinealoma
	Colloid cyst
	Intrinsic neoplasm (astrocytoma of septum and thalamus)
Foramina of Monro	Colloid cyst
	Ventriculitis
	Neoplasm (glioma, tuberous sclerosis)
Lateral Ventricles	Subependymal cyst Neoplasm Subependymal hemorrhage

which an obstruction can occur. Recent comprehensive reviews[6, 11, 19] that elaborate on all aspects of the subject are available, and the pathology of hydrocephalus has been discussed by Russell[24] and Alvord.[2] The manner in which hydrocephalus is classified varies from one author to another, but the one utilized by Milhorat[19] has merit from the clinical viewpoint. He makes two divisions on the basis of whether 1) the hydrocephalus is noncommunicating or communicating (see below) or 2) it is congenital or acquired. The following discussion will approach the topic on the basis of anatomy, i.e., the sites at which CSF flow may be blocked, and will mention selected examples of lesions that can cause these blocks.

Although some CSF is elaborated by the ependyma itself, the choroid plexus is believed by most to be its major source. Similarly, some reabsorption can occur through the ependyma, including that of the choroid plexus, but the largest portion of CSF is reabsorbed into the major venous sinuses from the subarachnoid spaces over the cerebral hemispheres. Any lesion that isolates the major sources of CSF from the major reabsorptive sites can lead to an excessive volume of fluid, clinically recognized as hydrocephalus. However, the block leading to hydrocephalus in most cases is likely to occur at one of the sites of normal narrowing of the ventricular system: the foramina of Monro, cerebral aqueduct or foramina of Luschka and Magendie. This type of hydrocephalus is commonly called *obstructive, noncommunicating*. The word "noncommunicating" implies only that the occluded lateral ventricles do not communicate with the lumbar subarachnoid space; this observation is derived from the old diagnostic study of injecting a dye into the lateral ventricle and subsequently performing a lumbar puncture. A block can also occur in the basal cisterns, preventing the flow of CSF over the cerebral hemispheres; this is *obstructive, communicating* hydrocephalus. A more distal block at the arachnoid villi also produces obstructive, communicating hydrocephalus. Multiple sites of CSF blockage are present in many cases, so that the diagnosis and treatment may be somewhat complicated. This is especially true in cases with a papilloma of the choroid plexus (see Chapter 6), or with infections producing ventriculitis and meningitis.

Abnormalities of the Subarachnoid Spaces

Unusual findings in the subarachnoid space have included hair (Fig. 7–4) and epithelial

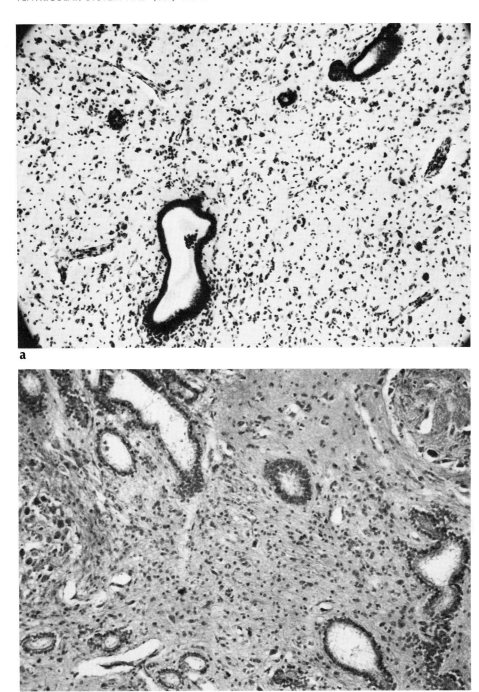

FIG. 7–5a and **b.** Two microscopic views from the same patient showing marked forking malformation of the aqueduct with complete rosettes. (From Alvord, 1961) (#D-658)

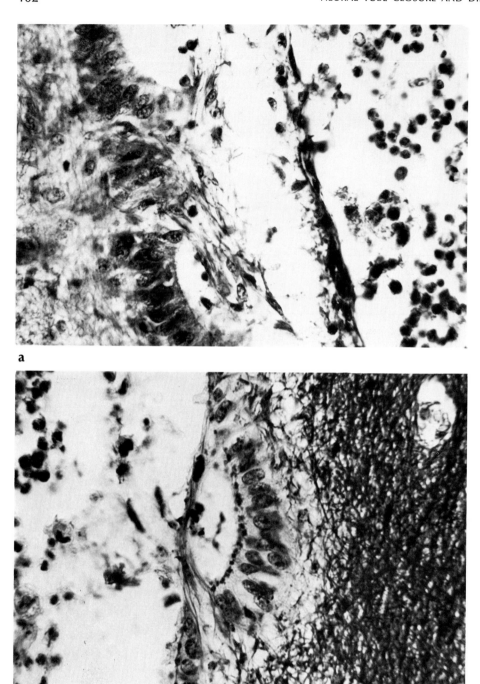

a

b

FIG. 7–6**a** and **b.** Two microscopic views of the same patient (who had an Arnold–Chiari malformation) showing acquired forking of the aqueduct with incomplete rosettes resulting from proliferation of subependymal astrocytes and lack of proliferation of the ependymal cells. (From Alvord, 1961) (#D-520)

debris in patients with meningomyeloceles.[14] The pathogenesis of this is not clear, but it probably represents a secondary inclusion of ectodermal tissue due to failure of the neural tube to close rather than an abnormal development of multipotent cells.

Cysts of the leptomeninges ("arachnoid") have been described in spinal and cranial regions (see Chapter 17); these can be due to inflammatory changes after infection or trauma but more commonly appear to be the result of a developmental anomaly with failure of the arachnoid trabeculae to become separated from each other or with splitting of the arachnoid membrane itself as it delaminates from the dura. Thoracic arachnoid cysts have been well described in the clinical literature and probably represent a failure of the primitive leptomeninges to dedifferentiate; dorsal to the spinal cord are created multiple pockets that become distended with CSF and can penetrate the dura or compress the spinal cord. Leptomeningeal cysts can occur within the dura without apparent connection to the subarachnoid space; these attest to the fact that some fluid secretion can occur from leptomeningeal cells themselves. Arachnoid cysts have also been noted over the cerebral hemispheres and in the posterior fossa. Some of these achieve considerable size and can compress the adjacent brain, distort skull growth and cause hydrocephalus.

The arachnoid villi that line the major sinuses are probably essential for the absorption of CSF, although they are sparsely present at the time of birth and develop in the first several years of life. Congenital anomalies of these structures have been described, but prenatal and perinatal infection or subarachnoid hemorrhage can also lead to their obliteration and the subsequent development of obstructive communicating hydrocephalus. We have observed one case in a child with bilateral subdural hemorrhages along the falx cerebri, effectively separating the arachnoid from the villi.

Other inflammatory processes occurring *in utero* or in the perinatal period can obliterate the outlet foramina of the fourth ventricle and cause obstructive noncommunicating hydrocephalus. As discussed in Chapter 10, congenital malformations such as the Arnold–Chiari can obliterate the outlet foramina of the fourth ventricle because of impaction of the caudal cerebellum into the foramen magnum, thus producing obstructive hydrocephalus. In the Dandy–Walker malformation there is usually atresia or failure of the foramina to form. However, foraminal occlusion is not always present with this malformation and the mechanism of obstruction may not be apparent; possibly the large fourth ventricle itself may act as a mass and block CSF flow. One should keep in mind the possibility that both the Arnold–Chiari and Dandy–Walker malformations may relate to abnormalities in the roof plate of the fourth ventricle (see Chapter 10).

Abnormalities in the Ventricular System

AQUEDUCTAL STENOSIS. The most common site of intraventricular blockage of CSF is at the aqueduct of Sylvius. There are multiple causes of this abnormality, and their differentiation is not always possible even on a histologic basis.[16] Many families have been reported with X-linked aqueductal stenosis.[13] Current estimates are that 2% of all patients with congenital hydrocephalus have the X-linked form.[11] Obliteration of the aqueduct is a common feature of the Arnold–Chiari malformation, and the genesis of this may in part be related to the overlying anomaly of the collicular plate. A frequent lesion leading to obstructive hydrocephalus is "forking" of the aqueduct with multiple blind pouches or diverticula. Forking can occur in the absence of any other CNS anomaly and may result from infection or abnormal glial proliferation; it may even be acquired after the insertion of a ventricular shunt to treat communicating hydrocephalus. Forking is classically differentiated from stenosis by the multiple channels, but either condition can occur with or without gliosis depending on the age at which the lesion develops. Most cases of forking (Fig. 7–5) are characterized by complete ependymal rosettes and by the absence of gliosis, indicating that the lesion developed before the periaqueductal astrocytes developed and while the ependymal cells could proliferate, but many cases of apparent forking have incomplete ependymal rosettes and abundant surrounding gliosis (Figs. 7–6 through 7–8), usually due to a superimposed infectious process.

Aqueductal occlusion can also be due to

FIG. 7–7

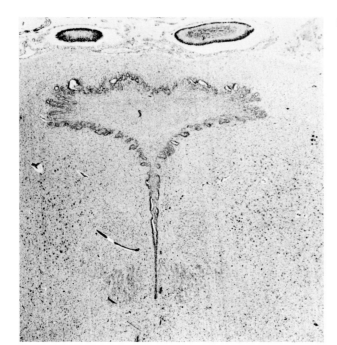

FIG. 7–8

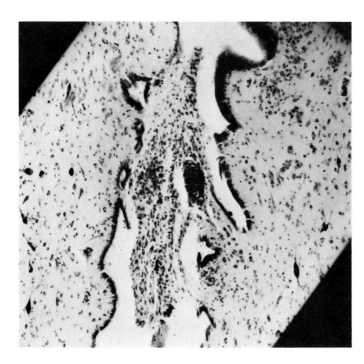

◀ FIG. 7–7. Photomicrograph showing total obliteration of the lumen of the aqueduct of Sylvius by an astrocytic scar. In this case there was an associated hydranencephaly (see Chapter 15), which could have resulted from an obstructive hydrocephalus *in utero*. (From Alvord, 1961)

◀ FIG. 7–8. Photomicrograph of acquired aqueductal forking revealing incomplete rosettes, *i.e.*, multiple channels partially lined by ependyma, interrupted by proliferation of subependymal astrocytes and chronic inflammation. (From Alvord, 1961)

FIG. 7–9. **a.** Posterior view of the brain demonstrating remains of a large cyst arising from a cerebellar folium and extending rostrally between the cerebellar and cerebral hemispheres. **b.** After transection of the midbrain and removal of the brain stem and cerebellum one can see the compression of the aqueduct by the cerebellar cyst in Fig. 7–9**a.** (From Alvord and Marcuse, 1962)

compression by other lesions, such as a cerebellar cyst (Fig. 7–9) or an aneurysm of the vein of Galen (Fig. 7–10). The latter may compress the aqueduct because of the mass of the blood vessels in the incisura of the tentorium, which is itself unyielding.

INFECTION AND HEMORRHAGE. The foramina of Monro or any other part of the ventricles may be occluded by glial membranes that are the result of infection or malformation (Fig. 7–11). These membranous structures can sometimes be due to subependymal cysts, probably resulting from viral infections *in utero* (see Chapter 23), raising the ependymal surface so as to occlude the otherwise normal ventricle. Hemorrhage within the ventricles can similarly act as a mass so as to prevent CSF egress.

TUMORS. Certain tumors characteristically block the flow of CSF because of their location. The colloid (neuroepithelial) cyst of the third ventricle is an example of this phenomenon; this tumor, which is more commonly symptomatic in adults than in children, can obstruct either the third ventricle or one or both of the foramina of Monro. A choroid plexus papilloma can also obstruct a ventricle by mass or produce leptomeningeal blocks by hemorrhage or shedding of tumor cells, but more commonly the papilloma secretes excessive amounts of CSF leading to communicating nonobstructive hydrocephalus. These two tumors are discussed in Chapter 6. A wide variety of other neoplasms, more fully described in Chapter 22, can cause hydrocephalus; these are usu-

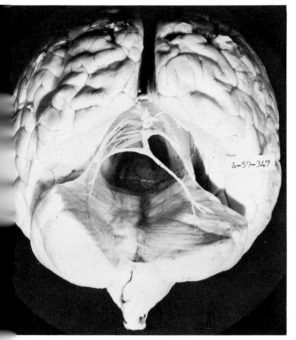

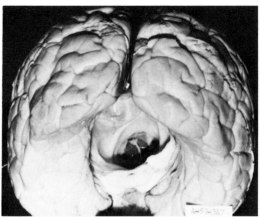

b

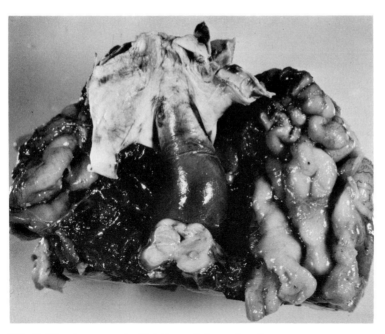

FIG. 7–10. Aneurysmal dilatation of the vein of Galen (see Chapter 20) compressing the aqueduct of Sylvius. (#Np 908)

FIG. 7–11. Coronal section of the brain of a 13-month-old boy with agenesis of the corpus callosum (see Chapter 16), unilateral arhinencephaly (see Chapter 14), contralateral occlusion of the foramen of Monro with unilateral ventricular dilatation. (From Loeser and Alvord, 1968. Reprinted with permission of the authors, from Neurology. Copyright The New York Times Media Co., Inc.) (#Np 541)

FIG. 7–12. Sagittal section of the brain of a 16-month-old boy with dilatation of all of the ventricles due to obstruction at the exit foramina of the fourth ventricle. The canals of Luschka were imperforate. The posterior medullary velum bulged widely into a retrocerebellar cyst lined partially by ependyma. Thus the foramen of Magendie did not form but developed into a cyst such as Blake (1900) described in subhuman forms. (#Np 775)

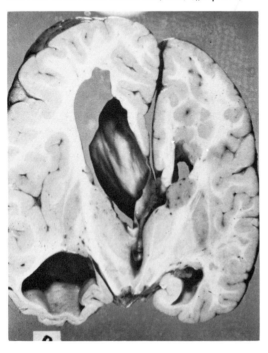

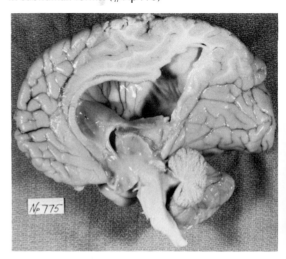

ally gliomas, especially pinealomas, which occasionally can be present *in utero*. It is essential to adequately study every child with hydrocephalus to ascertain the etiology.

CYSTS. A variety of nonneoplastic cysts can occur within the ventricular system and cause obstructive hydrocephalus.[3, 20, 21] The etiology of these cysts is diverse. Some may be the result of inflammatory changes; others are a malformation of choroid plexus or ependymal surface. Figure 7–12 shows the degree of hydrocephalus produced by a cyst of the posterior fossa that obstructed the outlet foramina of the fourth ventricle.

Some cysts containing ependyma and even choroid plexus do not have an apparent connection with the ventricular system. These have been reported above or below the tentorium and are often responsible for both local mass effect and obstructive hydrocephalus. Theories about the origin of such cysts are myriad, but it is our belief that the presence of a well-developed choroid plexus and ependyma without connection to the ventricle and without an underlying defective development of the normal cortex or ventricular system implies that ectopic differentiation (such as by the approximation of ependyma and mesenchyme) has occurred, rather than the displacement of normally formed structures and subsequent loss of continuity with the ventricular system. Experimental models for this process have been described by Birge.[7]

REFERENCES

1. Alexander L: Die Anatomie der Seitentaschen der vierten Hirnkammer. Z Anat 95:531–707, 1931

2. Alvord EC Jr: The pathology of hydrocephalus. Disorders of the Developing Nervous System. Edited by WS Fields and MM Desmond. Springfield, CC Thomas, 1961, pp. 343–412

3. Alvord EC Jr, Marcuse PM: Intracranial cerebellar meningoencephalocele (posterior fossa cyst) causing hydrocephalus by compression at the incisura tentorii. J Neuropathol Exp Neurol 21:50–69, 1962

4. Barr ML: Observations on the foramen of Magendie in a series of human brains. Brain 71:281–289, 1948

5. Bartelmez GW, Dekaban AS: The early development of the human brain. Contrib Embryol 37:13–32, 1962

6. Bell WE, McCormick WF: Increased Intracranial Pressure in Children. Philadelphia, WB Saunders, 1972

7. Birge WJ: Induced choroid plexus development in chick metencephalon. J Comp Neurol 118:89–96, 1962

8. Blake JA: The roof and lateral recesses of the fourth ventricle, considered morphologically and embryologically. J Comp Neurol 10:79–108, 1900

9. Brockelhurst G: The development of the human cerebrospinal fluid pathway with particular reference to the roof of the fourth ventricle. J Anat 105:467–475, 1969

10. Chamberlain JG: Early neurovascular abnormalities underlying 6-aminonicotinamide (6-AN) induced congenital hydrocephalus in rats. Teratology 3:337–388, 1970

11. Dignan PSJ, Warkany J: Congenital malformations: Hydrocephaly. *In* Mental Retardation (and Developmental Disabilities). Vol VI. Edited by Joseph Wortis. New York, Brunner/Mazel, 1974

12. Heuser CH, Corner GW: Developmental horizons in human embryos. Description of age group X, 4 to 12 somites. Contrib Embryol 36:29–39, 1957

13. Holmes LB, Nash A, Zu Rhein GM, Levin M, Opitz JM: X-linked aqueductal stenosis: clinical and neuropathological findings in two families. Pediatrics 51:697–704, 1973

14. Jacobs EB, Landing BH, Thomas W Jr: Vernicomyelia. Am J Pathol 39:345–353, 1961

15. Kalter H: Teratology of the Central Nervous System. Chicago, Univ Chicago Press, 1968

16. Lichtenstein BW: Atresia and stenosis of the aqueduct of Sylvius. J Neuropathol Exp Neurol 18:3–21, 1959

17. Loeser JD, Alvord EC Jr: Clinicopathological correlations in agenesis of the corpus callosum. Neurol 18:745–756, 1968

18. Margolis G, Kilham L: Experimental virus-induced hydrocephalus. J Neurosurg 31:1–9, 1969

19. Milhorat TH: Hydrocephalus and the Cerebrospinal Fluid. Baltimore, Williams & Wilkins, 1972

20. Peach B: Cystic prolongation of fourth ventricle: Anomaly associated with Arnold–Chiari malformation. Arch Neurol 11:609–612, 1964

21. Rand BO, Foltz EL, Alvord EC Jr: Intracranial telencephalic meningo-encephalocele containing choroid plexus. J Neuropathol Exp Neurol 23:293–305, 1964

22. Rasmussen AT: Additional evidence favoring the normal existence of the lateral apertures of

the fourth ventricle in man. Anat Rec 33:179–182, 1926

23. Rogers L, West CM: The foramen of Magendie. J Anat 65:457–467, 1931

24. Russell DS: Observations on the Pathology of Hydrocephalus. Med Res Council Report, #265, London, 1949

25. Streeter GL: Development of the nervous system. Manual of Human Embryology, vol. 2. Edited by F Keibel and FC Mall. Philadelphia, JB Lippincott, 1912, pp. 1–156

26. Streeter GL: Developmental horizons in human embryos. Contrib Embryol 31:27–63, 1945

27. Streeter GL: Developmental horizons in human embryos. Contrib Embryol 32:133–203, 1948

28. Streeter GL: Developmental horizons in human embryos. Contrib Embryol 34:165–196, 1951

29. Strong RM, Green LD, Oliverio JV: The lateral aperture of the fourth ventricle in man (abstracted). Anat Rec 32:223, 1926

30. Weed LH: Development of the cerebrospinal fluid spaces in pig and man. Contrib Embryol 5:1–16, 1917

31. Wilson JT: On the nature and mode of origin of the foramen of Magendie. J Anat 71:423–428, 1936

32. Wisniewski H, Weller RO, Terry RD: Experimental hydrocephalus produced by the subarachnoid infusion of silicone oil. J Neurosurg 31:10–14, 1969

33. Woodard JC, Newberne PM: The pathogenesis of hydrocephalus in newborn rats deficient in vitamin B_{12}. J Embryol Exp Morphol 17:177–187, 1967

SEGMENTAL STRUCTURES

chapter 8

BRAIN STEM AND CRANIAL NERVES

Since they are protrusions of the forebrain, as presented in Chapter 2, the development of cranial nerves I (olfactory) and II (optic) is covered in Chapters 13 and 14. The present chapter discusses the remaining cranial nerves III–XII, *i.e.*, those originating in brain stem segments. The interrelationships of the developing cranial nerves of human embryos between 4- and 14-mm CR (stages XII–XVIII) have been depicted by Streeter,[45–47] and except where otherwise noted, the following discussion is derived from these sources.

NORMAL DEVELOPMENT*

MIDBRAIN SEGMENT (FIG. 8–1)

Oculomotor Nerve (III)

The first indication of the third cranial nerve (CN-III) appears early in stage XIV (5- to 7-mm CR) when *pathfinder* axons are seen in the caudal third of the mesencephalon.[5] By the end of this stage small rootlets have converged to form the first nerve trunk, which becomes a well-defined nerve during stage XVI (10-mm CR).

Mann[27] and Pearson[35] have studied the development of the nuclei of CN-III. Although there are differences in their terminologies, the first indication of the chief (or lateral) nucleus appears in stage XXII (25-mm CR) when cellular groups arise in continuity with the ependymal floor. At 35-mm CR length the unpaired median nucleus of Perlia appears and connects the two lateral

* See Chapter 1 for background information on embryologic development and staging system.

groups. The Edinger–Westphal nucleus, arising from the dorsal component of the lateral group, forms at 48-mm CR length. The constantly changing nature of the various cellular groups during early fetal development causes some confusion, but at one time or another there are six different laterally placed groups in addition to the median nucleus, all showing increasing separation from each other between 75- and 100-mm CR length. The representation of the various extraocular muscles in the adult oculomotor nucleus has been established in experimental monkeys with a pattern of approximately parallel subnuclei.[52] It is interesting that Perlia's nucleus does not project outside the midbrain. Only the most caudal of the lateral nucleus, that which innervates the superior rectus muscle, shows partial crossing of their axons, a pattern carried to the extreme by the trochlear nerve, which crosses completely immediately caudally.

Kuntz[25] has extensively studied the autonomic components of the cranial nerves and found the primordium of the ciliary ganglion to be present in stage XVII (14-mm CR). The development of the extraocular muscles is described in Chapter 13.

Trochlear Nerve IV

The first fibers of the fourth cranial nerve (CN-IV) appear during stage XIV (5- to 7-mm CR) just caudal to the oculomotor nucleus. Between stages XVI and XIX (10- and 17-mm CR) the fourth nerve trunk becomes well defined and courses dorsally over the mesencephalic–metencephalic isthmus to cross the midline in the anterior medullary

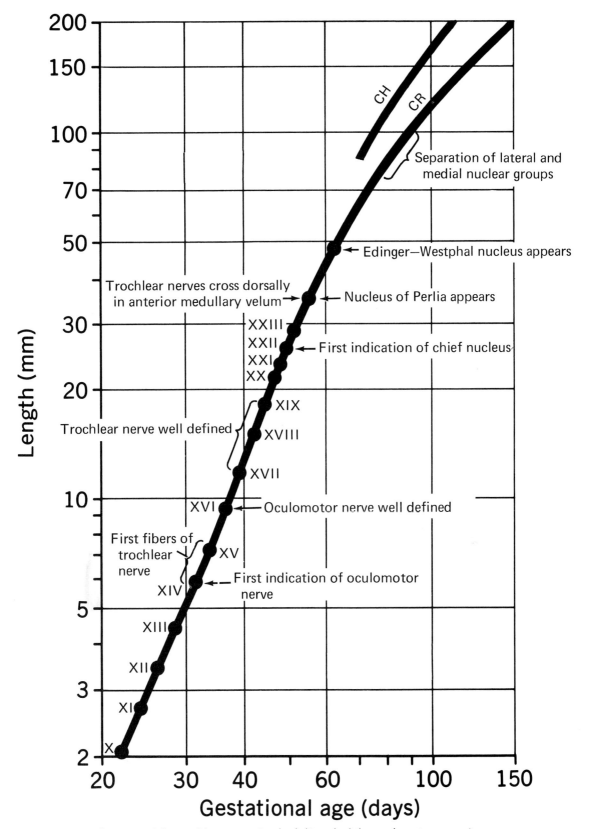

FIG. 8–1. Development of the trochlear nerve (to the left) and of the oculomotor nerve (to the right) correlated with gestational age and CR length.

velum.[5, 10, 34, 47] The nucleus consists of a main cell group and a small caudal group of cells.[34]

ANTERIOR HINDBRAIN SEGMENT (FIG. 8–2)

Trigeminal Nerve (V)

The trigeminal system arises in association with the first and second rhombic grooves. Table 8–1 summarizes the observations of Streeter[47] Windle and Fitzgerald,[53] Pearson,[38, 39] Brown,[7, 8] Bartelmez and Dekaban[5] and Humphrey.[23] The chief sensory nucleus is probably determined in stage XV (7- to 9-mm CR) when the mesencephalic root differentiates.

MIDDLE HINDBRAIN SEGMENT (FIGS. 8–3 AND 8–4)

Abducens Nerve (VI)

In stage XV (7- to 9-mm CR) several rootlets of the abducens nerve extend from the hindbrain and penetrate the mesodermal condensation that forms the lateral rectus muscle.[17] By stage XVI (10-mm CR) this nerve is seen as a single trunk arising from the fourth rhombic groove and bending rostrally at an angle of 90°, passing medial to the semilunar ganglion of CN-V.

Facial Nerve (VII)

The CN-VII arises in association with the third rhombic groove, rostral to CN-VI. During development the abducens (VI) moves rostrally, distorting the facial nerve to form the genu of the facial nerve. Table 8–2 summarizes the findings of Streeter,[47, 48] Pearson,[36, 37] Bartelmez and Dekaban[5] and Gasser.[16]

Acoustic and Vestibular Nerves (VIII)

The development of CN-VIII (in rhombomere 4) is exceedingly complex, and specific morphologic facts are somewhat limited. The best description is given in Figure 93 of Streeter,[47] who showed drawings of the ganglion acousticum and its branches in embryos of 4, 7, 9, 20 and 30-mm CR length. Additional features are provided by Streeter[48] and Bartelmez and Dekaban[5] and, for histologic changes in the vestibular nuclei, from Humphrey.[22] Table 8–3 summarizes these observations.

TABLE 8–1. ADDITIONAL FEATURES OF THE DEVELOPMENT OF THE TRIGEMINAL NERVE (see Fig. 8–2)

CR (mm)	Stage	Observations
2.5–4.5	XI	Large trigeminal "center" apparent
3–5	XII	Few neurons in semilunar ganglion
4–6	XIII	Three primary divisions of nerve recognizable
5–7	XIV	Afferent and efferent root fibers present; sensory fibers enter metencephalon opposite sulcus limitans (have short ascending and long descending tracts); semilunar ganglion large; motor nucleus appears
7–9	XV	Primordium of mesencephalic nucleus appears (differentiates in caudorostral direction)
8–11	XVI	First neurons of mesencephalic nucleus differentiate; ophthalmic division has frontal and nasociliary branches; mandibular division has lingual and inferior alveolar branches
11–14	XVII	Maxillary division shows branching
13–17	XVIII	All divisions have their major branches, which now show secondary branching; scattered fibers found in spinal tract of V down to middle of C1 segment
16–18	XIX	Mesencephalic root fibers extend into anterior medullary velum and mesencephalon (with nerve cells scattered along their course), some fibers cross with the decussation of CN-IV; spinal tract of V extends to C2 segment
23–28	XXII	Mesencephalic root fibers connect with motor and other sensory roots of CN-V, VII and VIII; peripheral components of all three divisions close to cutaneous surfaces
32		Spinal tract of V extends to C3 segment (with a few fibers to C4)
35		Mesencephalic root fibers enter cerebellum
45		Mesencephalic root fibers decussate in anterior medullary velum and central gray of aqueduct
120		Some mesencephalic root fibers form a flattened layer between fourth ventricle and vestibulocerebellar tract

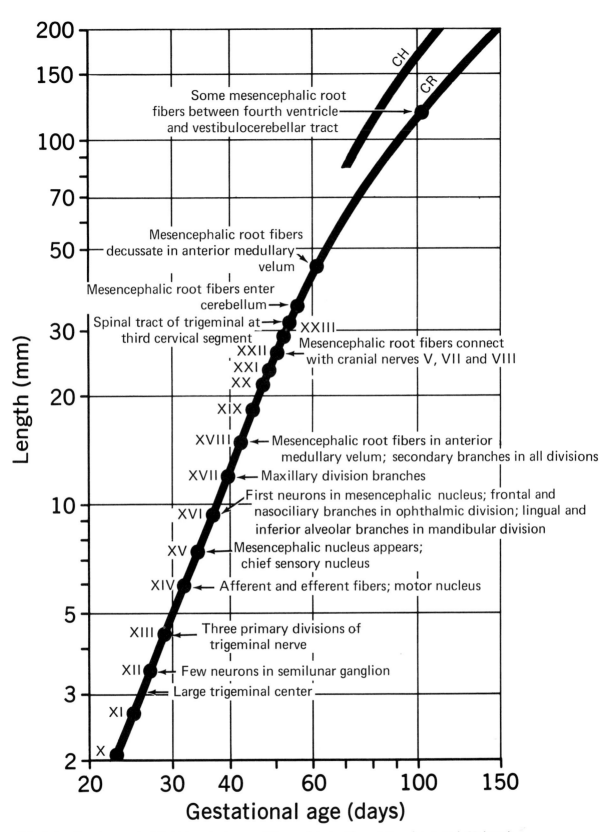

FIG. 8–2. Development of the trigeminal nerve (V) correlated with gestational age and CR length.

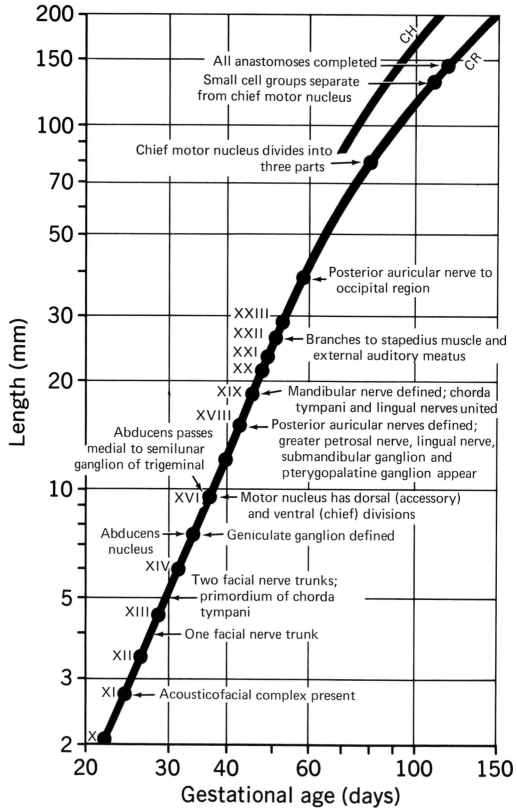

FIG. 8–3. Two features in prenatal development of the abducens nerve (VI) are noted at the lower left (stages XV and XVI). The remainder of the figure depicts the development of the facial nerve (VII).

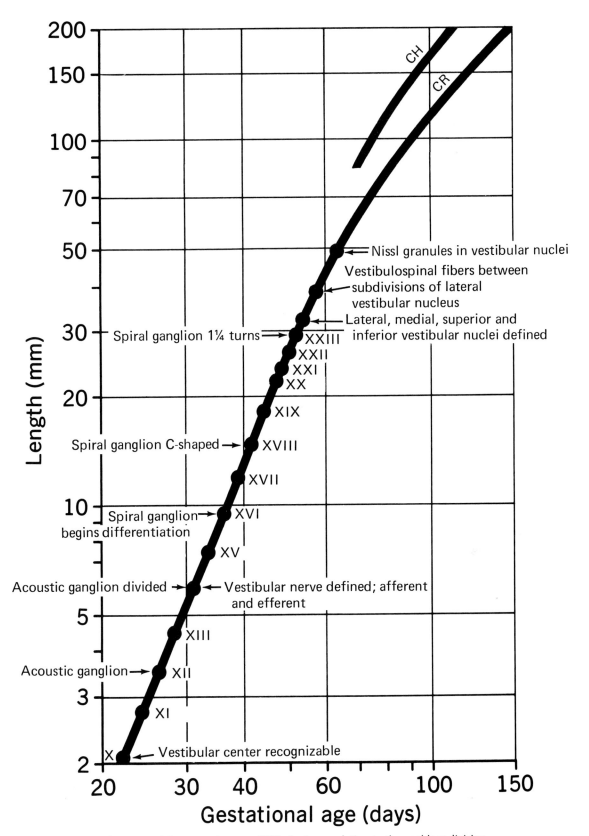

FIG. 8–4. Development of the acoustic nerve (VIII). Features relating to the cochlear division, left, and to the vestibular division, right.

TABLE 8–2. ADDITIONAL FEATURES OF THE
DEVELOPMENT OF THE
FACIAL NERVE (see Fig. 8–3)

CR (mm)	Stage	Observations
2.5–4.5	XI	Acousticofacial "complex" is surrounded by mesodermal elements
4–5	XIII	One facial nerve trunk at 4-mm CR, two trunks by 5-mm CR, the caudal being the main facial nerve; the rostral trunk enters the mandibular arch as the primordium of the chorda tympani (first branch to develop)
7–9	XV	Geniculate ganglion is definable; chorda tympani now well defined
8–11	XVI	Facial and acoustic complexes separate; motor nucleus has small dorsal or accessory portion and larger ventral "chief" nucleus
13–17	XVIII	Greater petrosal nerve (second recognizable branch); also submandibular ganglion, pterygopalatine ganglion and lingual nerve develop; the posterior auricular nerve appears late (first extracranial branch to develop); twigs to posterior digastric "premuscle" mass are found and the nervus intermedius is defined (fibers between CN-VII and VIII)
16–18	XIX	Chorda tympani and lingual nerve united; mandibular nerve defined; posterior auricular nerve divides into cranial and caudal branches, the latter communicating with nerves from C2 to C3; peripheral CN-VII divides into several "bundles"
23–28	XXII	Branches to stapedius muscle and external auditory meatus; communications established with infraorbital, buccal, auriculotemporal and mental branches of CN-V
37		Posterior auricular nerve courses to occipital region
80		Chief motor nucleus divides into dorsal, intermediate and ventral parts; all anastomoses of CN-VII are present except with zygomaticofacial, lacrimal, infratrochlear and external nasal nerves
130		Some cell groups separate from ventral and intermediate parts of chief motor nucleus
146		All anastomoses completed
240		All cell groups well defined (essentially as at birth)

TABLE 8–3. ADDITIONAL FEATURES OF THE
DEVELOPMENT OF ACOUSTIC AND
VESTIBULAR NERVES (see Fig. 8–4)

CR (mm)	Stage	Observations
2–3.5	X	Vestibular "center" first recognizable
2.5–4.5	XI	Acousticofacial "complex" present
3–5	XII	Acoustic ganglion with primordium of vestibular nerve
4–6	XIII	Some "sheath" cells of CN-VIII seen
5–7	XIV	Afferent and efferent fibers present; acoustic ganglion divides into pars superior and pars inferior; vestibular nerve very distinct from pars superior
8–11	XVI	Acoustic and facial complexes separate; spiral ganglion begins differentiation from pars inferior of acoustic ganglion; first cochlear nerve fibers from spiral ganglion; first fibers from pars superior and pars inferior seen
13–17	XVIII	Cochlear nerve very distinct beside vestibular nerve; spiral ganglion C-shaped; separate nerves (from pars inferior) to saccule and ampulla of posterior semicircular canal identifiable; a common trunk from the pars superior divides into three branches (one each to ampullae of superior and lateral semicircular canals and one to utricle)
27–31	XXIII	Spiral ganglion (now 1.25 turns) is completely separate from pars inferior
32		Lateral (LVN), medial (MVN), superior (SVN) and inferior vestibular (IVN) nuclei are recognizable; LVN has two subdivisions (medial and lateral)
37.5		A few vestibulospinal fibers are found between the subdivisions of LVN
44		Fibers separate neurons in lateral subdivision of LVN; basophilic granules present in neurons of MVN
48.5		Fibers separate neurons in medial subdivision of LVN; fine Nissl granules around nuclei in MVN
60.5		Some clumping of Nissl granules in LVN
90		Thin rodlike Nissl bodies extend into larger dendrites of LVN

Glossopharyngeal Nerve (IX)

In stage XI (3-mm CR) a few cells beneath the fifth rhombic groove can be recognized as comprising the center for CN-IX (Fig. 7–xi of Streeter[48]). Late in stage XII (3- to 5-mm CR) the petrosal ganglion is evident just caudal to the auditory placode, and in stage XIII (4- to 6-mm CR) there is differentiation between it and the superior ganglion. During stage XIII the trunks of both the lingual and pharyngeal nerves can also be seen. By stage XVI (8- to 11-mm CR) the nucleus ambiguus is present, and in stage XVII (11- to 14-mm CR) the tympanic branch is found arising from the petrosal ganglion.

Vagus Nerve (X)

During stage XI (3-mm CR) three small clusters of cells are seen to represent the primordium of CN-X. Initially in association with the sixth rhombic groove, with further differentiation its components become more widespread and closely associated with CN-IX, XI and XII. In stage XII (3- to 5-mm CR) the ganglion nodosum is apparent; it becomes loosely fused with the petrosal ganglion (CN-IX) during stage XIV (5- to 7-mm CR). Also during stage XIV the jugular ganglion is seen, and the spinal accessory nerve is found to be closely associated with the caudal aspect of both it and the ganglion nodosum. The main trunk of the vagus is quite large by this stage, containing both afferent and efferent fibers. Although rudimentary, the pharyngeal branch of CN-X is also present in stage XIV, as are fibers of the superior laryngeal nerve. The ventral motor nucleus of the vagus (nucleus ambiguus) appears during stage XVI (8- to 11-mm CR). Differentiation of the dorsal efferent and afferent nuclei (with fasciculus solitarius) is found by stage XVIII (13- to 17-mm CR).

Accessory Nerve (XI)

CN-XI is termed the *spinal accessory* nerve since its fibers are closely associated with the posterior hindbrain segmental nerves (especially the vagus), and since its nucleus lies within the first six cervical segments (1–6) of the spinal cord. Its first cells, continuous in a line with those of the ventral vagus, are seen in stage XI (3-mm CR). Its first fibers are found in stage XII (3- to 5-mm CR) and become well developed by stage XIV (5- to 7-mm CR). Pearson *et al.*[32,40] have provided detailed descriptions of the later development of this nerve with respect to course and surrounding structures.

Hypoglossal Nerve (XII)

The first rootlets of CN-XII, arising in from three to four separate groups, are seen late in stage XII (3- to 5-mm CR). During stage XIV (5- to 7-mm CR) these rootlets fuse into a common trunk and establish connections with the second and third cervical nerves as the ansa hypoglossi. The motor nucleus of the hypoglossal is apparent by stage XVI (8- to 11-mm CR), and by stage XXII (23- to 28-mm CR) it is seen as a prolongation of the cervical anterior gray column into the posterior hindbrain segment (situated just under the ependyma and extending from a little below the obex to the level of the highest root of CN-X). Pearson,[33] in a study of human embryos between 17- and 46-mm CR length, has provided a detailed discussion of the development of CN-XII. In a 45-mm CR length fetus, he saw the hypoglossal cell column dividing into dorsal and ventral portions with the cephalic end of the dorsal portion subdividing into medial and lateral parts.

ABNORMAL DEVELOPMENT

The incidence of congenital malformations of the cranial nerves is very small if the olfactory (CN-I) and optic (CN-II) are excluded (see Chapters 10 and 11). Even in cases of anencephaly, the cranial nerves are usually present, although their courses may be aberrant. Most disorders of the cranial nerves noted at birth appear to be due to focal necrosis, rather than to primary malformations, whereas most of the syndromes that arise postnatally (indeed, usually in adults) are secondary to neoplasms or infections.[18]

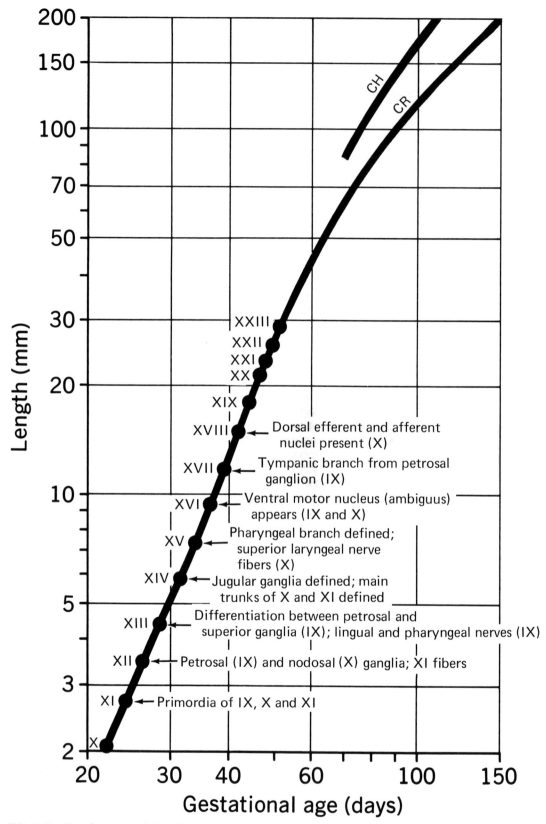

FIG. 8–5. Development of the glossopharyngeal (IX), vagus (X) and accessory nerves (XI) correlated with gestational age and CR length.

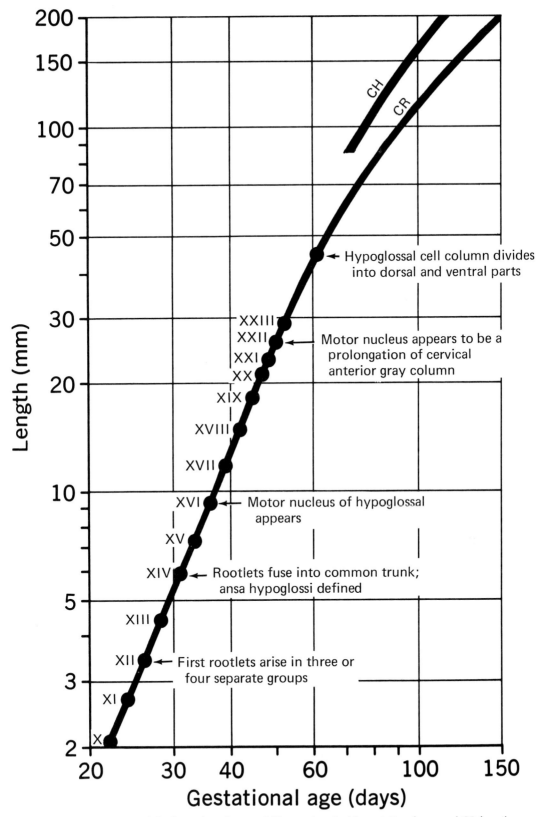

FIG. 8–6. Development of the hypoglossal nerve (XII) correlated with gestational age and CR length.

OCULOMOTOR (III) AND TROCHLEAR (IV) NERVES

"Involvement" of the oculomotor nerve can be seen in the Möbius syndrome (see Facial Nerve, below). Hypoplasia has been reported in de Lange syndrome. The trochlear nerve is usually spared in the former, but it can be involved in the latter syndrome.

TRIGEMINAL NERVE (V)

Anseth[4] reports one case of a child developing a unilateral corneal opacity and then ulceration at 21 months of age. A year later, anesthesia of both corneas was diagnosed. This was apparently the fifth such case reported, but the possibility of this being a primarily neurogenic lesion was not discussed, and no further details were given. The trigeminal nerve can also be involved in the Möbius syndrome and neurofibromatosis.

ABDUCENS NERVE (VI)

Although esotropia is not uncommon in infancy, it is not clear how often this is neurogenic (and developmental), rather than being secondary to "weakness" of the rectus lateralis. Primary involvement of the nerve or nucleus is frequently seen in the Möbius syndrome and less commonly in the Arnold–Chiari malformation.

FACIAL NERVE (VII)

Perhaps the best-known malformation of the facial nerve complex is found in the Möbius syndrome (also known as the congenital facial diplegia syndrome). Although usually sporadic, Van der Weil[50] reports its occurrence in six generations of one family (14 parents affected; 32 of 70 children affected), suggesting that autosomal dominant transmission can occur. Besides facial nerve palsy there is frequently palsy of the abducens nerve (CN-VI) and sometimes of the oculomotor (CN-III) and hypoglossal (CN-XII) nerves. Although all cranial nerves can be involved in a given case, the trochlear (CN-IV) and spinal accessory (CN-XI) are usually spared.[13] The neuropathology is variable, ranging from aplasia or hypoplasia of the facial nerve nuclei to hypoplasia of the entire brain stem.[21] The latter situation may

account for the "strikingly wide" posterior and basal cisterns found in one air study.[19] Associated anomalies of the pectoralis muscles and extremities, especially equino varus, are common.[19, 20] The underlying pathogenesis of the syndrome is unknown.

Facial nerve palsy of the lower motor neuron type has been found in association with congenital heart defects and other malformations.[3, 31] Paralysis of the nerve has also occurred in association with otic capsule abnormalities.[28]

Fowler[15] reviews seven variations of the course of the facial nerve through the temporal bone. Besides changes in angulation, it has also been described to bifurcate, to bifurcate and then rejoin (forming a loop) or to split into three parts. Many of the aberrant positions in which the facial nerve has been found are associated with anomalies of the first and second branchial arch. Bifurcation has also been reported just distal to the geniculate ganglion,[9] and bifurcations of its branches, such as the chorda tympani, have also been found.[12] Bifurcation of the facial nerve within the temporal bone was found in 3 of 500 bones randomly studied.[6] Anomalous origin of its branches can occur (e.g., the chorda tympani arising from the geniculate ganglion[15]), and sometimes branches are completely missing (e.g., lesser superficial petrosal nerve[1]). Other recent studies of similar facial nerve anomalies have been reported by Sando et al.,[43] Dickinson et al.[11] and Pou.[42] Although not common with respect to the other anomalies, both agenesis and anomalous bifurcation of CN-VII were found in some cases of thalidomide embryopathy.[29]

ACOUSTIC NERVE (VIII)

Table 8–4 summarizes the causes of congenital deafness. Altmann,[2] in addition to presenting an excellent resumé of inherited nerve deafness in subhuman species, reviews the histologic information in humans with "developmental anomalies." The spiral ganglion can show decreased numbers of ganglion cells and nerve fibers or may be completely absent in rare cases. The cochlear division of the acoustic nerve is often thin in inherited nerve deafness, and in at least two cases a reduction in ganglionic cells in the spiral ganglia was found. It is not clear whether or not the reduction in such cases is

TABLE 8–4. CAUSES OF CONGENITAL DEAFNESS[14]

Cause	No. Cases	%
Genetic	244	36
Anoxia	91	13.4
Hemolytic disease of newborn (Kernicterus)	83	12.2
Rubella	40	5.9
Other (thalidomide; congenital malformations)	12	1.7
Unknown	207	30.5
Total	677	99.7

due to a lack of initial development or is secondary to a degenerative process, such as can be produced by streptomycin.[44]

The lesions associated with deafness in rubella embryopathy involve the cochlea itself and not the nerve or nuclei. The histopathology of these lesions has been described in human embryos by Töndury and Smith[49] to consist of necrotic foci in the epithelium and atrophic changes in the stria vascularis.

Maniglia et al.[26] report a unique finding in a patient with trisomy 13 syndrome. On the vestibular branch to the horizontal ampulla they found a small mass of striated muscle and nerve fibers that they interpreted as being a teratoma. The organ of Corti was reduced to a clumped mound with no recognizable cells.

The acoustic nerve can also be involved in neurofibromatosis and its vestibular branch is the commonest cranial nerve to be involved in a tumor, usually a neurinoma (Schwannoma).

GLOSSOPHARYNGEAL NERVE (IX)

We are unable to identify reports of isolated anomalies of this nerve.

VAGUS NERVE (X)

Primary anomalies of the vagus nerve are apparently unusual. Plott[41] reports three siblings with laryngeal abductor paralysis (one with associated palsy of CN-VI) and postulates a dysgenesis of the nucleus ambiguus. Kirsch et al.[24] consider an aberration of the caudal portion of the nucleus ambiguus to be responsible for laryngeal palsy (abductor paralysis) in five cases with Arnold–Chiari malformation. The vagus nerve can also be involved in neurofibromatosis.

ACCESSORY NERVE (XI)

The pathogenesis of congenital torticollis (paralysis of the sternocleidomastoid muscle) seems to be variable, with good evidence that some of the cases occur prenatally.[51] However, it is uncertain whether primary malformation of the spinal accessory nerve accounts for any of these cases.

HYPOGLOSSAL NERVE (XII)

The hypoglossal nerve can be affected as part of the brain stem dysplasia in the Möbius syndrome (see Facial Nerve). It can also be involved in patients with neurofibromatosis. There are cases with hemiatrophy of the tongue that are present at birth due to vascular insufficiency of the vertebral artery with necrosis and gliosis of the posterior hindbrain (Fig. 8–7). Lastly, Opitz et al.[30] found abnormally small roots of the hypoglossal nerve in the Dq− syndrome (the other cranial nerves being normal).

FIG. 8–7. Low-power photomicrograph showing asymmetric gliosis (Holzer stain) of the paramedian gray matter of the caudal medulla of a 3-month-old boy with chronic respiratory difficulties, paralysis of the left vocal cord and atrophy of the left side of the tongue since birth. The left vertebral artery was absent. (#Np 3156)

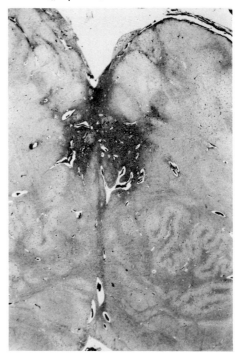

REFERENCES

1. Altmann F: Problem of so-called congenital atresia. Arch Otolaryngol 50:759–788, 1949

2. Altmann F: Histolgic picture of inherited nerve deafness in man and animals. Arch Otolaryngol 51:852–890, 1950

3. Anand JK, Butler LJ: The cardiofacial syndrome: Report of a case with severe facial palsy. Dev Med Child Neurol 15:69–71, 1973

4. Anseth A: Congenital bilateral corneal anesthesia. Acta Ophthal Rhinol Laryngol 46:909–911, 1968

5. Bartelmez GW, Dekaban AS: The early development of the human brain. Contrib Embryol 37:13–32, 1962

6. Basek M: Anomalies of the facial nerve in normal temporal bones. Ann Otol Rhinol Laryngol 71:382–390, 1962

7. Brown JW: The development of the nucleus of the spinal tract of V in human fetuses of 14 to 21 weeks of menstrual age. J Comp Neurol 106:393–423, 1956

8. Brown JW: The development of the subnucleus caudalis of the nucleus of the spinal tract of V. J Comp Neurol 110:105–133, 1958

9. Caparosa RJ, Klassen D: Congenital anomalies of the stapes and facial nerve. Arch Otolaryngol 83:420–421, 1966

10. Cooper ERA: The development of the nuclei of the oculomotor and trochlear nerves (somatic efferent column). Brain 69:50–57, 1946

11. Dickinson JT, Srinsomboon P, Kamerer DB: Congenital anomaly of facial nerve. Arch Otolaryngol 88:357–359, 1968

12. Durcan DJ, Shea JJ, Sleeckx JP: Bifurcation of the facial nerve. Arch Otolaryngol 86:619–631, 1967

13. Evans PR: Nuclear agenesis. Möbius' syndrome: The congenital facial diplegia syndrome. Arch Dis Child 30:237–243, 1955

14. Fisch L: The causes of congenital deafness. Public Health 83:68–74, 1969

15. Fowler EP Jr: Variations in the temporal bone course of the facial nerve. Laryngoscope 71:937–946, 1961

16. Gasser RF: The development of the facial nerve in man. Ann Otol Rhinol Laryngol 76:37–56, 1967

17. Gilbert PW: The origin and development of the human extrinsic ocular muscles. Contrib Embryol 36:59–78, 1957

18. Gorlin RJ, Pindborg JJ: Syndromes of the head and neck. New York, McGraw-Hill, 1964

19. Hellström B: Congenital facial diplegia. Acta Paediatr Scand 37:464–473, 1949

20. Henderson JL: The congenital facial diplegia syndrome; clinical features, pathology and aetiology. Brain 62:381–403, 1939

21. Hicks AM: Congenital paralysis of lateral rotators of eyes with paralysis of muscles of face. Arch Ophthalmol 30:38–42, 1943

22. Humphrey T: The embryologic differentiation of the vestibular nuclei in man correlated with functional development. International Symposium on Vestibular and Oculomotor Problems. Japan Society of Vestibular Research, pp. 51–56, 1965

23. Humphrey T: The development of trigeminal nerve fibers to the oral mucosa, compared with their development to cutaneous surfaces. J Comp Neurol 126:91–108, 1966

24. Kirsch WM, Duncan BR, Black FO, Stears JC: Laryngeal palsy in association with myelomeningocele, hydrocephalus and the Arnold–Chiari malformation. J Neurosurg 28:207–214, 1968

25. Kuntz A: The development of the sympathetic nervous system in man. J Comp Neurol 32:173–229, 1920–21

26. Maniglia AJ, Wolff D, Herques AJ: Congenital deafness in 13–15 trisomy syndrome. Arch Otolaryngol 92:181–188, 1970

27. Mann IC: The developing third nerve nucleus in human embryos. J Anat 61:424–438, 1927

28. Manning JJ, Adour KK: Facial paralysis in children. Pediatrics 49:102–109, 1972

29. Miehlke A: Normal and anomalous anatomy of the facial nerve and an embryological study of the thalidomide catastrophy in Germany. Trans Am Acad Ophthalmol Otolaryngol 68:1030–1044, 1964

30. Opitz JM, Slungaard R, Edwards RH, Inhorn SL, Muller J, de Venecia G: Report of a patient with a presumed Dq— syndrome. Birth Defects 5(5):93–99, 1969

31. Pape KE, Pickering D: Asymmetric crying facies: An index of other congenital anomalies. J Pediatr 81:21–30, 1972

32. Pearson AA: The spinal accessory nerve in human embryos. J Comp Neurol 68:243–266, 1938

33. Pearson AA: The hypoglossal nerve in human embryos. J Comp Neurol 71:21–39, 1939

34. Pearson AA: The trochlear nerve in human fetuses. J Comp Neurol 78:29–43, 1943

35. Pearson AA: The oculomotor nucleus in the human fetus. J Comp Neurol 80:47–63, 1944

36. Pearson AA: The development of the motor nuclei of the facial nerve in man. J Comp Neurol 85:461–476, 1946

37. Pearson AA: The roots of the facial nerve in human embryos and fetuses. J Comp Neurol 87:139–159, 1947

38. Pearson AA: The development and connections of the mesencephalic root of the trigeminal nerve in man. J Comp Neurol 90:1–46, 1949

39. Pearson AA: Further observations on the mesencephalic root of the trigeminal nerve. J Comp Neurol 91:147–194, 1949

40. Pearson AA, Sauter RW, Herrin GR: The ac-

cessory nerve and its relation to the upper spinal nerves. Am J Anat 114:371–391, 1964

41. Plott D: Congenital laryngeal–abductor paralysis due to nucleus ambiguus dysgenesis in three brothers. N Engl J Med 271:593–597, 1964

42. Pou JW: Congenital anomalies of the middle ear: presentation of two cases. Laryngoscope 81:831–839, 1971

43. Sando I, English GM, Hemenway WG: Congenital anomalies of the facial nerve and stapes: a human temporal bone report. Laryngoscope 78:316–323, 1968

44. Stevenson LD, Alvord EC Jr, Correll JW: Degeneration and necrosis of neurones in eighth cranial nuclei caused by streptomycin. Proc Soc Exp Biol Med 65:86–88, 1947

45. Streeter GL: The development of the cranial and spinal nerves in the occipital region of the human embryo. Am J Anat 4:83–116, 1904

46. Streeter GL: On the development of the membranous labyrinth and the acoustic and facial nerves in the human embryo. Am J Anat 6:139–165, 1906–07

47. Streeter, GL: The development of the nervous system. Manual of Human Embryology, vol. II. Edited by F Keibel and FP Mall. Philadelphia, JB Lippincott, 1912, pp. 1–156

48. Streeter GL: Developmental Horizons in Human Embryos. Age Groups XI–XXIII. Embryology Reprint, vol II, Washington DC, Carnegie Inst Wash, 1951

49. Töndury G, Smith DW: Fetal rubella pathology. J Pediatr 68:867–879, 1966

50. Van der Weil HJ: Hereditary congenital facial paralysis (abstracted). Acta Genet et Statistica Med 7:348, 1957

51. Warkany J: Congenital Malformations. Chicago, Year Book Med Publ, 1971

52. Warwick R: Representation of the extro-ocular muscles in the oculomotor nuclei of the monkey. J Comp Neurol 98:449–503, 1953

53. Windle WF, Fitzgerald JE: Development of the human mesencephalic trigeminal root and related neurons. J Comp Neurol 77:597–608, 1942

chapter 9

SPINAL CORD AND NERVES

NORMAL DEVELOPMENT*

SPINAL CORD

The development of the spinal cord and nerves varies at different levels. The landmarks presented in Figure 9–1 are only representative examples.

Stages of Development

The light and electron microscopic studies of Malínský and Malínská[47] provide one approach to staging spinal cord differentiation. Malínský and Malínská describe 15 stages based on "ovulation ages," the first 6 of which cover stages X–XXIII of the Carnegie System (see Chapter 1). Stage 7 is an overlap between an "old embryo and early fetus" as applied to the gestational information given in Chapter 1. We have applied approximate CR lengths to each of their subsequent stages, based on their ranges, fully realizing the probability of error in transforming this information—especially since it is not clear which segments were studied in each stage (Table 9–1).

Length of Cord

Bardeen[6] summarizes data on both total and regional lengths of spinal cords in 17 embryos and early fetuses between 7- and 50-mm CR length; Lassek and Rasmussen[41] present measurements of spinal cord lengths in 19 fetuses between 150- and 500-mm CH

* See Chapter 1 for background information on embryologic development and staging system.

length (corresponding to between 105- and 340-mm CR). The prenatal curves presented in Figure 9–2 are derived from these studies. Studies on adult spinal cord lengths show a marked variation depending on stature and sex.[6] Of more clinical interest than the overall length of the spinal cord is the level at which it terminates relative to the vertebrae. To avoid possible damage to the conus, lumbar puncture to obtain CSF should be made caudal to the termination of the cord. As discussed in Chapter 5, the end of the spinal cord extends well into the tail of the embryo until retrogressive differentiation begins at stages XVIII to XX. This process results in the formation of the filum terminale and the conus medullaris, the tip of which progressively assumes a higher position relative to the vertebral segments. The determination of the level of the conus has been studied during the first half of gestation by Kunitomo,[35] Streeter[68] and Barry[9] and thereafter by Barson.[10] The curve presented in Figure 9–3 is derived from these data and represents the means. The development of any one segment (and rarely two segments) can vary such that an "adult level" of L1–L2 can be reached as early as the 31st week of gestation.

Area of Cord

Cross-sectional area measurements of the spinal cord have been made on two stage XIV (5- and 6-mm CR) embryos,[43] on fetuses between 150- and 500-mm CH length[41] and on adults.[40] The latter two studies analyze the surface area of gray and white matter in the cervical, thoracic, lumbar and sacral regions (Table 9–2).

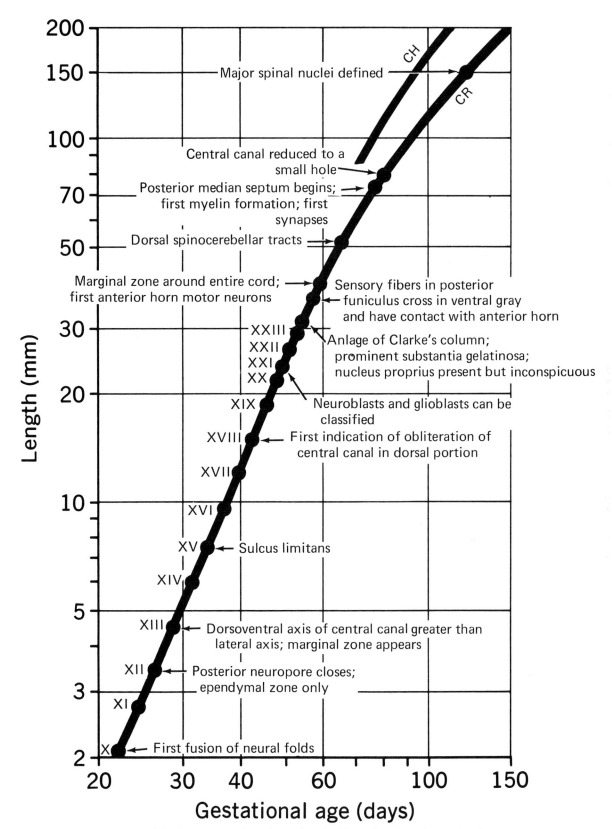

FIG. 9–1. Development of the human spinal cord correlated with CR length and gestational age.

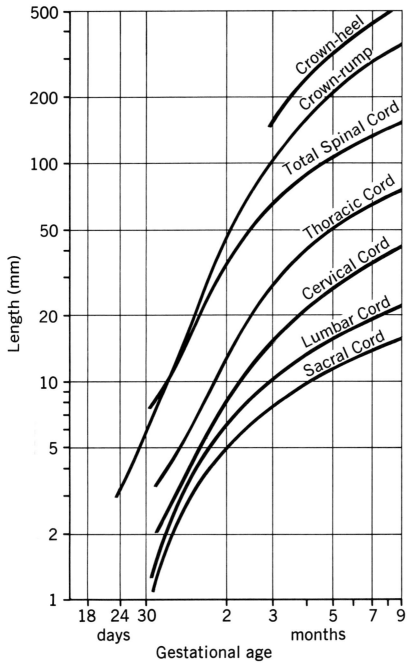

FIG. 9–2. Lengths of the spinal cord and its subdivisions as compared to CR and CH length at various gestational ages. (From Bardeen, 1905 and Lassek and Rasmussen, 1939)

Myelination

The differentiation of cell columns and tracts produces constantly changing relationships in the developing spinal cord. The central canal, initially large relative to the surround- ing neural tube, rapidly decreases in size so that by 80-mm CR length it is a small hole. This reduction is secondary to the growth of both gray and white matter, and as indicated in Table 9–2, white matter becomes more prominent with increasing gestational age

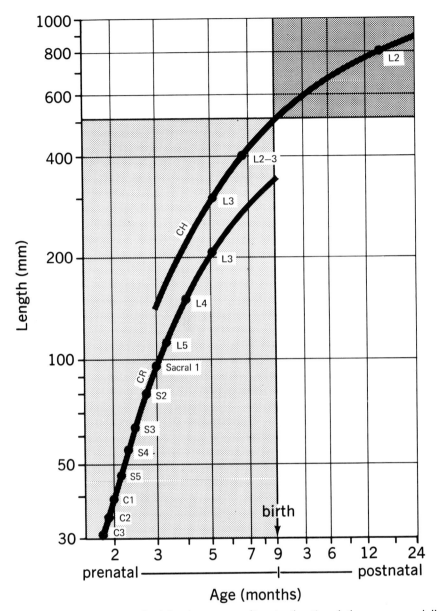

FIG. 9–3. Average vertebral level corresponding to the tip of the conus medullaris correlated with age (pre- and postnatal) and body lengths. Retrogressive differentiation of the caudal neural tube discussed in Chapter 5 is demonstrated.

except in the sacral cord. This reflects the increasing myelination of the numerous tracts. The first indication of myelin formation in the fetal cord is found between 75- and 105-mm CR length by electron microscopy; between 105- and 145-mm CR length myelin formation is found by light microscopy.[47] The spinothalamic and spinocerebellar tracts are well myelinated by the 28th gestational week, the rubrospinal and tectospinal by the 32nd week.[39] Somewhat different figures are given by Langworthy,[38] who found myelination of the cord to begin in the following sequence: ventral spinal roots at 16 weeks; dorsal spinal roots, dorsal spinocerebellar tract and ventral commissure at 20 weeks; vestibulospinal tract at 24 weeks; and corticospinal and tectospinal

TABLE 9–1. ADDITIONAL FEATURES OF THE DIFFERENTIATION OF THE HUMAN SPINAL CORD (see Fig. 9–1)

| Carnegie stage or CR length (mm) | Malinsky and Malinska[47] | | Cord Development |
	Stage	Age (days)*	
X	1	17–21	Ependymal zone only; neural groove and first fusion of neural folds
XI–XII	2	21–25	Neuropores close
XIII–XIV	3	25–29	Lateral walls thicken; dorsoventral axis of central canal greater than lateral; groups of cells in basal lamina begin to differentiate; marginal zone present
XV–XVII	4	29–35	Sulcus limitans divides ependymal zone into two symmetric halves; marginal zone present in several areas
XVIII–XX	5	35–41	Sulcus limitans more ventrally placed; first indication of obliteration of central canal in dorsal part
XXI–XXIII	6	41–49	Neuroblasts and glioblasts can be classified in the basal lamina; contralateral funiculi not yet fused in medial plane
26–38 mm	7	49–57	Marginal zone around entire cord with some glial cells migrating into it; first groups of large motor neurons in basal lamina
38–55 mm	8	57–67	Ependymal zone much thinner; central canal small and pentagonal
55–75 mm	9	67–77	Increase in marginal zone greater than increase in mantle zone; thin glial layer is first indication of posterior median septum
75–105 mm	10	77–91	Greater volume of white matter than gray matter; first myelin formation by EM; first synapses
105–145 mm	11	91–112	Posterior columns more flattened and elongated; myelin sheaths visible through light microscope
145–180 mm	12	112–140	Fetal cord has similar shape and ultrastructural features of postnatal cord
180–265 mm	13	140–189	Thoracic cord over 60% white matter
265–340 mm	14	189–term	All cells in gray and white matter can be classified
340	15	Newborn	—

* Discrepancies exist in the comparison between the ages and stages used by these authors and those used throughout this book (see Chapter 1).

tracts one month postnatally. These observations, although based on only four specimens (235-mm CR, 309-mm CR, a newborn and a two-month-old infant) nevertheless are well described and documented with excellent photographs. For information on the density of myelination of the various tracts, as well as their development after birth, the work of Yakovlev and Lecours[75] should be consulted (see Figs. 3–1 through 3–3).

Cell Groups

Elliott[22] studied the distribution of cell columns in fetal spinal cords in six specimens ranging from 90- to 250-mm CR

length. He found that compact cell clusters could be seen up to 150-mm CR length and that between 150- and 200-mm CR length these clusters subdivided into well-defined groupings. Beyond this period, all groups tended to become diffuse and overlap, making the recognition of individual columns difficult. Romanes[58] studied the spinal cell columns of the cervical and lumbar enlargements in a human fetus of "fourteen weeks" (CR length not given) and concluded that they had reached an adult arrangement by this time.

Hogg[29] describes the anlage (a group of three to four cells) of Clarke's column as being present at 32-mm CR length with a

TABLE 9–2. AMOUNT OF GRAY MATTER IN FETAL AND ADULT SPINAL CORD[40,41]

Prenatal CH Length (mm)	Gestational Age (Months)	Percentage of cross-sectional area			
		Cervical	Thoracic	Lumbar	Sacral
150	3	55	53	63	65
210	3.5	51	50	64	68
250	4.5	41	49	61	71
320	5.5	44	42	58	68
380	6	42	42	57	64
410	7	39	34	52	62
440	7.5	38	32	51	66
470	8	40	32	53	68
500	9	35	29	49	65
Adult		19	12	30	46

few fibers from them entering the lateral funiculus. He followed the development of this column and its relationship with other cord structures in 33 older fetuses until birth. Also seen at 32-mm CR length is a prominent substantia gelatinosa, an inconspicuous nucleus proprius and a few fibers of the dorsal component of the dorsal commissure.

By 36-mm CR length sensory fibers from the posterior horn cross in the ventral gray through the anterior commissure, and other fibers from the posterior horn establish contact with anterior horn cells. At 40-mm CR length the middle component of the dorsal commissure is present and most nuclear groups have increased numbers of neuroblasts. By 53-mm CR length the dorsal spinocerebellar tract can be identified.

The complexity of the cells in embryonic and fetal spinal cords is evidenced by the finding of isolated unipolar and bipolar sensory ganglion-type cells within the cord proper. Humphrey[30] describes such unipolar cells in specimens of 16-, 26-, 89- and 145-mm CR length; she found bipolar cells in 5-, 16-, 22- and 26-mm CR length embryos. Youngstrom[76] also reports finding cells of this type. These cells are transitory and may be equated with the Rohow–Beard cells found in lower vertebrates. Unipolar sensory ganglion cells also have been reported to occur within the central canal of the spinal cord in specimens of from 5- to 37-mm CR length. [31] These vary from 1 to 76 cells per embryo, are most prevalent (68%) in the lumbosacral region and are the equivalent of the mesencephalic trigeminal nucleus.

SPINAL NERVES

Numerous comprehensive studies have been made on the development of spinal nerves, but only representative examples will be selected due to the limited clinical applicability.

Spinal Ganglia

During stage XII (3- to 5-mm CR), neural crest cells are found to cluster in some regions, indicating the anlage of the spinal ganglia.[60] These gradually enlarge and over the next three stages (XIII–XV) migrate ventrally around the neural tube such that by stages XVI–XVII (8- to 14-mm CR) their ventral tips are at the level of the origins of the motor nerve roots. These ventral tips enter the intervertebral foramina in stage XVIII (13- to 17-mm CR) and are approximately one-half within these foramina by stage XXI (22- to 24-mm CR). At this time, these ganglia are completely invested with dura mater. Thereafter (stage XXIII) they lie completely within the intervertebral foramina.

Sensory Nerves (Fig. 9–4)

Whereas the spinal ganglia are easily identified on a morphologic basis, distinguishing sensory from motor nerve fibers is difficult during early development. The first fibers connecting the spinal ganglia to the spinal cord appear during stage XIV (5- to 7-mm CR) in the cervical region.[67] These fibers can be traced to cell bodies within the

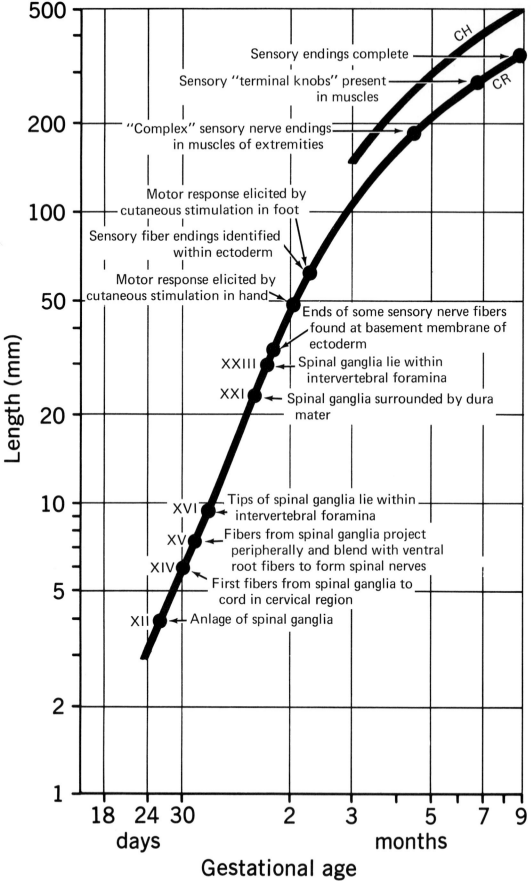

FIG. 9–4. Development of the sensory nerves of the human spinal cord correlated with CR length and gestational age.

ganglia, and by stage XV (7- to 9-mm CR) some fibers are present distal to the ganglia. These latter fibers blend with ventral (motor) root fibers to form the spinal nerves. Once these dorsal and ventral fibers have merged, it is difficult to separate them morphologically during the later embryonic period except at their cutaneous ends.

Hogg[28] studied the cutaneous distribution of sensory nerves in 19 specimens between 22- and 87-mm CR length, whose "physiological reactions" to stimuli had been tested prior to fixation. Motor responses to light cutaneous stimulation were found in the face at 25-mm CR length, in the hand at 48-mm CR length and in the foot at 61-mm CR length. Histologic examination during the "premotile period" (before 25-mm CR) revealed nerve fibers close to the epithelium, especially on the ventral surface of the embryo and the proximal flexor portions of the extremities. He noted that during this period there was a tendency for these fibers to form plexuses in the mesenchyme and not to enter the ectoderm. At 32-mm CR length, the ends of some fibers reached the basement membrane of ectodermal cells, but they did not pierce the membrane until 63-mm CR length. Invasion of hair follicles by nerve endings also occurred at this time.

Hewer[27] found "complex" sensory nerve endings in muscles of the extremities during the 20th gestational week and "terminal knobs" at 28 weeks. It was not until birth that the sensory endings were "finished." Keegan and Garrett[32] produced the most recent, if still controversial, dermatomal analysis of the segmental distribution of nerve endings in the adult.

Motor Nerves (Fig. 9–5)

The first ventral root fibers are seen in stage XIII (4- to 6-mm CR).[8,44] These develop rapidly, and by the end of stage XIV (7-mm CR) all motor roots through S2 are present and have intersegmental anastomoses.[65] As mentioned above, these blend with sensory root fibers during stage XV (7- to 9-mm CR) to form spinal nerves. Development beyond this time is complex, and the peripheral connections depend on the differentiation of specific muscles. The development of the motor end-plate is complex, going through

many stages as described by Cuajunco,[15] who traced the phases of muscle fiber development in the arm and correlated them with the connections by motor nerves between 38- and 362-mm CR length. Hewer[27] provides additional information about the development of nerve endings to muscles and tendons elsewhere in the body.

Lewis[44] follows the early development of the nerves and muscles of the arm in detail. During stage XIII (5-mm CR), the first indication of the cervical and brachial plexuses are present. These initially appear as "brush-like" endings on the spinal nerves from C1 to T3. By the end of stage XIV (7-mm CR), nerve fibers from the brachial plexus extend into the arm. During stage XVI (9 mm CR), the main portion of the brachial plexus appears as a continuous sheet of nerves from C4 to T1. As it enters the arm, it splits into a dorsal and ventral portion. The dorsal part is mainly the musculospiral nerve with a smaller component being the circumflex nerve. The ventral part subdivides into the suprascapular, musculocutaneous, ulnar and part of the median nerves; the last two extend to the distal end of the developing humerus. Some nerve fibers are present in the hand at this time. Shortly thereafter (10-mm CR), the axillary and radial nerves are identifiable.[66] In stage XVII (11-mm CR), the three major divisions of the brachial plexus are apparent, and there is further branching of the above nerves. By stage XX (20-mm CR), the major subdivisions of the brachial plexus are similar to those of an adult,[44] but the main plexus is still one fused mass.[8]

Nerves from the cervical and brachial plexuses supply other areas in addition to the arm. In stage XVI (9-mm CR), branches from C3–C7 can be traced to the levator scapulae and serratus anterior premuscle masses, a branch of C5 extends to the rhomboid premuscle mass, and branches from the brachial plexus reach to the anterior thoracic premuscle mass.[44] The C4 and C5 contributions to the phrenic nerve are also present at this time.

Bardeen and Lewis[7,8] have studied the development of the nerves to the leg. Late in stage XIV (7-mm CR), when the leg bud lies opposite the L5–S1 segments, bundles of nerve fibers from L2–L4 are found to extend

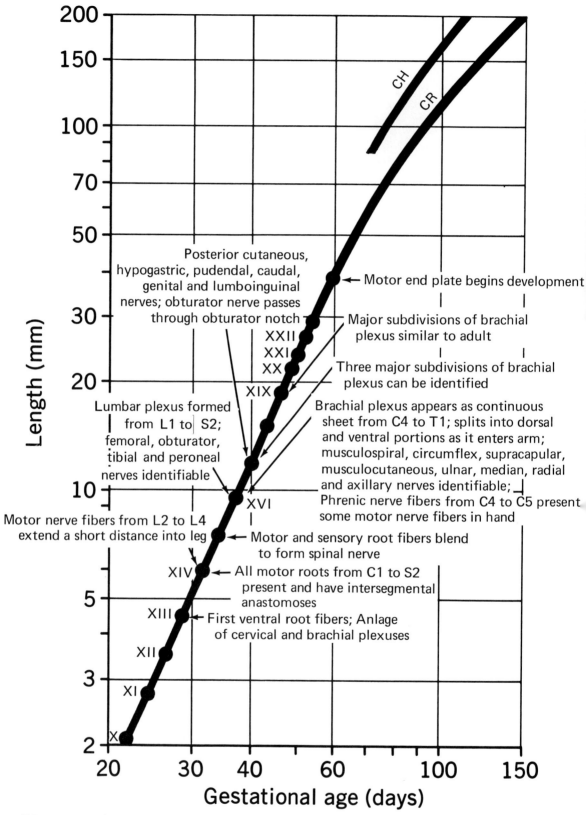

FIG. 9–5. Development of the motor nerves of the human spinal cord correlated with CR length and gestational age.

a short distance into it. In stage XVI (9-mm CR), fibers from L1–L5 and S1–S2 have anastomosed into the lumbar plexus, and the femoral, obturator, tibial and peroneal nerves arise from it. By 11-mm CR (late stage XVI, early stage XVII), nerves extend far into the developing leg. The posterior cutaneous, hypogastric, pudendal, caudal, genital and lumboinguinal nerves are also identifiable. The obturator nerve, now passing through the obturator notch, is found to branch, and the peroneal nerve gives off several branches to muscles.

The separation of the motor and sensory fibers of the developing lumbar plexus begins in stage XVIII (14-mm CR), when the lateral cutaneous nerve, arising from the main trunk of the femoral nerve, has endings that approach the ectoderm of the thigh. The saphenous nerve reaches the subcutaneous tissue near the knee after passing through the anlage of the sartorius and gracilis tendons. The sural nerve, arising from the tibial nerve, is also found at this time. By stage XX (20-mm CR), cutaneous branches of the tibial, sural and peroneal nerves are found. Except for later shifting, the nerves of the leg at this time are similar to those of the adult.

The developing spinal nerves have been the subject of many other studies that are useful references. Day[16] analyzes the blood supply to the lumbar and sacral plexuses in 18 stillborn fetuses ranging from the 18th week of gestation until term, in 1 neonate and in 1 adult. Barry[9] studied the angles at which spinal nerves exit from the cord in 10 specimens from 19- to 345-mm CR length. Electron microscopic studies on the nerves of 7 fetuses between 38- and 200-mm CR length have been made by Gamble.[24] The interrelationships between cervical nerves and the spinal accessory nerve have been studied in 25 embryos and fetuses by Pearson et al.[51]

AUTONOMIC NERVES (FIG. 9–6)

Although the sympathetic and the caudal parasympathetic nerves are associated with the spinal nerves, the autonomic system is generally regarded as being functionally different (being under involuntary control) and originating partly from motor neurons (preganglionic) in the CNS and partly from neural crest cells (postganglionic) in the periphery.

Sympathetic Chain

The primordia of the sympathetic trunks, appearing along the dorsolateral aorta as minute groups of cells, are seen in stage XIII (5-mm CR) in the lower thoracic and upper abdominal regions.[36] During stage XIV (6-mm CR), they are found to extend from the lower cervical to the sacral segments, becoming a continuous sheet of cells at 7-mm CR length late in the same stage. In stage XVI (8- to 11-mm CR), the sympathetic trunk extends to the upper cervical region and becomes segmented in some areas.The segmental nature of the trunk is quite prominent in the thoracic and abdominal regions of stage XVIII (15-mm CR) embryos.

Pearson and Eckhardt[50] studied the development of the rami communicantes between segments C7 and S5 between 4- and 35-mm CR length. The first white rami communicantes (preganglionic) were found in stage XIV, being present in segments T3–T8 in a 6-mm CR length embryo and in segments T2–T9 at 6.5-mm CR length. In all embryos of 9-mm CR (stage XVI) and greater, they were found caudal to L2 (83%) or L3 (17%), these being the same as in postnatal life. Gray rami communicantes (postganglionic) appear later than the white and are first present at 10-mm CR (stage XVI) in segments C8 and T1. During stage XVIII (13- to 17-mm CR), they extend from C7 (uppermost segment studied) to T5. They extend progressively caudally in stage XIX (18-mm CR) to T9, in stage XX (20-mm CR) to L3, in stage XXII (25-mm CR) to S3 and in stage XXIII (29-mm CR) to S5.

Esophageal and Cardiac Plexuses

Vagal nerve fibers with ganglion cells at their ends are found just beyond the tracheal bifurcation during stage XIII (5-mm CR). These extend to the tips of the developing lung buds and to the cardia of the stomach in stage XIV (6-mm CR) as the primordium of the esophageal plexus is very conspicuous. During stage XVIII (14-mm CR), the primordium of the cardiac plexus is present.[36]

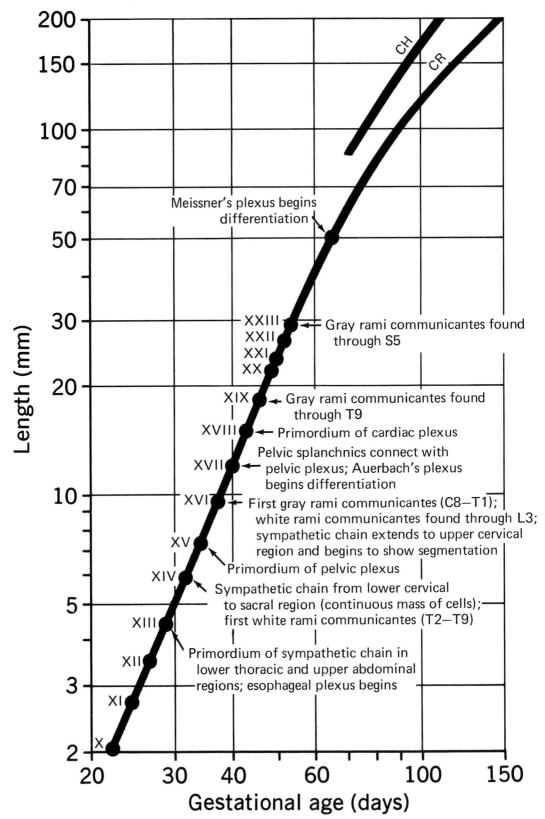

FIG. 9–6. Development of the spinal autonomic nerves correlated with CR length and gestational age.

134

Pelvic Plexus

Although Kuntz[36] believed that the primordium of the pelvic plexus was not present until stage XVII (12-mm CR), Kimmel and McCrea[33] found it during stage XV (7.5-mm CR) as a few primitive neural cells posterolateral to the rectum and urogenital sinus that were traceable as sympathetic neuroblasts in older specimens. During stage XVI (10-mm CR), pelvic splanchnic nerves (from segments S2 to S4) were found in close proximity to the pelvic plexus, and by stage XVII (12-mm CR), these fibers connected with the plexus. They also found a few fibers from the hypogastric plexus connecting with the pelvic plexus at this time. Smith[62] noted neuroblasts between the muscle layers of the colon in a stage XVII (12-mm CR) embryo and identified them as the first indication of Auerbach's plexus (numerous neuroblasts were present by 25-mm CR length). This closely agrees with the observations of Kimmel and McCrea[33] that in stage XXI (23-mm CR) the walls of the developing pelvic gut and bladder are invaded by nerve fibers and cells. However, they[33] believed that these represented rudiments of both the submucosal (Meissner) and myenteric (Auerbach) plexuses, whereas Smith[62] did not find neuroblasts in the submucosal layer until 50-mm CR length.

Other Observations

Hewer[27] identified nerve endings in the sinoatrial node, interatrial septum and epithelium of the lung at 10 weeks; in the lingual glands at 20 weeks; in the sweat glands at 22 weeks (fibers, but no "endings"); and in the media of blood vessels at from 26 to 28 weeks of gestational age. Unfortunately Hewer gave no CR lengths or other data to correlate with his estimates of gestational age.

ABNORMAL DEVELOPMENT

SPINAL CORD

Some major malformations of the spinal cord are discussed in Chapters 4 and 5 because their pathogenesis relates more to those topics of normal development. The entities considered in the present chapter are somewhat less well defined.

Occult Myelodysplasia

Myelodysplasia has been applied to a variety of malformations of the spinal cord, including meningomyelocele. As Warkany[71] stated, "spinal dysraphism is a myelodysplasia, but not all myelodysplasias are dysraphic." We use the term occult myelodysplasia for anomalies in the arrangement of gray or white matter in segments of neural tubes that have no associated surface abnormalities and do not have syringomyelia.

The incidence of myelodysplasia is not known, and clinically the symptoms are variable. In mild cases, there may be no symptoms, or there may be sphincter weakness, sensory abnormalities in the lower extremities, abnormal DTR or clefts in the vertebral spinous processes. However, myelodysplasia is also found in association with more severe disorders e.g., the Klippel–Feil syndrome[5] and familial osseous atrophy;[70, 71] as an entity in itself it may be severe (cases 2 and 3 of Lichtenstein[45]).

The lesions are variable, there always being neural defects and sometimes mesodermal defects. There may be no central canal, the ependyma being on the exterior surface of the cord,[5] or there may be several ependyma-lined central canals within a single cord.[45] There may be hydromyelia of one or more of these canals. In other cases, the dura mater may be present or absent dorsal to the cord; in the latter, vertebral clefts may be present. Duplication (see Diastematomyelia, Chapter 5) or "pseudoduplication"[45] of the cord may occur. The anomalous arrangements of gray and white matter are numerous, sometimes being so severe that there is a complete loss of architecture.[12] The spinal ganglia can be ectopic.

The pathogenesis of occult myelodysplasia is unclear because of the varying morphology. By limiting the definition to those cases in which there is intact skin over the lesion, it can be separated from the spectrum of meningomyeloceles (see Chapters 4 and 5). In many cases of myelodysplasia, the primary fault can possibly be attributed to a dorsal neural cleft, i.e., either the neuroecto-

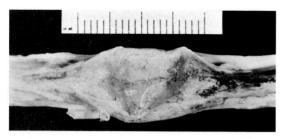

FIG. 9–7. Portion of the spinal cord of an 8-month-old girl with lumbar meningomyelocele, Arnold–Chiari malformation and thoracic hydromyelia. The hydromyelic portion lies just below the ruler and extends for approximately 2 cm. (#Np 3597)

FIG. 9–8. Cross section of the spinal cord from a 3-year-old boy with thorocolumbar meningomyelocele, Arnold–Chiari malformation and thoracic diastematomyelia with syringomyelia. (#Np 2268)

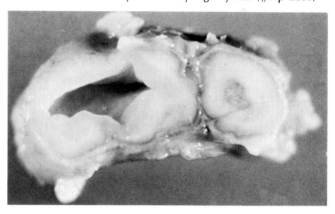

derm did not properly fuse, or "neuroschisis" has occurred.[48, 49]

Hydromyelia and Syringomyelia (Figs. 9–7 to 9–10)

Hydromyelia refers to an abnormal dilatation of the central canal. In one form, myelocystocele, it is frequently associated with cloacal extrophy. Lassman *et al.*[42] report six cases and provide a brief review. Hydromyelia may be associated with Arnold–Chiari malformation, diastematomyelia, kyphoscoliosis or myelodysplasia, or it may be completely asymptomatic. Pathologically, these ependyma-lined dilatations may occur in isolated segments or may involve the entire length of the cord.

In contrast to hydromyelia, in which the central canal is dilated, syringomyelia is an anomalous cavitation within the spinal cord that does not involve the central canal at many levels. The two conditions are frequently found together, and in some cases there is a direct connection between them. Whereas the hydromyelic cavity is lined by ependyma, the syringomyelic cavity is surrounded by gliosis and may be lined by collagenous connective tissue.

The pathogenesis of syringomyelia that occurs on a developmental basis is not known. Good reviews of the older hypotheses are provided by Riley[57] and by Scott *et al.*[59] Gardner[25] suggests that syringomyelia develops from hydromyelia by a break in the ependyma with further dissection of the cavity in the gray matter outside the central canal. Not all cases are of "developmental" origin, some being secondary to trauma, hemorrhage or infection. The association of syringomyelia and various types of spinal cord tumors (gliomatosis, ependymoma and angioma) is well known.[59]

The onset of symptoms most frequently

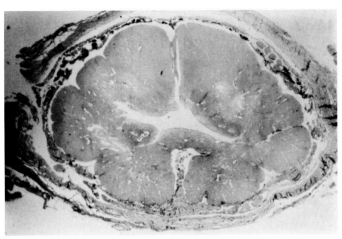

FIG. 9–9. Low-power photomicrograph of another case of Arnold–Chiari malformation with hydrosyringomyelia. (#Np 3930)

occurs in the second or third decades, with sensory loss (numbness, tingling, decreased pain and temperature), muscular atrophy and difficulty with coordination. Syringomyelia has been found in association with Sprengel's deformity.[20]

Since the cavities are most frequent in the cervical region, the typical syringomyelic pattern of loss of pain–temperature senses occurs bilaterally in the arms, but the cavity can be anywhere, either isolated or interconnected in the lower spinal cord and even the brain stem. Duffy and Ziter[19] report the case of a five-week-old male with apneic spells and stridor but no other findings; autopsy revealed syringobulbia similar to that shown in Fig. 9–10.

SPINAL NERVES

Anomalies of the Sensory System

Five separate developmental clinical syndromes are associated with dysfunction of the sensory system: 1) congenital indifference to pain, 2) congenital sensory neuropathy, 3) familial sensory neuropathy with anhidrosis, 4) hereditary sensory radicular neuropathy and 5) familial dysautonomia (which, though it also has sensory deficits, mainly involves the autonomic system; see Anomalies of the Autonomic System, below).

CONGENITAL INDIFFERENCE TO PAIN. *Congenital indifference to pain* is a term applied when there is a generalized absence or decreased sensation to painful stimuli, but no other findings. Temperature and touch are normal, and no consistent lesion is noted on biopsy.[74] These patients have normal development and intelligence. Although previous reports had occurred, Dearborn[17] brought attention to this condition in a thoroughly delightful, if unscientific, case study.

CONGENITAL SENSORY NEUROPATHY. Cases of *congenital sensory neuropathy* have an incomplete distribution of loss of pain. In addition, temperature and touch sensations are absent. Injuries are frequent, and delayed healing of wounds occurs. Credit for delineating this syndrome is usually given to Winkelmann *et al.*,[74] who presented findings in the case of a 9-year-old boy and provided a classification of the various syndromes involving loss of sensation. These patients may have normal or dull intelligence. The syndrome is probably transmitted as an autosomal recessive.[26] Biopsy reveals the absence of peripheral neural structures[46] in addition to a lack of myelination of sensory nerves.[74]

FAMILIAL SENSORY NEUROPATHY WITH ANHIDROSIS. *Familial sensory neuropathy with anhidrosis*[53] or congenital insensitivity to

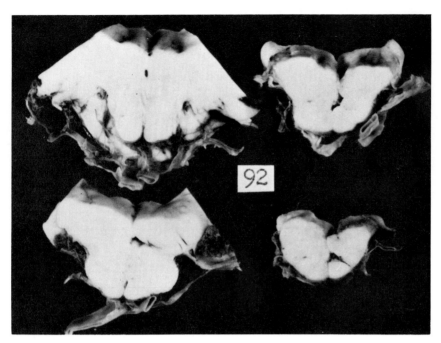

a

b

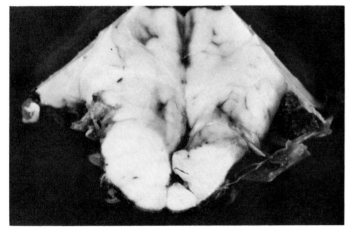

FIG. 9–10.   **a.** Cross sections of various levels of the brain stem from a case of syringobulbia. **b.** Reconstruction of Figure 9–10**a** showing the syringobulbia communicating with the fourth ventricle. (#NINDB-92)

pain,[69] is transmitted as an autosomal recessive and was separated as a distinct entity by Pinsky and DiGeorge.[53] These patients have mental retardation and a tendency to self-destructive behavior. Pain sensation is absent throughout the body and temperature sensation reduced but touch is present. Neuropathologic examination in one case by

Swanson *et al.*[69] revealed thickened dura mater with cavitation, adhesions of the arachnoid and dura and absence of Lissauer's tract (dorsolateral fasciculus) and the associated small, thinly myelinated dorsal root fibers and ganglion cells. In contrast to those cases with *congenital sensory neuropathy,* these patients have anhidrosis and normal dermal nerve networks. In contrast to *familial dysautonomia* (see Anomalies of the Autonomic System, below), these patients have normal lacrimation (and anhidrosis rather than hyperhidrosis). Although sweat glands are present, they do not respond to chemical or electrical stimulation.

HEREDITARY SENSORY RADICULAR NEUROPATHY. *Hereditary sensory radicular neuropathy* is transmitted as an autosomal dominant. Intelligence is normal. Pain, temperature and touch sensations are lost in the distal extremities. Warkany[71] discusses this condition under familial osseous atrophy since the patients develop perforating cutaneous ulcers that eventually lead to the destruction of the underlying bone. Neuropathologic examination in one case revealed loss of myelin in the dorsal columns and loss of peripheral and dorsal root nerve fibers in addition to numerous other changes.[18, 55]

Anomalies of the Motor System

Malformations or syndromes involving motor nerves are not so clearly defined as those involving sensory nerves. However, there are a number of conditions where anomalies of the motor nerves exist, although usually on a secondary basis and frequently with changes in the sensory nerves as well.

In the sacs of meningomyeloceles, both motor and sensory nerves have aberrations of number and course. The resulting motor and sensory levels have been correlated with the type of cord lesion.[64]

Webber[72] carefully dissected the lumbar nerves in a patient with six lumbar vertebrae. There were anomalous courses and anastomoses of motor, sensory and autonomic nerves.

Kristensson *et al.*[34] studied the cord and spinal nerves in one case of Tay–Sachs and three cases of Batten–Spielmeyer–Vogt disease. In the former, the motor neurons of the cord had distended cytoplasm, and the sciatic nerve had almost total destruction of myelin sheaths. The axons showed irregular elongated thickenings. There was a deficiency of neurons in the dorsal root ganglia. In the cases of Batten–Spielmeyer–Vogt disease, many of the anterior horn neurons were lost, and others had storage of lipo-

fuscin. The sciatic nerve showed myelin sheath destruction, and there was a loss of neurons in the dorsal root ganglia.

Anomalies of the Autonomic System

FAMILIAL DYSAUTONOMIA. *Familial dysautonomia* (Riley–Day) syndrome is characterized by early feeding difficulties, inability to produce overflow tears, indifference or insensitivity to pain, absent fungiform papillae on tongue, absent corneal reflex, hyporeflexia, postural hypotension, abnormal sweating, episodic fever, episodic vomiting and bowel disturbances. It mainly occurs in Ashkenazic Jews and has an autosomal recessive inheritance pattern.[13, 56]

The neuropathologic findings in familial dysautonomia have been inconsistent. Aring and Engel[4] describe one case with a "small cystic cavity within the dorsomedial and lateral nuclei of the thalamus." This was associated with demyelinization of fibers from the dorsomedial nucleus. The reticular formation showed a slight decrease in nerve fibers and myelin sheaths, and portions of the spinal cord had similar changes. Their case was diagnosed retrospectively as having had familial dysautonomia and is the only such case reported with a thalamic lesion.

Swollen fibers and myelin fragments were found in the reticular substance of the pons and medulla in a case reported by Cohen and Solomon.[14] Neurons in the nuclei of the vagus and spinal accessory nerves were shrunken. The posterior vermis of the cerebellum was incomplete, and some of the cerebellar folia were "denuded" of Purkinje cells.

Solitare and Cohen[63] describe distorted nuclei and vacuolated cytoplasm in the myenteric and submucosal plexuses of the gut. Similar cytoplasmic changes were found in the cells of the inferior cervical ganglion.

Pearson *et al.*[52] report degenerative changes in somatic sensory, sympathetic and parasympathetic ganglia associated with an absolute reduction of the nerve cells. There was also sponginess of the central segmental tract and a reduction of nerve fibers in the submucosa of the tongue.

Tabular summaries of autopsy reports provided by Riley and Moore,[56] Fogelson *et al.*[23] and Brunt and McKusick[13] show pathologic changes in the reticular formation in about 40% of cases, this lesion thus representing the most common finding in familial dysautonomia. Just how much of the syndrome is explained by this lesion is not clear. The recent report by Aguayo *et al.*[1] emphasizes the marked reduction in number of unmyelinated fibers in a sural nerve biopsy, and these authors speculate that a selective "developmental arrest during early differentiation of neurons in the neural crest could explain many of the cardinal features of the Riley–Day syndrome."

CONGENITAL MEGACOLON. *Congenital megacolon* (Hirschsprung disease) usually presents at birth or within the first few months after birth. Males are affected more often than females. The typical patient has stool retention and abdominal distension. The anomaly is more common in Down syndrome than in the general population.

Whitehouse and Kernohan[73] studied the myenteric plexuses in 11 cases of congenital megacolon. Ganglion cells were present in all segments through the descending colon, but there were none in the rectum and usually none in the distal sigmoid. They found a definite transitional zone in the proximal sigmoid in most cases, *i.e.*, a reduction but not an absence of ganglion cells. Closely packed bundles of nonmyelinated nerve fibers in connective tissue sheaths were present between the muscle layers of the aganglionic segments, but were not found in controls. They regarded this as an additional pathologic change. Whether those ganglion cells of the myenteric plexus that are normally identifiable late in the embryonic period were ever present, or whether they secondarily degenerated in congenital megacolon, is not known. Megacolon can occur secondary to other diseases postnatally.[71, 73]

Whether preganglionic elements are also absent is not known, since only one case has been examined.[2]

AUTONOMIC DYSFUNCTION. The Holmes–Adie syndrome, characterized by pupillotonia, hyporeflexia and segmental hypohydrosis, is regarded as a disorder of *autonomic function*. Although usually found asymptomatically in adults, at least one case has been reported in a child.[21]

Autonomic dysfunction has also been found in a patient with "cerebral gigantism."[3] The patient, a 19-month-old mentally retarded girl, had persistent fevers (to 40°C) and difficulty with sweating, beginning the second week after birth. Based on clinical studies, the authors believed that the patient had a hypothalamic lesion. Pneumoencephalography revealed cortical atrophy and enlarged interpeduncular cisterns, but no anatomic study has been presented.

The coexistence of anomalies involving autonomic nerves with other lesions is well known. Shocket and Teloh[61] report an 18-year-old male with congenital megacolon (diagnosed at age 2 years) who had a coexisting neurofibroma at the aortic bifurcation and a pheochromocytoma of the right adrenal. Potter and Parrish[54] studied a 1385 g, 375-mm CR length fetus of about 29 weeks gestation with numerous sympathetic tumors throughout the thorax and abdomen. In addition to a neoplasm involving the vagus nerve, there was hypertrophy of the nerve fibers themselves. The possibility of multifocal interactions between peripheral subcutaneous nerves (*i.e.*, subcutaneous "metastases") and neuroblastoma in some newborns has been suggested by Beckwith and Martin[11] (see Chapter 22).

REFERENCES

1. Aguayo AJ, Nair CPV, Bray GM: Peripheral nerve abnormalities in the Riley–Day syndrome. Arch Neurol 24:106–116, 1971

2. Alvord EC Jr, Stevenson LD, Dooley SW: Developmental anomaly with reduction of lateral horns of the spinal cord in a case of congenital megacolon (Hirschsprung's disease). J Neuropathol Exp Neurol 8:240–245, 1949

3. Appenzeller O, Snyder RD: Autonomic failure with persistent fever in cerebral gigantism. J Neurol Neurosurg Psychiatry 32:123–128, 1969

4. Aring CD, Engel GL: Hypothalamic attacks with thalamic lesion. II. Anatomic considerations. Arch Neurol Psychiatr 54:44–50, 1945

5. Avery LW, Rentfro CC: The Klippel–Feil syndrome: A pathologic report. Arch Neurol Psychiatr 36:1068–1076, 1936

6. Bardeen CR: Studies on the development of the human skeleton. Am J Anat 4:265–302, 1905

7. Bardeen CR: Development and variation of the nerves and musculature of the inferior extrem-

ity and of the neighboring regions of the trunk in man. Am J Anat 6:259–390, 1906–1907

8. Bardeen CR, Lewis WH: Development of the limbs, body-wall and back in man. Am J Anat 1:1–35, 1901

9. Barry A: A quantitative study of the prenatal changes in angulation of the spinal nerves. Anat Rec 126:97–110, 1956

10. Barson AJ: The vertebral level of termination of the spinal cord during normal and abnormal development. J Anat 106:489–497, 1970

11. Beckwith JB, Martin RF: Observations on the histopathology of neuroblastomas. J Pediatr Surg 3:106–110, 1968

12. Benda CE: Dysraphic states. J Neuropathol Exp Neurol 18:56–74, 1959

13. Brunt PW, McKusick VA: Familial dysautonomia. A report of genetic and clinical studies with review of the literature. Medicine (Baltimore) 49:343–374, 1970

14. Cohen P, Solomon NH: Familial dysautonomia; case report with autopsy. J Pediatr 46:663–670, 1955

15. Cuajunco F: Development of human motor end plate. Contrib Embryol 30:127–152, 1942

16. Day MH: The blood supply of the lumbar and sacral plexuses in the human foetus. J Anat 98:105–116, 1964

17. Dearborn GVN: A case of congenital general pure analgesia. J Nerv Ment Dis 75:612–615, 1932

18. Denny-Brown D: Hereditary sensory radicular neuropathy. J Neurol Neurosurg Psychiatry 14:237–252, 1951

19. Duffy PE, Ziter FA: Infantile syringobulbia: A study of its pathology and a proposed relationship to neurogenic stridor in infancy. Neurology (Minneap) 14:500–509, 1964

20. Du Toit F: A case of congenital elevation of the scapula (Sprengel's deformity) with defect of the cervical spine associated with syringomyelia. Brain 54:421–429, 1931

21. Easterly NB, Cantolino SJ, Alter BP, Brusilow SW: Pupillotonia, hyporeflexia and segmental hypohydrosis: Autonomic dysfunction in a child. J Pediatr 73:852–859, 1968

22. Elliott HC: Studies on the motor cells of the spinal cord: II. Distribution in the normal human fetal cord. Am J Anat 72:29–38, 1943

23. Fogelson MH, Rorke LB, Kaye R: Spinal cord changes in familial dysautonomia. Arch Neurol 17:103–108, 1967

24. Gamble HJ: Further electron microscope studies of human foetal peripheral nerves. J Anat 100:487–502, 1966

25. Gardner WJ: Hydrodynamic mechanism of syringomyelia: its relationship to myelocele. J Neurol Neurosurg Psychiatry 28:247–259, 1965

26. Haddow JE, Shapiro SR, Gall DG: Congenital sensory neuropathy in siblings. Pediatrics 45:651–655, 1970

27. Hewer EE: The development of nerve endings in the human foetus. J Anat 69:369–379, 1935

28. Hogg ID: Sensory nerves and associated structures in the skin of human fetuses of 8 to 14 weeks of menstrual age correlated with functional capability. J Comp Neurol 75:371–410, 1941

29. Hogg ID: The development of the nucleus dorsalis (Clarke's column). J Comp Neurol 81:69–95, 1944

30. Humphrey T: Primitive neurons in the embryonic human central nervous system. J Comp Neurol 81:1–45, 1944

31. Humphrey T: Sensory ganglion cells within the central canal of the embryonic human spinal cord. J Comp Neurol 86:1–35, 1947

32. Keegan JJ, Garrett FD: The segmental distribution of the cutaneous nerves in the limbs of man. Anat Rec 102:409–437, 1948

33. Kimmel DL, McCrea E: The development of the pelvic plexuses and the distribution of the pelvic splanchnic nerves in the human embryo and fetus. J Comp Neurol 110:271–298, 1958

34. Kristensson K, Olsson Y, Sourander P: Peripheral nerve changes in Tay–Sachs and Batten–Spielmeyer–Vogt disease. (A preliminary report). Acta Pathol Microbiol Scand 70:630–632, 1967

35. Kunitomo K: The development and reduction of the tail and of the caudal end of the spinal cord. Contrib Embryol 8:161–198, 1918

36. Kuntz A: The development of the sympathetic nervous system in man. J Comp Neurol 32:173–229, 1920–21

37. Kuntz A: Origin and early development of the pelvic neural plexuses. J Comp Neurol 96:345–357, 1952

38. Langworthy OR: Development of behavior patterns and myelinization of the nervous system in the human fetus and infant. Contrib Embryol 24:1–57, 1933

39. Larroche JC: The development of the central nervous system during intrauterine life. Human Development. Edited by F Falkner. Philadelphia, WB Saunders, 1966, pp. 257–276

40. Lassek AM, Rasmussen GL: A quantitative study of the newborn and adult spinal cords of man. J Comp Neurol 69:371–379, 1938

41. Lassek AM, Rasmussen GL: A regional volumetric study of the gray and white matter of the human prenatal spinal cord. J Comp Neurol 70:137–151, 1939

42. Lassman LP, James CCM, Foster JB: Hydromyelia. J Neurol Sci 7:149–155, 1968

43. Lemire RJ, Shepard TH, Alvord EC Jr: Caudal myeloschisis (lumbosacral spina bifida cystica) in a five millimeter (Horizon XIV) human embryo. Anat Rec 152:9–16, 1965

44. Lewis WH: The development of the arm in man. Am J Anat 1:145–183, 1902

45. Lichtenstein BW: "Spinal Dysraphism"; spina

bifida and myelodysplasia. Arch Neurol Psychiatr 44:792–810, 1940

46. Linarelli LG, Prichard JW: Congenital sensory neuropathy. Am J Dis Child 119:513–520, 1970

47. Malínský J, Malínská J: Developmental stages of prenatal spinal cord in man. Folia Morphol (Praha) 18:228–235, 1970

48. Padget DH: Spina bifida and embryonic neuroschisis; a causal relationship. Johns Hopkins Med J 123:233–252, 1968

49. Padget DH: Neuroschisis and human embryonic maldevelopment. J Neuropathol Exp Neurol 29:192–216, 1970

50. Pearson AA, Eckhardt AL: Observations on the gray and white rami communicantes in human embryos. Anat Rec 138:115–127, 1960

51. Pearson AA, Sauter RW, Herrin GR: The accessory nerve and its relation to the upper spinal nerves. Am J Anat 114: 371–391, 1964

52. Pearson J, Feingold MJ, Budzilovich G: The tongue and taste in familial dysautonomia. Pediatrics 45:739–745, 1970

53. Pinsky L, DiGeorge AM: Congenital familial sensory neuropathy with anhidrosis. J Pediatr 68:1–13, 1966

54. Potter EL, Parrish JM: Neuroblastoma, ganglioneuroma and fibroneuroma in a stillborn fetus. Am J Pathol 18:141–151, 1942

55. Reimann HA, McKechnie WG, Stanisavljevic S: Hereditary sensory radicular neuropathy and other defects in a large family. Am J Med 25: 573–579, 1958

56. Riley CM, Moore RH: Familial dysautonomia differentiated from related disorders: case reports and discussions of current concepts. Pediatrics 37:435–446, 1966

57. Riley HA: Syringomyelia or myelodysplasia. J Nerv Ment Dis 72:1–27, 1930

58. Romanes GJ: Cell columns in the spinal cord of a human foetus of fourteen weeks. J Anat 75:145–152, 1941

59. Scott E, LeFever H, Oliver M: Syringomyelia and syringobulbia. Ohio State Med J 30:213–223, 1934

60. Sensening EC: The early development of the meninges of the spinal cord in human embryos. Contrib Embryol 34:145–157, 1951

61. Shocket E, Teloh HA: Aganglionic megacolon, pheochromocytoma, megaloureter, and neurofibroma. Am J Dis Child 94:185–191, 1957

62. Smith B: Pre- and postnatal development of the ganglion cells of the rectum and its surgical implications. J Pediatr Surg 3:386–391, 1968

63. Solitare GB, Cohen GS: Peripheral autonomic nervous system lesions in congenital or familial dysautonomia. Neurology (Minneap) 15:321–327, 1965

64. Stark GD, Baker GCW: The neurological involvement of the lower limbs in myelomeningocele. Dev Med Child Neurol 9:732–744, 1967

65. Streeter, GL: The development of the cranial and spinal nerves in the occipital region of the human embryo. Am J Anat 4:83–116, 1904

66. Streeter GL: The peripheral nervous system in the human embryo at the end of the first month (10 mm). Am J Anat 8:285–301, 1908

67. Streeter GL: The development of the nervous system. Manual of Human Embryology, vol. II. Edited by F Keibel and FP Mall. Philadelphia, JB Lippincott, 1912, pp. 1–156

68. Streeter GL: Factors involved in the formation of the filum terminale. Am J Anat 25:1–11, 1919

69. Swanson AG, Buchan GC, Alvord EC Jr: Anatomic changes in congenital insensitivity to pain: Absence of small primary neurons in ganglia, roots and Lissauer's tract. Arch Neurol 12:12–18, 1965

70. Tocantins LM, Reimann HA: Perforating ulcers of feet with osseous atrophy. J Am Med Assoc 112:2251–2255, 1939

71. Warkany J: Congenital Malformations. Chicago, Year Book Med Publ, 1971

72. Webber RH: The lumbar nerves in a body with six lumbar vertebrae. Anat Rec 126:123–126, 1956

73. Whitehouse FR, Kernohan JW: The myenteric plexus in congenital megacolon. Arch Intern Med 82:75–111, 1948

74. Winkelmann, RK, Lambert EH, Hayles AB: Congenital absence of pain. Arch Dermatol 85: 325–339, 1962

75. Yaklovlev PI, Lecours AR: The myelogenetic cycles of the regional maturation of the brain. Regional Development of the Brain in Early Life. Edited by A Minkowski. Oxford, Blackwell, 1967, pp. 3–70

76. Youngstrom KA: Intramedullary sensory type ganglion cells in the spinal cord of human embryos. J Comp Neurol 81:47–53, 1944

SUPRASEGMENTAL STRUCTURES

chapter 10

CEREBELLUM

The unique form of the adult human cerebellum develops according to the general principle of ontology recapitulating phylogeny. During the transformation of the undifferentiated rhombic roof to the highly complicated suprasegmental organ that is intimately involved in practically all aspects of motor and sensory activity, the human cerebellum resembles that of lower animals. Because of this, it is possible to make reasonable guesses about the embryogenesis and morphogenesis of the human cerebellum even though the definitive embryologic studies have not always been carried out in homo sapiens. Emphasis will be placed upon the origin of the neurons that make the cerebellar cortex and nuclei and upon those morphologic changes in the region of the rhombic roof which eventually lead to the formation of the cerebellum. The description of the morphogenesis of the cerebellum (Fig. 10–1) is based upon the studies of Streeter,[46-50] Bartelemez and Dekaban,[4] Bradley,[7] Ingvar,[25] Langelaan,[30] Larsell[32-34] and Bolk.[6]

NORMAL DEVELOPMENT*

GROSS MORPHOGENESIS

In embryos of seven somites (stage X; 2- to 3.5-mm CR), two constrictions appear in the brain portion of the developing neural tube and divide it into prosencephalon, mesencephalon and rhombencephalon. As the neural tube closes, this segmentation be-

* See Chapter 1 for background information on embryologic development and staging system.

comes more prominent; it is quite obvious by stages XI and XII (2.5- to 5-mm CR). At this time the rhombencephalon is by far the largest portion of the developing brain, and the major flexures of the cephalic end of the neural tube begin to form.

The cephalic flexure that causes the forebrain to be at a right angle to the hindbrain is the first to form. A bulge marking the future site of the pontine flexure develops on the ventral surface of the rhombencephalon. The cephalic flexure increases to an acute angle, the pontine and cervical flexures begin to form, and the roof of the rhombencephalon becomes attentuated (Fig. 10–2). It is worth emphasizing that the cephalic and cervical flexures are related to changes in orientation of the remainder of the head and neck structures of the embryo, but the pontine flexure is unique to the neural tube. By the end of the first month of gestation (stage XIII; 4- to 6-mm CR), the lumen of the rhombencephalon is the widest portion of the neural tube. The alar plates are laterally flared because of the widening of the tube at the rhombencephalon. The portion of the alar plate rostral to the developing trigeminal sensory nerve is destined to become the major portion of the cerebellum, but at one month gestation it looks no different from the caudal portion of the rhombencephalic alar plate, which does not undergo such spectacular development.

The floor of the rhombencephalon contains the anlage of the fifth, sixth, seventh, eighth, ninth and tenth cranial nerves; these are identified during the third week of gestation by the six rhombic grooves. The most-rostral groove (related to the trigeminal

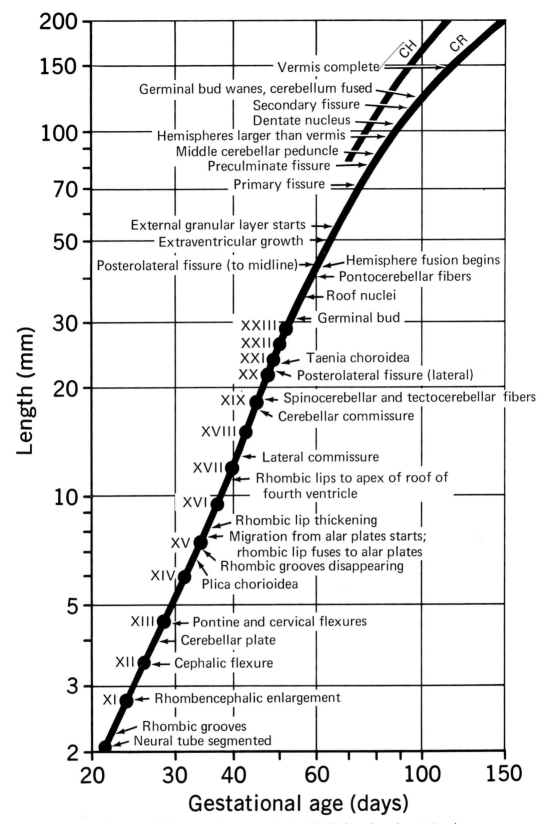

FIG. 10–1. Development of the cerebellum correlated with CR length and gestational age.

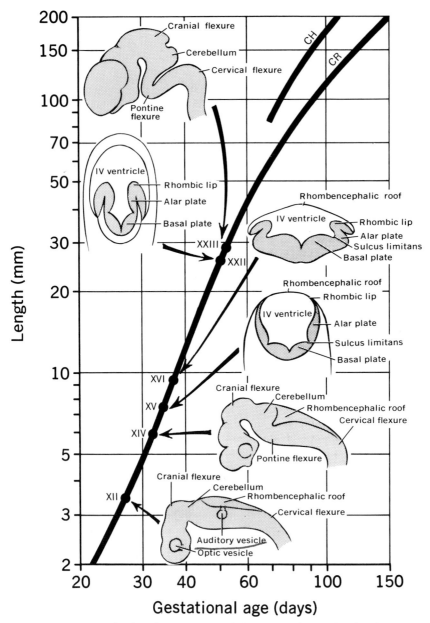

FIG. 10–2.   Longitudinal and cross sectional diagrams relating the development of flexures of the brain with some important landmarks for cerebellar morphogenesis.

nerve) lies at the level of the pontine flexure; the remainder of the grooves lie caudal to this landmark. The grooves disappear in the human embryo by stage XV (7- to 9-mm CR); the brain stem nuclei have developed many of their neuroblasts by this time and the external form of the rhombencephalic floor and roof begins to change rapidly.

The first critical step that occurs in the development of the rhombencephalon is the establishment of the pontine flexure during stages XIII–XVI (4- to 11-mm CR). This probably results from differential growth within the rhombencephalon, as it has no counterpart in the surrounding mesenchymal or ectodermal structures. The thin rhombic roof is transversely creased by the pontine flexure, and the greatest dimension of the roof changes from the longitudinal to the horizontal. Within the transverse crease (plica chorioidea), the choroid plexus will develop by the apposition of mesoderm to ependyma. It is important to note that the choroid plexus initially has a horizontal orientation corresponding eventually to the foramina of Luschka. The subsequent location of the choroid plexus is a map of the changes that will occur in the rhombic roof. It is also important to note that the cerebellum is destined to form rostral to the plica chorioidea. The rhombic lips are modified by the pontine flexure so that they now run in an oblique line towards the midline both rostrally and caudally from the pontine flexure and are no longer parallel to the longitudinal axis of the neural tube. The ependymal lining of the caudal portion of the rhombic roof looks inert histologically and is distinctly different from the cellular lining of the more active rostral and lateral roof region.

At the most lateral extent of the fold in the rhombencephalic roof, the alar plate is the site of intense neuroblastic activity during the fourth week. It rapidly hypertrophies to form the thickened rhombic lips that are the precursors of the cerebellum (Fig. 10–2). The cellular differentiation of the rhombic lips from the alar plates proceeds from the level of the vestibular nuclei rostrally until the rostral end of the rhombic roof is reached at stage XVII (11- to 14-mm CR), just caudal to the isthmus. The continued development of the pontine flexure, the migration of neuroblasts into the rhombic lips and mitotic activity within the lips cause the lips to fuse secondarily to what was formerly the ventricular surface of the alar plate. The development of the rostral portion of the rhombic lips leads to the formation of paired bilateral cerebellar primordia, consistent with the general rule that the dorsal midline of the neural tube is not a site of neuroblastic activity.

The rhombic lips at the level of the vestibular nuclei initially form the most primitive portions of the cerebellum: the flocculus and nodulus. The remainder of the cerebellum is derived later through the migration and proliferation of neuroblasts from the alar plate and rhombic lips.

The cerebellum lies completely within the fourth ventricle during the first two months of embryonic life; during the third month (40- to 90-mm CR length) it acquires neuroblasts at such a rate that it begins to bulge extraventricularly (Fig. 10–3). The growth of the cerebellum posterior to the contour of the rhombic roof creates the posterolateral fissure early in the third month (50-mm CR length). This is the most important fissure embryologically, as it separates the vestibular portion of the cerebellum (flocculonodular lobe) from the trigeminal–spinal portion of the cerebellum (lingula through uvula, part of the hemispheres, tonsils). The primary fissure, actually the second fissure to appear at 75-mm CR length, separates the culmen from the declive. The time of appearance of the vermian fissures and lobules is given in Table 10–1. The middle regions of the cerebellum proliferate more extensively than the rostral or caudal extremes, resulting in the change of a simple linear structure into one that is mushroom-shaped.

In general, the fissures and lobules in the vermis and flocculonodular lobules develop earlier than in the hemispheres; again, this is in keeping with their phylogenetic ages. Although the cerebellar hemispheres are larger than the vermis at 100-mm CR length, the

TABLE 10–1. FIRST APPEARANCE OF LOBULES AND FISSURES IN THE HUMAN CEREBELLAR VERMIS

Structure	CR Length (mm)
Anterior medullary velum	60
Lingula	105
Precentral fissure	105
Centralis	105
Preculminate fissure	78
Culmen	78
Primary fissure	72
Declive	130
Posterior superior fissure	130
Folium vermis	130
Horizontal fissure	132
Tuber vermis	132
Prepyramidal fissure	87
Pyramis	105
Secondary fissure	105
Uvula	105
Posterolateral fissure	45
Nodulus	105
Taenia chorioidea	22
Posterior medullary velum	127

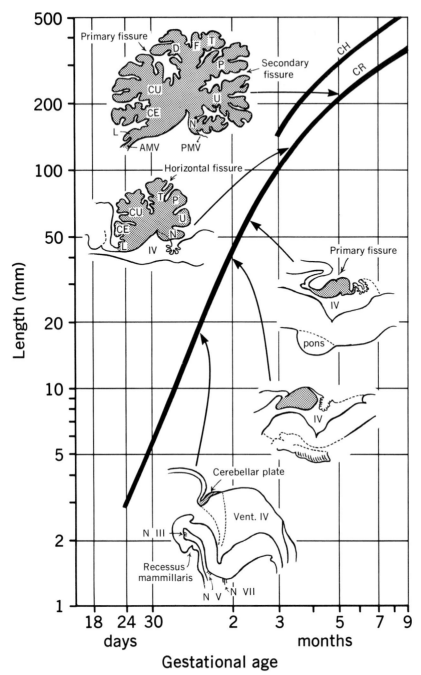

FIG. 10-3. Morphogenesis of the cerebellum correlated with gestational age and CR length. Note that early cerebellar development is exclusively intraventricular and that it is not until the development of the primary fissure at approximately 65-mm CR length that the cerebellum begins to develop extraventricularly.

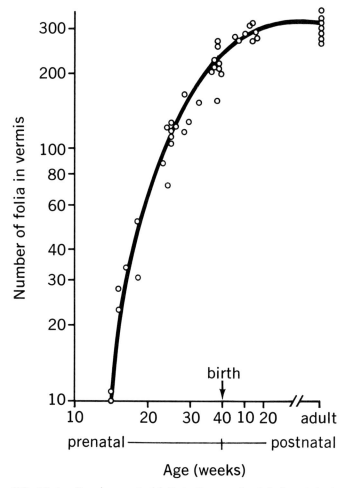

FIG. 10–4. Development of folia in the vermian lobules of the human cerebellum. (Adapted from Loeser et al., 1972)

fissures and lobules of the hemispheres actually appear from 30 to 60 days later than those of the vermis. Eventually the hemispheral growth all but obscures the vermis and causes a shifting in the paravermian lobules to accommodate the hemispheral bulk. The individual vermian lobules can be identified by 150-mm CR length; folia begin to be present in the vermis at this time and gradually increase in number; the middle vermian lobules take longer to reach full size (Figs. 10–4 and 10–5). The marked proliferation of the cerebellar cortex in association with the relative inactivity of the fastigium (that portion of the roof of the fourth ventricle lying ventral to the cerebellum) causes the fastigium to develop from a flat surface into an inverted "V" when viewed sagittally;

just as a kernel of popcorn explodes and inverts part of its former shell (Fig. 10–3). This causes an apparent "tucking in" of the nodulus, which comes to lie adjacent to the fastigial apex. No such migration of the nodulus occurs in fact; actually the overgrowth of the remainder of the cerebellar vermian lobules causes this important morphologic change. The nodulus is just rostral to the taenia, which is connected via the area membranacea superior (AMS) of the posterior medullary velum to the choroid plexus. The choroid plexus lies between the AMS and the area membranacea inferior (AMI). In the full term infant the choroid plexus can be seen coursing from the lateral recesses (the derivatives of the widest portion of the rhombic roof at the pontine flexure) towards

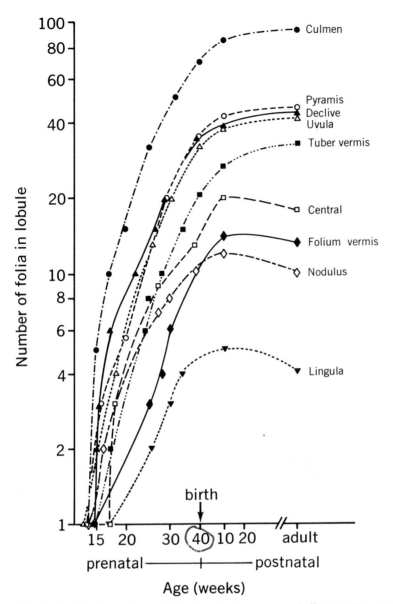

FIG. 10–5. Total number of folia in the human cerebellar vermis correlated with age. (Adapted from Loeser e *tal.*, 1972)

the midline, swinging caudally at the fastigium and running into the cisterna magna through the foramen of Magendie on the remnants of the posterior medullary velum. The importance of this growth pattern is that the extraventricular overgrowth of the cerebellum displaces a portion of the originally rostral roof of the fourth ventricle caudal to the derivatives of the transverse fold that demarcated the dorsal aspect of the pontine

flexure. These major steps in the early development of the cerebellum are illustrated in Figure 10–1.

The human cerebellum at birth is morphologically identical to that of the adult except for size. Cellular differentiation and migration as well as myelinization continue after birth and greatly enlarge the cerebellum (Table 10–2) without much change in its external appearance.[16]

TABLE 10–2. SURFACE AREA OF THE HUMAN
CEREBELLAR CORTEX[56]

	Fetal Age			
	16 weeks	24 weeks	Term Infant	Adult
Hemisphere				
Area (mm²)	86	448	15,200	57,620
% of Adult	0.15	0.77	22.2	100
Vermis				
Area (mm²)	68	142	2400	8840
% of Adult	0.85	1.6	27.1	100

HISTOGENESIS

The cerebellum develops from the alar plates of the rostral portion of the rhombencephalon, which are sites of intense neuroblastic activity. Some neuroblasts migrate laterally and dorsally to form the thickened rhombic lips from which neuroblast migration proceeds into the cerebellar plate, i.e., the thickening of the rostral portion of the rhombic roof. Neuroblasts from similar areas in the alar plates—and to a lesser extent in the basal plates—migrate ventrally to form pontine and inferior olivary nuclei.[30] Although Cooper[10] indicated that these nuclei originate from the midventral proliferation, the radioautographic study of Ellenberger et al.[15] is much more convincing, and it seems likely that the collection of cells which Cooper[10] identified as the midventral proliferation has migrated ventromedially in less discrete clusters from the alar plates.

The cerebellar plate then differentiates into a primitive ependymal zone, mantle zone, molecular layer and rudimentary external granular layer. This process starts at the widest portion of the rhombencephalon adjacent to the primordia of the vestibular nuclei and proceeds rostrally and medially until the apex of the rhombencephalic roof is reached. The earliest neuroblasts form the paired flocculonodular lobes. The neuroblasts derived from the cerebellar plate dominate the early development of the cerebellum, but the later cortical growth is related to another type of cellular proliferation.

The source of the neurons that form the various parts of the cerebellum has been a matter of debate for over a hundred years, and the final answers are still not completely available. There is little question that those neuroblasts which form the deep cerebellar nuclei and the Purkinje cells originate from the primitive ependyma in the alar plate of the cerebellum; initially this region has the typical ependymal, mantle and marginal zones. However, a large portion of the cerebellar cortex does not spring from this source but is derived from neuroblasts that migrate from the rhombic lips towards the midline and thence rostrally over the entire extraventricular cerebellar surface. This process leads to the formation of a "germinal bud" that lies caudal to the nodulus and is a site of intense neuroblastic activity lasting from 30- to 120-mm CR length. The ependymal cells in the rhombic lip itself remain mitotically active long after the remainder of the ependyma in the rhombencephalon and lead to the formation of the external granular layer.[18,38,54] The great majority of the extraventricular growth of the cerebellum is derived from these neuroblasts, which migrate from the rhombic lips to the germinal bud and thence over the cerebellum, forming the external granular layer. It first appears at about 8.5 weeks (40-mm CR length), covers the entire cortex by 14 weeks and achieves its maximum cellular proliferation and thickness by 24 weeks. The external granular layer is a transient morphologic feature that in man begins to disappear by 30 weeks gestation and is usually completely absent 2 years after term. The fate of these cells has not been conclusively determined in the human, but it is apparent in other mammals that they divide several times, migrate inward and differentiate into both glia and small neurons, which come to reside in the molecular and especially in the internal granular layers. The development of the cortical layers is plotted in Figs. 10–6 and 10–7.

Some mitotic activity is also seen in cells that have migrated from the ependymal surface into the internal granular layer. The tremendous proliferation of cells in the internal and external granular layers is largely responsible for the development of folia in the cerebellar cortex.

Woodard[58] claims that the external granular layer is derived from the rhombic roof and comes to lie upon the deeper cerebellar cortex by apposition of the rhombic roof to the burgeoning intraventricular cerebellum. It is clear that some apposition of rhombic lips to the alar plates occurs laterally, but we

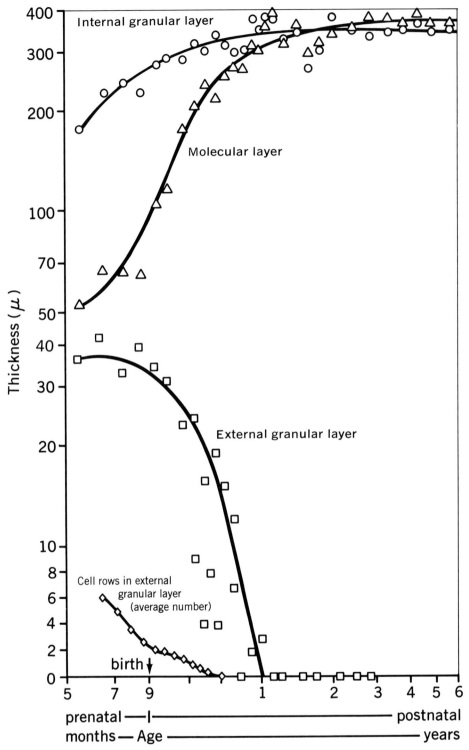

FIG. 10–6.   Cellular differentiation in the human cerebellar cortex. The thicknesses in microns of the internal granular layer, molecular layer and external granular layer are plotted as a function of age. In the bottom left the number of cell rows in the external granular layer is also plotted. (Adapted from Raaf and Kernohan, 1944)

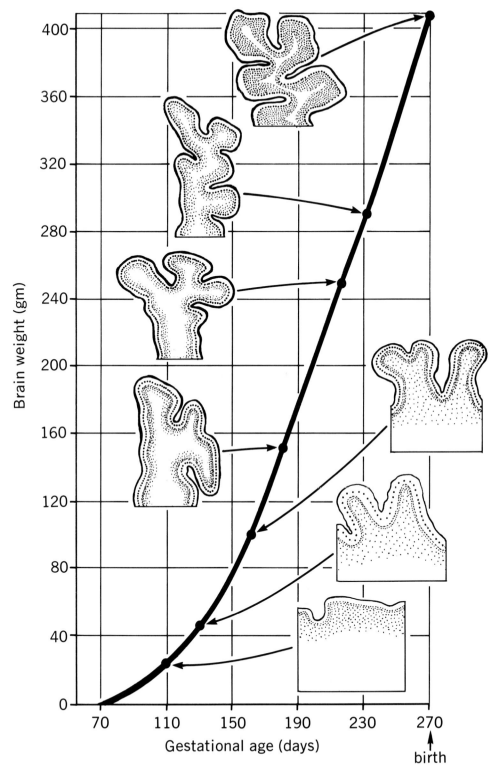

FIG. 10–7. Histologic appearances of the cerebellar cortex correlated with CR length and gestational age. (Adapted from Larroche, 1966)

153

cannot verify Woodard's concept that the external granular layer is totally derived from the rhombic roof, a tissue with no mitotic activity. There is clearly a region of intense neuroblast activity at the germinal bud and the external granular layer is first seen in this area. Woodard states that the roof plate adheres to the cerebellum between 10 and 14 weeks and forms the external granular layer, but no other worker has observed this phenomenon, which seems quite unlikely without mitotic activity in the roof plate.

The deep cerebellar nuclei form by migration of neuroblasts from the alar plates via the rhombic lips. The globose, emboliform and fastigial nuclei can first be identified at 35-mm CR length; the dentate nucleus and its efferent fibers to the red nucleus can first be seen at 100-mm CR length. Once again the phylogenetically newer structures develop after the older ones. The deep nuclei all originate in the rostral portion of the cerebellum and appear to migrate gradually to the middle portion overlying the fastigium. By 150-mm CR length the deep nuclei are separated from the cerebellar cortex by the developing white matter. By 280-mm CR length the deep cerebellar nuclei are similar in topography to those of the adult. The efferent tracts from the cerebellar nuclei can be detected at the same time as the nuclei become discrete entities. The deep nuclei, although morphologically similar in the fetus and the adult, achieve most of their volume after birth (Table 10–3).

Crossing fibers that are first seen in the rhombic roof in stage XVII (11- to 14-mm CR) constitute the lateral commissure, which is a part of the vestibular system.

TABLE 10–3. VOLUME OF THE HUMAN CEREBELLAR NUCLEI[56]

Nucleus	Fetal Age 24 weeks	Term Infant	Adult
Dentate			
Volume (mm³)	13.1	89.4	230
% of Adult	5.6	39	100
Intermediate			
Volume (mm³)	1.9	12.0	38.5
% of Adult	4.8	32	100
Fastigial			
Volume (mm³)	1.3	7.6	20.3
% of Adult	6.4	37	100

Additional neuroblasts migrate rostral to the original commissural fibers and cause the roof of the rhombencephalon to be progressively thickened in a rostrocaudal direction. By stage XVIII (17-mm CR), a second group of commissural fibers can be identified; those are derived especially from the trigeminal but also from the spinal, tectal and pontine nuclear systems. This group, the cerebellar commissure, is phylogenetically more recent than the lateral commissure. Although few commissural fibers are obvious in the mature cerebellum, the cerebellar commissure serves as the basis for the development of the largest portion of the human cerebellum, in fact, all of the cerebellum except the flocculonodular lobes. At a similar age, it is also possible to identify fibers of the ventral and dorsal spinocerebellar and tectospinal tracts; but pontocerebellar fibers are not present until after 40-mm CR length. These and other fiber systems do not complete their development until several years after birth; myelination occurs later in fetal and postnatal life.

Cellular differentiation and migration do not occur synchronously in all portions of the cerebellum. In general, the anterior and posterior ends of the vermis reach mature lamination and cellular differentiation prior to the middle vermian lobules. The vermis precedes by from six to eight weeks the lateral hemispheres in cortical development, and this again reflects both the phylogenetic and clinical features of cerebellar function.

ABNORMAL DEVELOPMENT

The cerebellum may undergo abnormal development because of intrinsic failures of morphogenesis in the neural tube or as a reflection of abnormalities in the surrounding mesenchymal and ectodermal structures.

Several types of environmental teratogens (e.g., toxins, vitamin deficiencies and irradiation) in experimental animals can lead to abnormalities in the cerebellum and are often associated with hydrocephalus. Little is known about the etiology of cerebellar anomalies in man, and the animal studies shed little light upon the mechanisms that could explain the majority of human malformations. Kalter[28] summarizes these studies.

OSSEOUS ANOMALIES

Of considerable clinical importance are platybasia and basilar impression, both of which can lead to medullary and cerebellar compression and displacement. The pathologic process in both of these malformations lies in the maldevelopment of the osseous structures about the foramen magnum. There is little evidence to support the contention that either of these anomalies is related directly to the development of the rhombencephalon, even though both may be associated with symptoms of cerebellar dysfunction and compression of the contents of the posterior fossa.

Similarly, congenital brevicollis (Klippel–Feil syndrome) can be associated with cerebellar anomalies, but this represents an error in cartilage and bone development, not in neural development primarily. The same can be said for osteogenesis imperfecta, which is often associated with severe reduction in the size of the posterior fossa and cerebellar dysfunction. *brevicollis*

ENCEPHALOCELES, MENINGOCELES AND DERMOID CYSTS

A variety of anomalies in the posterior fossa can be considered as the results of defects in the midline dorsal to the neural tube. Skin-covered defects in the posterior fossa often present as problems to the clinician. Included in this group are encephaloceles, meningoceles and dermoid cysts and sinuses. These lesions usually occur in the dorsal midline and may be associated with overlying ectodermal dysplasias, such as hair tufts, hyper- or hypopigmentation, hemangioma or lipoma.

An occipital encephalocele, if not necrotic or infected, can be seen to consist of skin, galea, dura, arachnoid and neural tissue. It is, of course, associated with a defect in the cranium that may vary widely in size. Whereas some encephaloceles contain minimal amounts of neural tissue and may be simply removed by transecting the stalk and repairing the dura, skull and skin, others may contain large amounts of essential neural structures (such as the medulla, cerebellum and collicular plate), rendering excision unfeasible. Some of these lesions include both infra- and supratentorial structures and are rarely compatible with normal extrauterine life. All six of our cases include the roof of the diencephalon with varying proportions of occipital lobes, colliculi, cerebellum and brain stem (Shaw, personal communication). Encephaloceles are often associated with hydrocephalus; the significance of this relationship is not clear, but the management of a child with an encephalocele should include careful consideration of this additional problem.

Cerebellar encephaloceles need not deform the dura or skull but can remain intracranial, appearing as thin-walled cysts that must be differentiated from arachnoid cysts.[1] They appear to develop as "blisters" from cerebellar folia and may or may not become symptomatic depending on size and location. When occurring at the foramen of Magendie, they (and arachnoid cysts) must also be differentiated from the Dandy–Walker syndrome by the second membrane separating the fourth ventricle from the cisterna magna (see Dandy–Walker Malformation, below).

Dermoid cysts and epidermoid sinuses can occur in the region of the cerebellum but obviously do not involve the cerebellum itself (see Chapter 5). These probably represent inclusions of ectodermal cells within the developing neuroectoderm rather than dedifferentiation of neuroectoderm itself. They can be associated with skull defects and with considerable destruction of cerebellar tissue. Secondary infection is always a hazard when a dermal sinus is present. Not all of the dermoid and epidermoid tumors occur in the midline. Some are not associated with a cutaneous defect and can present as a posterior fossa tumor; in fact, the typical epidermoid tumor presents as a diffuse pearly leptomeningeal mass ventral to the brain stem (see Chapter 22). Rupture of a dermoid or epidermoid tumor into the subarachnoid space is frequently associated with chemical meningitis.

AGENESIS

Complete agenesis of the cerebellum has been described in man and many other species.[2] It is a very uncommon anomaly, may occur in families[27] and has always been associated with major abnormalities in the nuclei of the pons and the medulla, especially the inferior olives. Several cases have been described in which the cerebellum consists of an undifferentiated roof plate with only a few islands of cerebellar tissue near the lateral recesses. Since the pontine and

olivary nuclei also originate in the alar plate of the rhombencephalon, it is not surprising that they are absent when there is no cerebellum.[13]

Unilateral agenesis of the cerebellum is somewhat less rare[51] and is associated with absence of the contralateral inferior olivary nucleus, pontine nucleus and red nucleus. This asymmetry can hardly be explained by the failure of one alar plate to develop since the neuroblasts do not migrate across the midline. More likely, there is a sequential failure of development of those nuclei dependent on the agenetic side of the cerebellum, corresponding to early atrophy of the von Gudden type. Figures 10–8 and 10–9 are examples of unilateral agenesis of the cerebellum.

Both types of cerebellar agenesis are often associated with mental retardation, which must be explained in terms of associated cerebral malformations, as in the case illustrated in Fig. 10–9, but these cerebral malformations have not been extensively documented.[13]

HYPOPLASIA

Hypoplasia of the cerebellum has been described in a variety of forms, some affecting the entire organ and others affecting only parts. The causes of this anomaly are probably diverse and vary from focal trauma or ischemic lesions to generalized neuroblastic

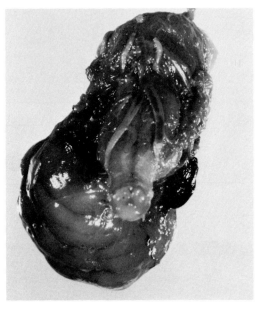

FIG. 10–8. Unilateral agenesis of the left cerebellar hemisphere in a newborn. (#D 732)

FIG. 10–9. Unilateral agenesis of the left cerebellar hemisphere in a 14-year-old, microcephalic (580g) girl. The cerebral cortex showed diffuse polymicrogyria. (#Np 462)

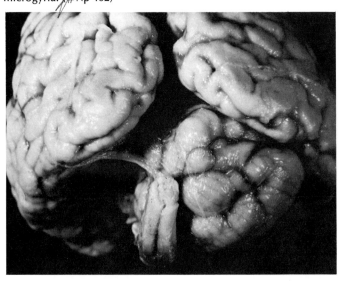

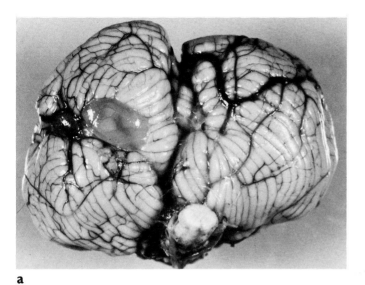

a

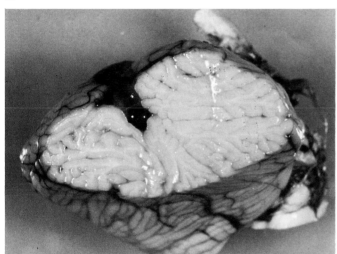

b

FIG. 10–10. **a.** A cyst of the cerebellar hemisphere of a 10-month-old boy who died of congenital heart disease. The cerebellar cyst originated in a folium and was covered by a thin gliotic membrane. There was also a subependymal cyst, a third abnormality suggesting a viral infection *in utero*. (#Np 3637) **b.** Cross section of the cerebellum with the cyst shown in Figure 10–10**a.**

dysfunction. In experimental animals, hydrocephalus can distend the cerebellar plate and lead to attenuation of the vermis. We have seen several examples of hypoplasia affecting the vermis far more than the hemispheres in the absence of any signs of hydrocephalus. Failure of fusion of the two sides may vary in degree and may be considered either hypoplasia of the vermis, or more logically, failure of fusion to form a vermis, the elements of which are still represented bilaterally. The Dandy–Walker malformation typically has hypoplasia of the vermis, diffusely and not just posteriorly (see Dandy–Walker Malformation, below).

CYSTS

Cystic structures within the posterior fossa may be related to the cerebellum and pre-

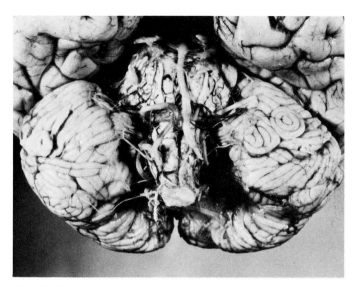

FIG. 10–11. Abnormal folial patterns on the surface of the left cerebellar hemisphere of a 57-year-
old man with incidental communicating hydrocephalus (probably posttraumatic) and imperforate
canals of Luschka. The flocculi were markedly hypoplastic.

FIG. 10–12. Horizontal section through the rostral
pons and anterior cerebellum demonstrating an
accessory left cerebellar lobe with its rudimentary
dentate nucleus and superior cerebellar peduncle
in an 81-year-old man. Note also malformed vermian cortex. This was an incidental observation at
autopsy. (#D 926)

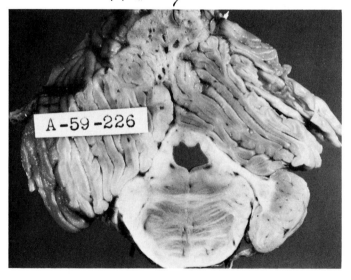

sent well-recognized clinical problems. Their
etiologies and types are diverse; they probably originate at many points in embryogenesis and in fetal and postnatal life. Some
cysts are clearly related to infarction and
degeneration within the cerebellar parenchyma; one of our cases was associated with
subependymal germinolysis[45] (see Chapter
23). Others appear to be more expansile and
possibly derive from intracerebellar hemorrhages or edema.[1] Figures 7–9 and 10–10
show cysts originating from the folia of the
cerebellum. Other cysts may represent arachnoidal inclusions or diverticula of the roof of
the fourth ventricle.[8] Another rare type of
cyst that can present near the cerebellum is

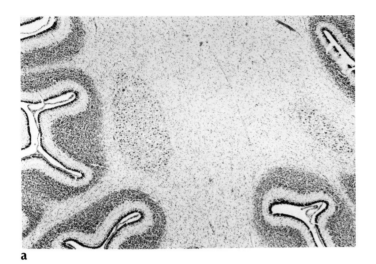

a

b

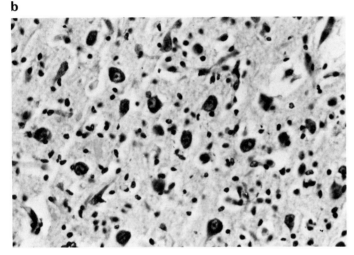

FIG. 10–13. **a.** Low power photomicrograph of nuclear heterotopias in the cerebellar white matter of a one-month-old girl with trisomy 18. (#Np 815) LFB–Nissl stain. **b.** Higher power photomicrograph of the cerebellar heterotopia shown in Fig. 10–13**a.** The neurons in this heterotopia are similar to Purkinje cells or those neurons found in the deep cerebellar nuclei.

the infratentorial extension of a supratentorial ventricular dilatation. The Dandy–Walker malformation, characterized by a cystlike dilatation of the fourth ventricle, will be discussed below.

DYSPLASIAS AND HETEROTOPIAS

There is a plethora of descriptions of cerebellar lobular, folial and nuclear dysplasias and heterotopias (Figs. 10–11 to 10–13).

These are often of no clinical significance unless large portions of the cerebellum are involved. Dysplasias and heterotopias, which are commonly found in association with the Arnold–Chiari malformation (see below) and in the trisomy syndromes (see Chapter 24), are readily induced by several teratogens in experimental animals.

ARNOLD–CHIARI MALFORMATION

The most common anomaly involving the cerebellum is the Arnold–Chiari malformation. It is almost constantly present in patients with meningomyelocele, but it may not always be clinically apparent. The essential feature of this common malformation is the elongation of the cerebellar vermis with

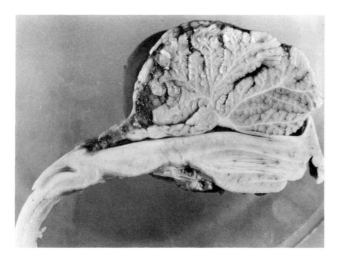

FIG. 10–14. Midsagittal section of a typical Arnold–Chiari malformation from a 3-year-old boy with a thoracolumbar meningomyelocele. Notice that the caudal cerebellar vermis is elongated and protrudes over the lower brain stem. There is a dorsal kink in the medulla, and the obex is everted. The caudal portions of the cerebellum are necrotic due to compression by herniation through the foramen magnum. The anterior lobe of the cerebellum appears to be more normally formed than the middle or posterior lobes. (#Np 2268)

failure of the nodulus to lie adjacent to the fastigium. In most cases the caudal vermis is herniated through the foramen magnum and lies over a dorsally kinked medulla and upper cervical spinal cord. Frequent concomitants of the Arnold–Chiari malformation are polymicrogyria, subependymal heterotopias, beaked collicular plate, aqueductal stenosis, hydrocephalus, impaction of cerebellar tonsils into the foramen magnum often with infarction, and syringobulbia-syringomyelia (Figs. 10–14 and 10–15).

The origin of the Arnold–Chiari malformation would appear to be independent of the cerebellum itself, which is well-formed except for the caudal vermis. Several hypotheses have been postulated regarding the pathogenesis of this malformation.[39] One hypothesis, known as the "traction theory," proposed that the developing spinal cord is tethered to the vertebrae at the site of the accompanying meningomyelocoele and cannot normally ascend by the process of retrogressive differentiation (see Chapter 5). As development proceeds, traction occurs, and the medulla and cerebellum are displaced caudally through the foramen magnum.[3] If

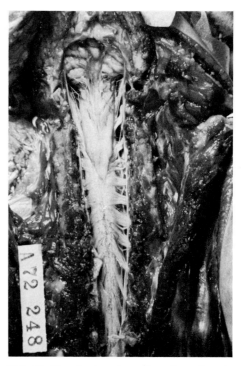

FIG. 10–15. Postmortem dissection of an Arnold–Chiari malformation in a 4-year-old girl viewed posteriorly. The herniated cerebellar vermis can be seen to extend over C2, and the dorsally kinked medulla to C5. The upper cervical roots run rostrally to exit through their dural sheaths. The cerebellar tonsils are not herniated. (#Np 3740)

this hypothesis is correct, the spinal nerves should course abnormally rostrally, but Barry et al.[3] have shown in two fetuses with Arnold–Chiari malformation that while the

falx

nerves in the cervical region have rostral displacement, those in the thoracic region run a normal course. Whatever "traction" occurs is lost within a few segments of the meningomyelocoele and some other mechanism must be postulated for the abnormal course of the cervical nerve roots. Another feature against the traction hypothesis is the rare occurrence of Arnold–Chiari malformation in the absence of a meningomyelocoele. In addition, the experimental study by Goldstein and Kepes,[22] who failed to produce the Arnold–Chiari malformation by postnatal suturing of the cord in newborn rats and opossums, adds no support for the theory, and perhaps some evidence against it. Finally, it would seem impossible for the spinal cord to pull the posterior vermis of the cerebellum without pulling the inferior cerebellar peduncles first!

The possibility that the Arnold–Chiari malformation may be secondary to hydrocephalus is another popular hypothesis—the pressure from above pushing the cerebellum caudally through the foramen magnum. That this hypothesis is not an acceptable explanation in all cases is evidenced by the fact that some patients with the Arnold–Chiari malformation do not develop significant hydrocephalus. The hypothesis also implies a downward flow of CSF, whereas the findings of squamous cells and lanugo hair in the subarachnoid space and central canal of patients with the Arnold–Chiari malformation[26] implies an upward flow. Furthermore, the opposite hypothesis has been proposed by Cameron[9]—that leakage from the meningomyelocoele is the pathogenetic factor; Emery and MacKenzie[17] support this view, finding a correlation between the severity of the leakage and the severity of the medullocervical kinking.

In contrast to the above two hypotheses suggesting that the Arnold–Chiari malformation arises secondary to other influences, there are other hypotheses related to primary disturbances in the development of hindbrain structures themselves. Daniel and Strich[12] suggested that part of the primary fault might exist in failure of the pontine flexure to form, which would lead to an elongated brain stem. At a later time, when the cervical flexure straightens, the medulla would "kink" over the upper cervical cord. Peach[41] extended this hypothesis and postu-

lated that a developmental arrest of the entire CNS occurs prior to the development of the pontine flexure. He relates each of the findings in the Arnold–Chiari malformation to the consequences of such an arrest in development.

Several fetuses with the Arnold–Chiari malfunction have been studied.[14] Van Hoytema and van den Berg[55] postulated that the posterior medullary velum remains intact, attached to the upper spinal cord, prohibiting inward rotation of the cerebellar vermis; with further growth of the cerebellar tonsils the vermis is displaced downward through the foramen magnum. Padget[40] believed that the Arnold–Chiari malformation arose from premature approximation or fusion of the cerebellar primordia in a small posterior fossa. Barry et al.[3] postulated that overgrowth of the cerebellum and medulla occurring in a small posterior fossa forced their gradual protusion through the foramen magnum.

Since all of these hypotheses have points which can be raised against them, the complex can be regarded as a multifocal abnormality, involving telencephalon (with subependymal heterotopias and microgyria), the diencephalon (with an enlarged massa intermedia), the mesencephalon (with aqueductal forking), the rhombencephalon (with elongated caudal brain stem), the spinal cord (with lumbosacral meningomyelocele), and even the mesoderm (with Lückenschädel, hypoplastic falx and tentorium, and a posterior fossa which is too small because the tentorium lies too low and the bony part is too small). Why most of these form a reasonably constant constellation is not easy to understand, but each can occur almost independently in rare cases.

Dr. Shaw has studied one case with almost complete agenesis of the cerebellum, the caudal hernia consisting of a thick roof plate and kinked medulla. Since the caudal vermis is the earliest part of the cerebellum to differentiate, the basic lesion may lie in the caudal portion of the rhombic roof, which does not attenuate in its normal fashion during stage XX (18- to 22-mm CR). This could result in the secondary approximation of the nodulus to the obex because of the abnormal persistence of the thick posterior medullary velum. This is not a primary hydrocephalic process such as Gardner[20, 21] has postulated,

obex

and is independent of the patency of the lateral foramina of the fourth ventricle, although the foramen of Magendie does not form. Such a failure of degeneration of the caudal rhombic roof could also explain the dorsal eversion of the obex, as this is the site of attachment of the caudal end of the rhombic roof.

Our unpublished studies of the cerebellum in Arnold–Chiari malformation show that the numbers of folia per lobule in the vermis have a somewhat greater than normal variation. The caudal end of the vermis is always involved; the uvula and pyramis may also be affected if the nodulus is severely distorted. The exact status of the flocculus is frequently not described, but it appears generally to be present, much less malformed than the nodulus, and typically wrapped ventrally almost completely around the pontomedullary junction.

This malformation seems to be based upon unusual events in the dorsal midline of the rhombic roof caudal to the plica chorioidea (area membranacea inferior). The cerebellum is not a midline structure, and we can find no report of a unilateral Arnold–Chiari malformation. Since the cerebellar vermis is always intact, even though caudally malformed and malpositioned, this anomaly is not one of failure of fusion of the cerebellum. However, as shown by Dr. Shaw's case described above, what we began by defining as the "essential feature" of the Arnold–Chiari malformation may be absent, thus proving how little we really understand about this very common anomaly.

DANDY–WALKER MALFORMATION

The Dandy–Walker malformation—as well as the Arnold–Chiari malformation—has long been of interest to surgeons, pediatricians, embryologists and pathologists.[5, 8, 11, 19, 23, 24, 44, 57] Patients with the Dandy–Walker malformation usually present clinically with the signs and symptoms of hydrocephalus, but surprisingly they may be older children and even teenagers. A noticeable bulging of the occipital region is frequently present, and transillumination of the head reveals increased light in the posterior fossa. Pneumoencephalography and angiography[35] are useful in differentiating Dandy–Walker mal-

formation from arachnoid cysts of the posterior fossa (see Chapter 17).

The neuropathology of Dandy–Walker syndrome is variable but the criteria utilized by Hart et al.[24] are useful: 1) hydrocephalus, 2) partial or complete absence of the cerebellar vermis, and 3) posterior fossa cyst continuous with the fourth ventricle. The hydrocephalus usually involves all ventricles. The cystic dilatation of the fourth ventricle is associated with marked but usually incomplete separation of the cerebellar hemispheres, the vermis usually being present anteriorly but reflected rostrally over the colliculi, so that it may appear to be absent when viewed from the fourth ventricle. The caudal part of the vermis is always absent, but remnants of cerebellar cortex are frequently detectable in the membrane which forms the cyst and which must be the persistent posterior medullary velum, as though the developing posterior vermian neuroblasts got lost in a posterior medullary velum which was too voluminous. The resulting cystic dilatation of the fourth ventricle causes elevation of the tentorium. Patency of the outlet foramina (Luschka and Magendie) is difficult to establish in many cases; they have been reported as being all closed, all open or one open and one closed.[43, 52] Hart et al.[24] recorded additional CNS anomalies in 19 of their 28 cases. Nonspecific and specific gyral anomalies and heterotopias were found in 12, agenesis of the corpus callosum in 4 and anomalies of the inferior olivary nuclei in 4 cases. One of the cases was a 7-year-old child with de Lange syndrome.

The pathogenesis of Dandy–Walker malformation is not known, but several hypotheses have been advanced.[5, 8, 20, 21, 40, 52] The popular suggestion that atresia of the foramina of Luschka and Magendie is responsible[52] is invalidated in some cases by the demonstration of their patency. In those cases where they are anatomically closed it is difficult to say whether or not they were physiologically closed during life, since dialysis of CSF across the large area of the cyst might well have been adequate to compensate for the obstruction. At present this hypothesis, while perhaps applicable to most cases, does not appear to be the only mechanism. Brodal and Hauglie-Hanssen,[8] on the

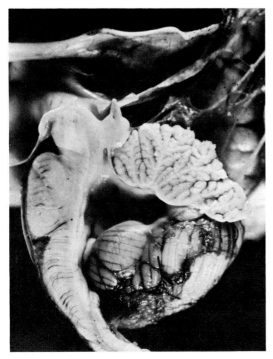

FIG. 10–16. Midsagittal section of the brain stem and cerebellum from a patient with Dandy–Walker malformation with marked hydrocephalus. The anterior portion of the cerebellum is everted over the colliculi, and the caudal vermian lobules are absent. The lateral cerebellar structures are hypoplastic. The thin cystlike extension from the caudal cerebellar vermis was destroyed during removal of the specimen. (#MCV A-410-66. Courtesy Dr. Margaret Jones)

basis of comparative findings in mice, concluded that the basis of the Dandy-Walker syndrome was "increased intraventricular pressure, the reasons of which remain unknown."

From study of our own cases (unpublished data), we see that the cerebellum seems to be mainly an intraventricular structure with paired laterally placed lobes, the caudal vermis thinning out into the roof of the markedly dilated fourth ventricle (Fig. 10–16). This malformation may be the result of partial failure of secondary formation of the rhombic lips from the alar plate, with a general deficiency of neurons in the cerebellum and a hypoplasia and gross alteration in cerebellar form. The aberrations in medullary nuclei that have been recently reported in association with the Dandy–Walker malformation are another manifestation of errors in migration of neuroblasts from the rhombic lips.[23]

In summary then, both the Dandy–Walker and the Arnold–Chiara malformations implicate an anomaly of the posterior medullary velum, being too voluminous in one and too thick in the other. It seems doubtful, however, that these are the only anomalies, and a satisfactory hypothesis remains to be developed.

MEDULLOBLASTOMA

Medulloblastomas can be considered a malformation related to the abnormal migration of neuroblasts from the germinal bud in the rhombic lips.[29] As discussed in more detail in Chapter 22, this tumor may represent the escape of the pluripotential cells of the germinal bud from their normally controlled replication. This type of tumor is most common in the cerebellum, but can occasionally occur at other sites of germinal matrix cells which will differentiate into glia and neurons.

REFERENCES

1. Alvord EC Jr, Marcuse PM: Intracranial cerebellar meningoencephalocele (posterior fossa cyst) causing hydrocephalus by compression at the insura tentorii. J Neuropathol Exp Neurol 21:50–69, 1962

2. Baker RC, Graves GO: Cerebellar agenesis. Arch Neurol Psychiatr 25:548–555, 1931

3. Barry A, Patten BM, Stewart BH: Possible factors in the development of the Arnold–Chiari malformation. J. Neurosurg 14:285–301, 1957

4. Bartelmez GW, Dekaban AS: The early development of the human brain. Contrib Embryol 37:13–32, 1962

5. Benda CE: The Dandy–Walker syndrome or the so-called atresia of the foramen Magendie. J Neuropathol Exp Neurol 13:14–29, 1954

6. Bolk L: Das Cerebellum der Saugetiere. Jena, Gustav Fischer, 1906

7. Bradley OC: On the development and homology of the mammalian cerebellar fissures. J Anat Physiol 37:448–475, 1903

8. Brodal A, Hauglie-Hanssen E: Congenital hydrocephalus with defective development of the cerebellar vermis (Dandy–Walker Syndrome). J Neurol Neurosurg Psychiatry 22:99–108, 1959

9. Cameron AH: The Arnold–Chiari and other neu-

roanatomical malformations associated with spina bifida. J Pathol 73:195–211, 1957

10. Cooper ERA: The development of the substantia nigra. Brain 69:22–33, 1946

11. D'Agostino AN, Kernohan JW, Brown JR: The Dandy–Walker syndrome. J Neuropathol Exp Neurol 22:450–470, 1963

12. Daniel PM, Strich SJ: Some observations on the congenital deformity of the central nervous system known as the Arnold–Chiari malformation. J Neuropathol Exp Neurol 17:255–266, 1958

13. Dow RS, Moruzzi G: The Physiology and Pathology of the Cerebellum. Minneapolis, Univ Minnesota Press, 1958

14. Duckett S: Foetal Arnold–Chiari malformation. Acta Neuropathol 7:175–179, 1966

15. Ellenberger C Jr, Hanaway J, Netsky MG: Embryogenesis of the inferior olivary nucleus in the rat: A radioautographic study and re-evaluation of the rhombic lip. J Comp Neurol 137:71–88, 1969

16. Ellis RS: Norms for some structural changes in the human cerebellum from birth to old age. J Comp Neurol 32:1–33, 1920

17. Emery JL, Mackenzie N: Medullo-cervical dislocation deformity (Chiari II deformity) related to neurospinal dysraphism (meningomyelocele). Brain 96:155–162, 1973

18. Fujita S: Autoradiographic studies on histogenesis of the cerebellar cortex. Neurobiology of Cerebellar Evolution and Development. Edited by R Llinas. Chicago, American Med Assoc, 1969, pp. 743–747

19. Gardner E, O'Rahilly R, Prolo D: The Dandy–Walker and Arnold–Chiari Malformations. Arch Neurol 32:393–407, 1975

20. Gardner WJ: The Dysraphic States: From Syringomyelia to Anencephaly. Excerpta Medica Amsterdam, p. 201, 1973

21. Gardner WJ, Smith JL, Padget DH: The relationship of Arnold–Chari and Dandy–Walker malformations. J Neurosurg 36:481–486, 1972

22. Goldstein F, Kepes JJ: The role of traction in the development of the Arnold–Chiari malformation. An experimental study. J Neuropathol Exp Neurol 25:654–666, 1966

23. Hanaway J, Netsky MG: Heterotopias of the inferior olive: Relation to Dandy–Walker malformation and correlation with experimental data. J Neuropathol Exp Neurol 30:380–389, 1971

24. Hart MN, Malamud N, Ellis WG: The Dandy–Walker syndrome. A clinicopathological study based on 28 cases. Neurology (Minneap) 22:771–780, 1972

25. Ingvar S: Zur Phylo-und Ontogenese des Kleinhirns. Folia Neuro-Biol 11:205–495, 1918

26. Jacobs EB, Landing BH, Thomas W Jr: Vernicomyelia: Its bearing on theories of genesis of the Arnold–Chiari complex. Am J Pathol 39:345–353, 1961

27. Joubert M, Eisenring JJ, Robb JP, Andermann F: Familial agenesis of the cerebellar vermis: A syndrome of episodic hyperpnea, abnormal eye movements, ataxia and mental retardation. Neurology (Minneap) 19: 813–825, 1969

28. Kalter H: Teratology of the Nervous System. Chicago, Univ Chicago Press, 1968

29. Kershman J: The medulloblast and the medulloblastoma. Arch Neurol Psychiatr 40:937–967, 1938

30. Langelaan J: On the development of the external form of the human cerebellum. Brain 42: 130–170, 1919

31. Larroche JC: Development of the nervous system in early life. Part II: The development of the central nervous system during intrauterine life. In Human Development. Edited by F Falkner. Philadelphia, Saunders, 1966

32. Larsell O: Morphogenesis and evolution of the cerebellum. Arch Neurol Psychiatr 31:373–395, 1934

33. Larsell O: The development of the cerebellum in man in relation to its comparative anatomy. J Comp Neurol 87:85–129, 1947

34. Larsell O: Development of the tonsilla, accessory paraflocculus and biventral lobule in man (abstracted). Anat Rec 133:302, 1959

35. La Torre E, Fortuna A, Occhipinti E: Angiographic differentiation between Dandy–Walker cyst and arachnoid cyst of the posterior fossa in newborn infants and children. J Neurosurg 38:298–308, 1973

36. Lichtenstein, BW: Distant neuroanatomic complications of spina bifida (spinal dysraphism): Hydrocephalus, Arnold–Chiari deformity, stenosis of the aqueduct of Sylvius etc.; Pathogenesis and pathology. Arch Neurol Psychiatr 47: 195–214, 1942

37. Loeser JD, Lemire RJ, Alvord EC Jr: The development of the folia in the human cerebellar vermis. Anat Rec 173:109–114, 1972

38. Maile IL, Sidman RL: An autoradiographic analysis of histogenesis in the mouse cerebellum. Exp Neurol 4:277–296, 1961

39. Milhorat TH: Hydrocephalus and the Cerebrospinal Fluid. Baltimore, Williams & Wilkins, 1972, pp. 97–102

40. Padget DH: Development of so-called dysraphism; with embryologic evidence of clinical Arnold–Chiari and Dandy–Walker malformations. Johns Hopkins Med J 130:127–165, 1972

41. Peach B: The Arnold–Chiari malformation: Morphogenesis. Arch Neurol 12:527–535, 1965

42. Raaf J, Kernohan JW: A study of the external granular layer in the cerebellum. Am J Anat 75:151–172, 1944

43. Raimondi AJ: Atresia of the foramina of Luschka and Magendie: Dandy–Walker cyst. J Neurosurg 31:202–216, 1969

44. Sahs AL: Congenital anomaly of the cerebellar vermis. Arch Pathol 32:52–63, 1941

45. Shaw CM, Alvord EC, Jr: Subependymal germinolysis. Arch Neurol 31:374–381, 1974

46. Streeter GL: The development of the nervous system. Manual of Human Embryology, vol II. Edited by F Keibel. Philadelphia, JB Lippincott, 1912, pp. 1–156

47. Streeter GL: Developmental horizons in human embryos. Description of age group XI, 13 to 20 somites, and age group XII, 21 to 29 somites. Contrib Embryol 30:211–245, 1942

48. Streeter GL: Developmental horizons in human embryos. Description of age group XIII, embryos about 4 or 5 millimeters long, and age group XIV, period of indentation of the lens vesicle. Contrib Embryol 31:27–63, 1945

49. Streeter GL: Developmental horizons in human embryos. Description of age groups XV, XVI, XVII, XVIII, being the third issue of a survey of the Carnegie collection. Contrib Embryol 32:133–203, 1948

50. Streeter GL, Heuser CH, Corner GW: Developmental horizons in human embryos. Description of age groups XIX, XX, XXI, XXII and XXIII, being the fifth issue of a survey of the Carnegie collection. Contrib Embryol 34:165–196, 1951

51. Strong OS: A case of unilateral cerebellar agenesis. J Comp Neurol 25:361–391, 1915

52. Taggart JK Jr, Walker AE: Congenital atresia of the foramens of Luschka and Magendie. Arch Neurol Psychiatr 48:583–612, 1942

53. Trowbridge WV, French JD: Benign arachnoid cysts of the posterior fossa. J Neurosurg 9:398–404, 1952

54. Uzman LL: The histogenesis of the mouse cerebellum as studied by its tritiated thymidine uptake. J Comp Neurol 114:137–149, 1960

55. van Hoytema GJ, van den Berg R: Embryological studies of the posterior fossa in connection with Arnold–Chiari malformation. Dev Med Child Neurol (Suppl) 11:61–76, 1966

56. Verbitskaya LB: Some aspects of the ontophylogenesis of the cerebellum. Neurobiology of Cerebellar Evolution and Development. Edited by R Llinas. Chicago, American Med Assoc, 1969, pp. 859–874

57. Vuia O, Pascu F: The Dandy–Walker syndrome associated with syringomyelia in a newborn infant. Confin Neurol 33:33–40, 1971

58. Woodard JS: Origin of the external granule layer of the cerebellar cortex. J Comp Neurol 115:65–73, 1960

Rd. 2/5/88

chapter 11

COLLICULI

There is little information available on the normal development of the colliculi, also referred to as the tectum, or corpora quadrigemia (Fig. 11–1). These important suprasegmental structures, concerned with both visual (superior colliculi) and auditory (inferior colliculi) pathways, develop from the alar plate of the midbrain (mesencephalon). They overlie the cerebral aqueduct and extend caudally from the level of the posterior commissure to the dorsal decussation of the trochlear nerve (CN-IV). The following information is mainly derived from the study of Bartelmez and Dekaban[1] and a few notations provided by Streeter.[9]

NORMAL DEVELOPMENT*

During stage X (2- to 3.5-mm CR), when the neural folds are first fusing, the initial demarcation of forebrain, midbrain and hindbrain is seen. The rostral demarcation of the midbrain is the prosmesencephalic sulcus, which is an abrupt narrowing of the neural folds just caudal to the optic primordium. During this stage there is only a single midbrain segment. Early in stage XI (2.5- to 4.5-mm CR), the rostral neural folds fuse to the level of the midbrain, thus establishing the primordium of the collicular plate. Fusion of the neural folds continues and the anterior neuropore closes later in this stage. About this time there is definition of two midbrain neuromeres, the rostral of which is quite large while the caudal one is

less distinct. Bartelmez and Dekaban[1] equate these with the pretectal and collicular areas of Streeter[9] and believe that he was wrong in assuming that the former did not contribute to the superior colliculus. Just caudal to the second midbrain neuromere, the first indication of the mesmetencephalic sulcus is seen externally. As it further indents, it is known as the isthmus.

In stage XII (3- to 5-mm CR), the cranial (cephalic) flexure appears at the level of the two midbrain neuromeres. The prosmesencephalic sulcus (separating forebrain and midbrain) develops into a deep narrow constriction in contrast to the isthmus (separating midbrain and hindbrain), which is much broader. Bartelmez and Dekaban[1] comment on and illustrate a "thin spot" in the roof of the midbrain appearing in stage XIII (4- to 6-mm CR), but they do not discuss its significance. During this or the next stage the sulcus limitans appears and separates the tectum (colliculi) from the tegmentum. Stage XIV (5- to 7-mm CR) is characterized by "rapid growth in the region of the isthmus," and in stage XV (7- to 9-mm CR) the roof thickens and the collicular plate is approximately equal throughout.

During stage XVI (8- to 11-mm CR), both the posterior commissure and the dorsal decussation of the trochlear nerve are found, thus precisely defining the rostral and caudal boundaries of the tectum. In stage XVII (11- to 14-mm CR), the collicular plate increases in thickness, and in stage XVIII (13- to 17-mm CR), the primordia of the superior and inferior colliculi are distinct.

The further differentiation of the colliculi cannot be presented sequentially due to in-

* See Chapter 1 for background information on embryologic development and staging system.

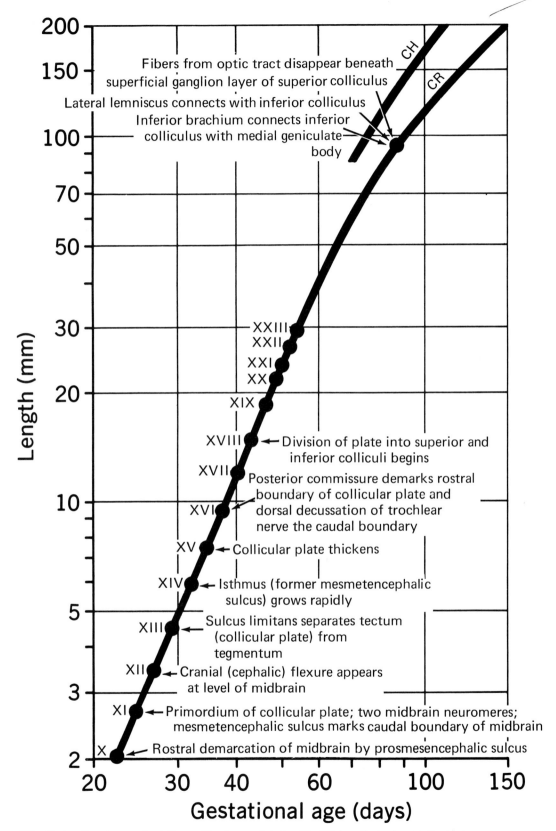

FIG. 11–1. Development of the colliculi correlated with CR length and gestational age.

sufficient information. Streeter,[8] in reference to a 95-mm CR length fetus, states that "the fibers from the optic tract and lateral lemniscus can be plainly traced to the colliculi . . . the optic fibers disappear beneath the superficial ganglion layer of the superior colliculus, while the lateral lemniscus spreads over the surface of the inferior colliculus. About the same time, the inferior brachium connecting the inferior colliculus with the median geniculate body can be recognized." The frequently quoted study of Shaner[7] on the development of nuclei and tracts of the midbrain deals with pigs.

ABNORMAL DEVELOPMENT

Primary malformations of the colliculi are exceedingly unusual in humans, and most reports of their secondary involvement are only briefly mentioned in neuropathologic descriptions. Probably the "beaked tectum" found in 75% of cases of Arnold–Chiari malformation[6] is the most common anomaly. Daniel and Strich[2] compare its appearance

to that of fetuses of 50-mm CR length and believe, as does Peach,[6] that it supports a hypothesis of early development of the Arnold–Chiari malformation. An opposing viewpoint is that the hydrocephalic forebrain has secondarily compressed the collicular plate.

Examples of less-known entities in which the colliculi might be considered anomalous include hereditary anophthalmia, where an autopsy revealed the superior colliculi to be flattened and the inferior colliculi to be "not as large as normal" (Mann,[4] p. 62); cases where pineal "rests" are found in the colliculi;[10] and the Dq– syndrome, where one patient was found to have fusion of the superior colliculi and well-separated inferior colliculi.[5]

Kalter[3] provides examples of tectal malformations in animals, either occurring sporadically or induced by teratogens. These generally accompanied more-severe CNS defects and included hypoplasias, lack of separation of superior and inferior colliculi and complete absence of the colliculi in polydactylous guinea pigs.

REFERENCES

1. Bartelmez GW, Dekaban AS: The early development of the human brain. Contrib Embryol 37:13–32, 1962

2. Daniel PM, Strich SJ: Some observations on the congenital deformity of the central nervous system known as the Arnold–Chiari malformation. J Neuropathol Exp Neurol 17:255–266, 1958

3. Kalter H: Teratology of the Central Nervous System. Chicago, Univ Chicago Press, 1968

4. Mann I: Developmental Abnormalities of the Eye, ed 2. Philadelphia, JB Lippincott, 1957

5. Opitz JM, Slungaard R, Edwards RH, Inhorn SL, Muller J, de Venecia G: Report of a patient with a presumed Dq– syndrome. Birth Defects 5:93–99, 1969

6. Peach B: The Arnold–Chiari malformation. Arch Neurol 12:527–535, 1965

7. Shaner RF: Development of nuclei and tracts of mid-brain. J Comp Neurol 55:493–511, 1932

8. Streeter GL: The development of the nervous system. Manual of Human Embryology, vol. II. Edited by F Keibel and FP Mall. Philadelphia, JB Lippincott, 1912, pp. 1–156

9. Streeter, GL: Developmental Horizons in Human Embryos. Age Groups XI–XXIII. Embryology Reprint, vol II. Washington DC, Carnegie Inst Wash, 1951

10. Wurtman R, Axelrod J, Kelly DE: The Pineal. New York, Academic Press, 1968

Rd. 2/6/88

12

DEEP CEREBRAL NUCLEI

The *deep cerebral nuclei* include all of the structures that develop from the diencephalon and some of the structures from the adjacent telencephalic and mesencephalic regions/ Classic neuroanatomists and others have had difficulty in deciding whether to include the latter with the *basal ganglia* or not, depending on whether they thought that the basal ganglia should be of "motor," "telencephalic" or other function or origin! We shall attempt a more inclusive compromise, based initially on the difficulty inherent in defining any suprasegmental structure as motor or sensory and finally on the difficulty that persists in defining the origin of at least one of the major nuclei/

The developing diencephalon is defined by the relationships of its major subdivisions to certain ventricular sulci, some of which are transient, and to certain fiber laminae, some of which appear different in different planes of sections. These factors have led to a rather complicated and confusing terminology, and the argument whether the globus pallidus is of diencephalic or telencephalic origin only compounds the difficulty. In general, we shall follow the outline of Cooper[12] with specific additions and modifications as noted/

NORMAL DEVELOPMENT*

EPITHALAMUS, DORSAL THALAMUS, VENTRAL THALAMUS AND HYPOTHALAMUS

The major subdivisions of the diencephalon are the epithalamus, dorsal (or main)

* See Chapter 1 for background information on embryologic development and staging system/

thalamus, ventral thalamus and hypothalamus (Figs. 12–1 to 12–5). The epithalamus, ventral thalamus and hypothalamus differentiate first, but after stage XX (22-mm CR) most of the subsequent development of the diencephalon is overshadowed by the growth of the main thalamus. This accounts for much of the shift of the epithalamus caudally and of the ventral thalamus laterally. Major reorientation of the geniculate bodies occurs still later in fetal life.

Although the epithalamus, dorsal thalamus, ventral thalamus and hypothalamus may be identified quite early, by stage XV (8.5-mm CR), it is not until slightly later, in stage XVIII (15- to 16-mm CR), that the major ventricular sulci (dorsalis, medius and hypothalamicus) are present and separate the four nuclear masses (Fig. 12–6). With the growth of the dorsal thalamus and the displacement of the ventral thalamus laterally, the sulcus medius and sulcus hypothalamicus fuse to form the hypothalamic sulcus characteristic of the adult brain/

Certain fiber laminae arising at specific times (Fig. 12–6) further aid in the delineation of the different nuclear groups. The first of these is the ventral medullary lamina (zona limitans intrathalamica) passing laterally from the sulcus hypothalamicus. The lateral (or external) medullary lamina arises next and initially separates the lateral and ventral thalamic nuclei. Later it bounds the ventral thalamic nuclei laterally. The appearance of the medial medullary lamina at 40-mm CR length demarcates the centrum medianum. Ascending somatic afferent fibers form part of the lateral and medial medullary laminae. Much later the incorporation of the developing mammillothalamic tract into

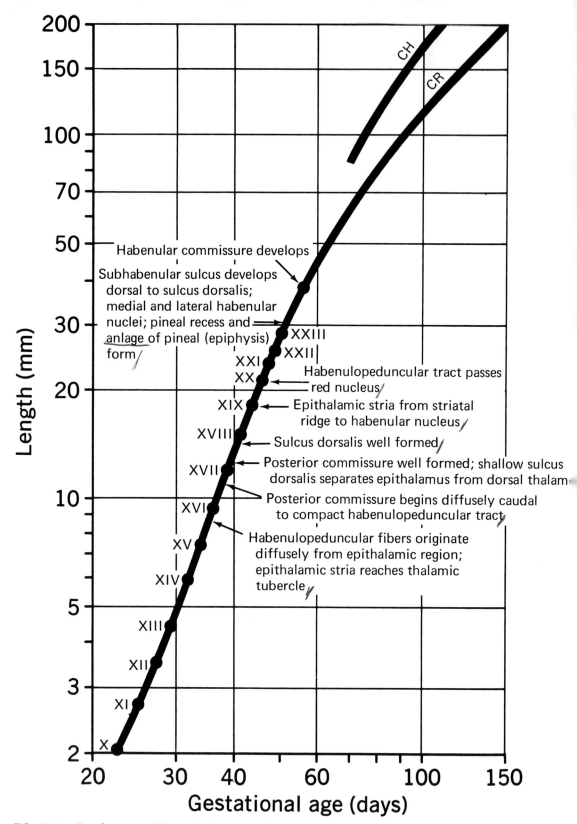

FIG. 12–1. Development of the epithalamus correlated with CR length and gestational age.

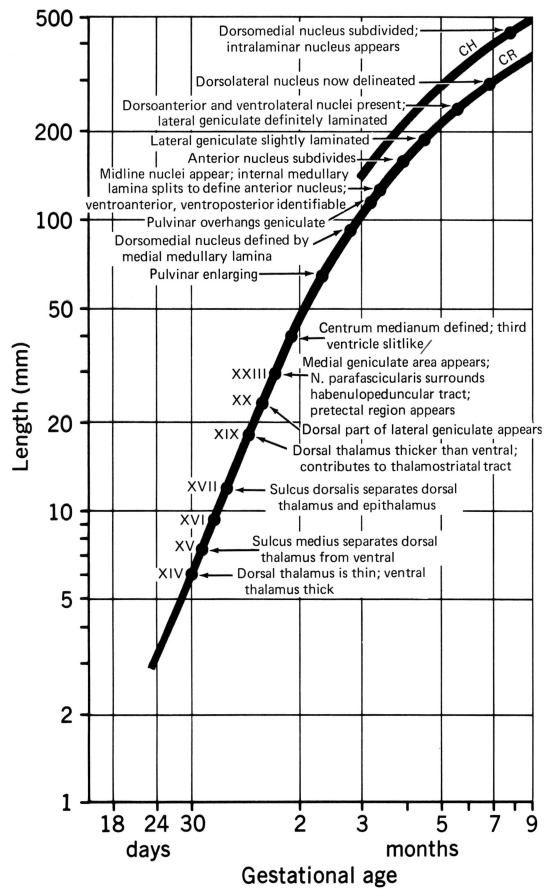

FIG. 12–2. Development of the dorsal (main) thalamus correlated with CR length and gestational age.

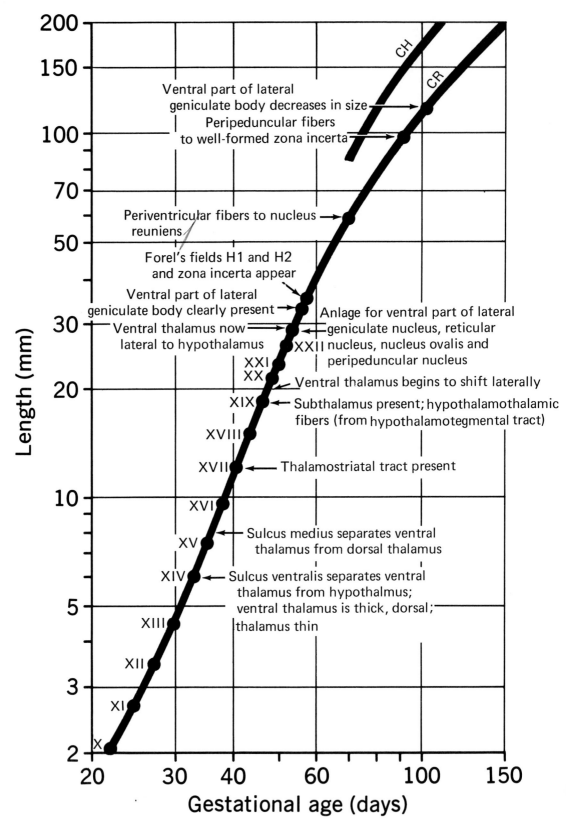

FIG. 12–3. Development of the ventral thalamus correlated with CR length and gestational age.

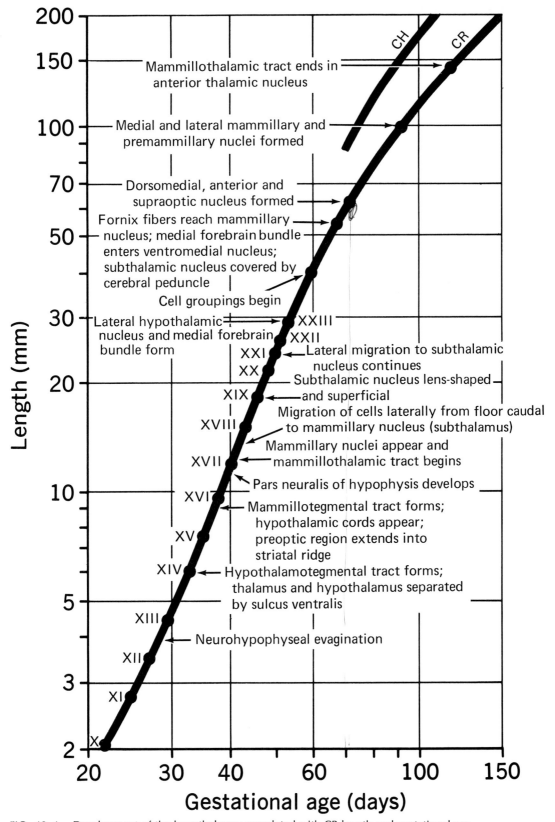

FIG. 12–4. Development of the hypothalamus correlated with CR length and gestational age.

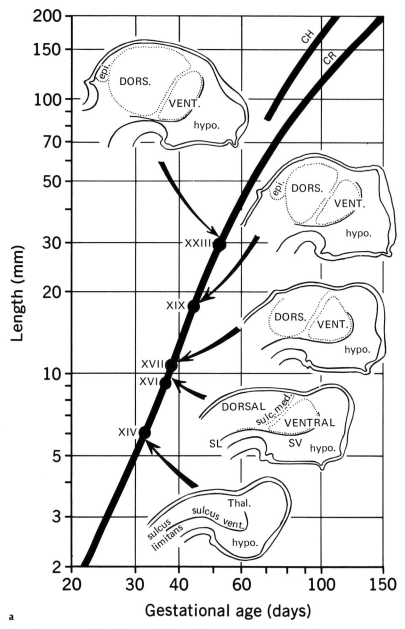

FIG. 12–5. **a.** Development of the diencephalic sulci as seen in midsagittal reconstructions during the embryonic period, correlated with CR length and gestational age. (Adapted from Gilbert, 1935) **b.** Development of the diencephalon during early fetal period correlated with CR length and gestational age. The lower two are midsagittal reconstructions. (Adapted from Gilbert, 1935) The upper three are cross sections. (Adapted from Cooper, 1950) The oldest specimen was sectioned horizontally (in the plane of the optic tract), whereas the two younger specimens were sectioned coronally. The center median (*CM*), medial (*M*), dorsal (*D*), ventral (*V*) and lateral (*L*) thalamic nuclei are separated by the medial (*MML*), ventral (*VML*) and lateral medullary laminae (*LML*); lateral geniculate nucleus (*LG*), medial geniculate nucleus (*MG*), mammillothalamic tract (*MTT*), red nucleus (*RN*), ventral part of lateral geniculate nucleus (*VLG*).

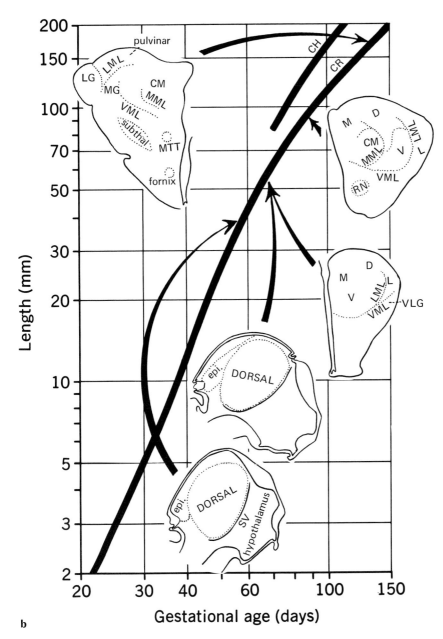

the anterior growth of the medial medullary lamina forms the internal medullary lamina. With the formation of the internal medullary lamina the rostral thalamus is subdivided into its medial and lateral parts with the anterior thalamic nuclei lying in the bifurcation.

Thus, as defined by the various sulci and laminae, the following major derivatives of the four major subdivisions of the diencephalon are noted:[12]

A. Epithalamus
    habenular nucleus
    nucleus parataenialis
B. Dorsal thalamus
    anterior nuclear group (medialis, ventralis, dorsalis)
    intralaminar
    medial and midline nuclei
    dorsomedial thalamic nucleus
    lateral nuclear group (dorsolateral, posterolateral, pulvinar)

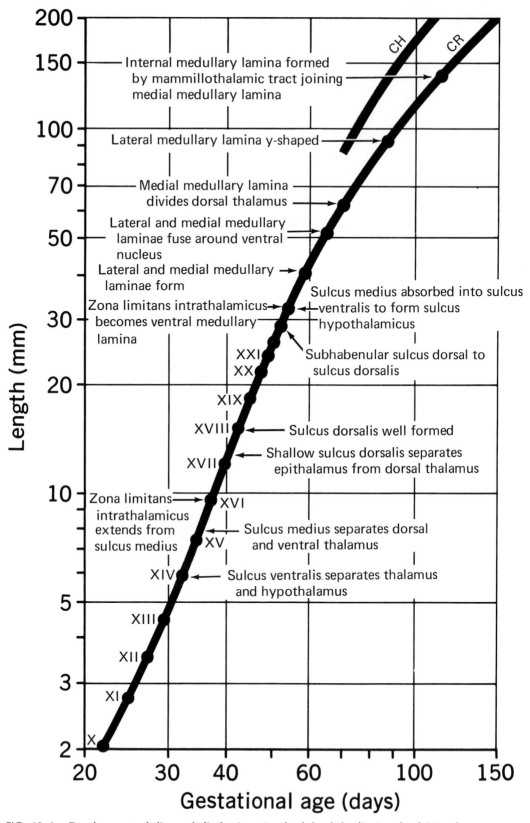

FIG. 12–6. Development of diencephalic laminae (to the left of the line) and sulci (to the right of the line) correlated with CR length and gestational age.

ventral nuclear group (anterior, lateral,
    posterior)
medial geniculate body
lateral geniculate body (pars dorsalis)
C. Ventral thalamus
    lateral geniculate body (pars ventralis)
    reticular nuclei
    zona incerta
    subthalamus (? from dorsal hypothal-
        amus, with globus pallidus)
D. Hypothalamus
    mammillary bodies
    lateral and medial hypothalamic nuclei
    supraoptic nucleus

According to Dekaban[15] few alterations
occur in the diencephalic wall until stage
XXII (25-mm CR). However, according to
both Gilbert[22] and Cooper[12] several significant structures can be detected before that
time. The sulcus ventralis (hypothalamicus)[12] is detected in embryos during stages
XIV and XV (6- to 9.5-mm CR), and the
dorsal thalamus, ventral thalamus and hypothalamus are discernible by stage XV (8.5-
mm CR). The first tract detected in the
diencephalon is the hypothalamotegmental
tract (stage XVI).[22] The mammillary
nuclei appear in the hypothalamus during
stages XVI and XVII (8- to 14-mm CR)
with fibers from that nucleus joining the
hypothalamotegmental tract. The habenular
nuclei, habenulopeduncular tract and posterior commissure develop during the same
period,[12, 22] although Dekaban[15] did not see
the habenular nuclei until stage XXIII
(27- to 31-mm CR).
In stage XVIII (13- to 17-mm CR) all of
the ventricular sulci are present. The fiber
tract (the zona limitans intrathalamicus)
that separates the dorsal and ventral thalamus was identified earlier by Gilbert[22] as
lying subjacent to the sulcus medius. The
sulcus medius leads from the interventricular foramen of Monro to merge with the
posterior part of the sulcus hypothalamicus
at the diencephalomesencephalic junction
(Fig. 12-5). The sulcus hypothalamicus
runs from the optic recess toward the sulcus
limitans, but according to most investigators
there is never a true junction of any of the
diencephalic sulci with the sulcus limitans.
Thus, there is no real basis for agreement
concerning the relationships of the seg-

mental alar (association) and ventral
(motor) plates to the diencephalic zones. In
stage XVII (11-mm CR) embryos, Gilbert[22]
identifies the striotegmental tract running
over the lateral surface of the diencephalon
and the thalamostriatal tract joining the
striatal ridge and ventral thalamus. These
two tracts are considered homologous with
the lateral forebrain bundle of lower vertebrates.
Between stages XX and XXI (18- to 24-
mm CR), the dorsal thalamus begins its
burgeoning growth and causes gradual shifts
of the epithalamus caudally and of the ventral thalamus laterally. The habenular nuclei
are well defined at this time. The subthalamic nucleus (corpus Luysii) appears
first at the surface and then later beneath the
cerebral peduncles. According to Gilbert[22]
and Kuhlenbeck,[36] the subthalamic nucleus
is derived from the hypothalamus, and according to Kuhlenbeck and Haymaker,[37] the
globus pallidus is similarly derived from the
dorsal hypothalamus. By accepting homology, if not actual continuity, between the
sulcus hypothalamicus and the sulcus limitans, one can see the basis for the opinion
that the subthalamic nucleus, globus pallidus and hypothalamus are basal (motor)
plate derivatives, such as one might expect
of a motor extrapyramidal system. On the
other hand, the subthalamus is regarded as a
part of the alar plate by Cooper,[12] who
further regards the globus pallidus as of
telencephalic origin. We see no easy way of
resolving this controversy, except possibly by
accepting all of the forebrain as suprasegmental, arising in the midline as a crescent
about and above the mesencephalic alar
plate, much like the rhombic lips about the
rhombencephalon contribute to the development of the cerebellum (see Chapter 10).
Such a concept would also fit with certain
ideas regarding the maldevelopment, holoprosencephaly (see Chapter 14).
Fibers of the striae medullares (epithalamic striae) reach the habenular nuclei during stage XX (18-mm CR).[22] By stage
XXIII (30-mm CR), most of the fibers of the
thalamostriatal tract arise from the dorsal
thalamus, whereas previously the ventral
thalamus had contributed the greater part.
In the hypothalamus, the lateral hypothalamic nucleus is identified with the first component of the medial forebrain bundle, the

olfactohypothalamic tract, which arises in the olfactory bulb and passes through the striatal ridge and preoptic region. During this same period, from 30- to 37-mm CR length, the anlage of the pineal body is cupping the pineal recess in the dorsal midline, while the habenular complex is splitting into its medial and lateral parts.

With the continued growth of the dorsal thalamus, the third ventricle is reduced to a slitlike cavity, the sulcus medius is compressed toward the sulcus hypothalamicus, and the ventral thalamus is displaced lateral to the hypothalamus and away from the ventricle.

As thalamic fibers run laterally, the zona limitans intrathalamica is reinforced so that a well-defined ventral medullary lamina is formed. Within this zone the fasciculus thalamicus (Forel's field H1) develops. A less conspicuous zone that separates the ventral thalamus from the caudal hypothalamus will become the fasciculus lenticularis (Forel's field H2). Between these two laminae will develop the zona incerta.[36] Caudally the lateral medullary lamina extends from the ventral medullary lamina parallel to the lateral edge of the thalamus and defines a narrow strip of thalamus as the lateral thalamic nucleus (Fig. 12–5).[12] According to Cooper,[12] the lateral thalamus differentiates only into the lateral geniculate body in response to entering optic tract fibers, so that Cooper's lateral thalamus differs from that of other observers.[15, 22] As the dorsal part of the lateral geniculate body is appearing in the lateral thalamus, the ventral part of the lateral geniculate body and portions of the reticular nucleus are appearing in the ventral thalamus. Also appearing in this period, from 30- to 39-mm CR length, is the medial medullary lamina, a cell-free band curving dorsally in a C-shaped manner to demarcate the center median nucleus (Fig. 12–5). Within the ventral, lateral and medial medullary laminae, the ventral thalamic nucleus is in the hind part of the diencephalon. The developing ventral thalamic nucleus gives rise to nuclei ventralis posteromedialis and ventralis posterolateralis.[12] By 34-mm CR length the habenular commissure is present,[22] and a few fornix fibers are detected in the striatal ridge.

Thus, by from 50- to 60-mm CR length, although parts of the major subdivisions (particularly of the dorsal thalamus, ventral subthalamus and hypothalamus) have appeared, the cephalic part of the dorsal thalamus is still not differentiated. By 54-mm CR length fornix fibers reach the mammillary nuclei, the ventromedial hypothalamic nucleus and medial forebrain bundle are well defined, and the subthalamic nucleus is encapsulated by fibers of the cerebral peduncles.[22] The supraoptic nucleus is present by 60-mm CR length, as are the ventromedial, ventrolateral and anterior hypothalamic nuclei.

The dorsal thalamus becomes more prominent with the appearance of the pulvinar (70- to 90-mm CR length) carrying the geniculate bodies caudally. The medial geniculate body begins to assume its normal orientation medial to the lateral geniculate body. The medial medullary lamina is prolonged dorsally so that the dorsomedial thalamic nucleus begins to separate from the dorsal thalamus. The posteromedial and posterolateral nuclei appear in the ventral thalamic nucleus, and as these alterations are taking place, the mammillothalamic tract reaches the level of the main thalamus. Dekaban[4] notes the appearance of the center median nucleus at 104-mm CR length by a splitting of the internal medullary lamina (identified above by Cooper at from 30- to 39-mm length with the appearance of the medial medullary lamina). Thus, according to Dekaban,[15] the center median nucleus is the first of the intralaminar nuclei to appear, and the remainder with the midline nuclei appear at 145-mm CR length. According to Cooper,[12] the internal medullary lamina is formed later (140- to 150-mm CR length) by joining of the mammillothalamic tract with the anteriorly growing medial medullary lamina (originally identified at 30- to 39-mm CR). Thus, according to Cooper,[12] there is no splitting of the internal medullary lamina around the center median nucleus, but rather an addition of fibers. As the mammillothalamic tract grows more rostrally, the anterior thalamic nuclear group is delineated by this capsule of fibers from the dorsal and ventral thalamic nuclei.

The zona incerta develops from the peripeduncular nucleus between the reticular nucleus and the thalamic peduncle at about 100-mm CR length. The ventral anterior and ventral posterior nuclei may be identified by

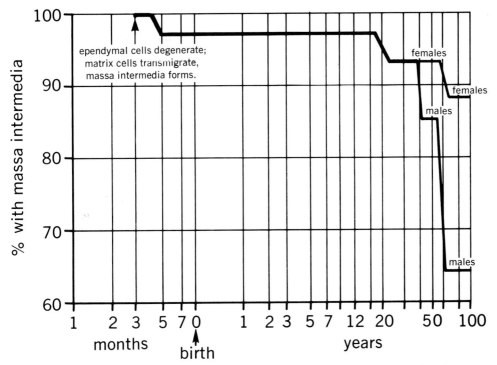

FIG. 12–7. Development and disappearance of the massa intermedia correlated with age. (Adapted from Rosales et al., 1968)

118-mm CR length, and at 145-mm CR length the future intralaminar and midline nuclei appear next to the wall of the third ventricle. The parataenial and paraventricular nuclei appear at about the same time.[15] According to Rosales et al.[56] the massa intermedia is formed after the medial walls of the third ventricle touch (12 weeks gestation), when the cuboidal epithelial cells degenerate and matrix cells transmigrate (13 weeks gestation). By 14–15 weeks gestation the massa intermedia is always present and relatively large, almost filling the third ventricle. As Fig. 12–7 shows, the massa intermedia is present in 97% of brains between 17 weeks gestation and 19 years after birth, but decreases markedly thereafter, especially in men.

Between 110- and 130-mm CR length the pulvinar and ventral thalamic nuclei grow rapidly such that the pulvinar overhangs the geniculate bodies and the original dorsal and lateral thalamic nuclei are shifted backward. By from 160- to 170-mm CR length the internal medullary lamina includes transverse fibers of the thalamocortical radiation, and the subdivisions of the anterior thalamic nuclei are organized.[12] The parafascicular nucleus may be delineated from the center median nucleus at 175-mm CR length. According to Dekaban[15] subdivisions of the anterior nucleus do not appear before 216-mm CR length, 23–24 weeks gestation (Fig. 12–5), when the dorsal anterior and ventral lateral nuclei may be recognized. The dorsolateral nucleus is not clearly delineated until three weeks later.

The first lamination of the lateral geniculate body appears at 185-mm CR length, and definite vertical laminations are seen by 216-mm CR length. As the geniculate bodies are displaced caudally and ventrally, the lateral geniculate bodies rotate such that by 250-mm CR length they are in their final place and position.

Although most of the major nuclear subdivisions are readily discernible by midgestation, even at term it is still impossible to clearly separate the subdivisions of the ventral nuclear group, although subdivisions can be seen in the dorsomedial nucleus and within the intralaminar nuclei.

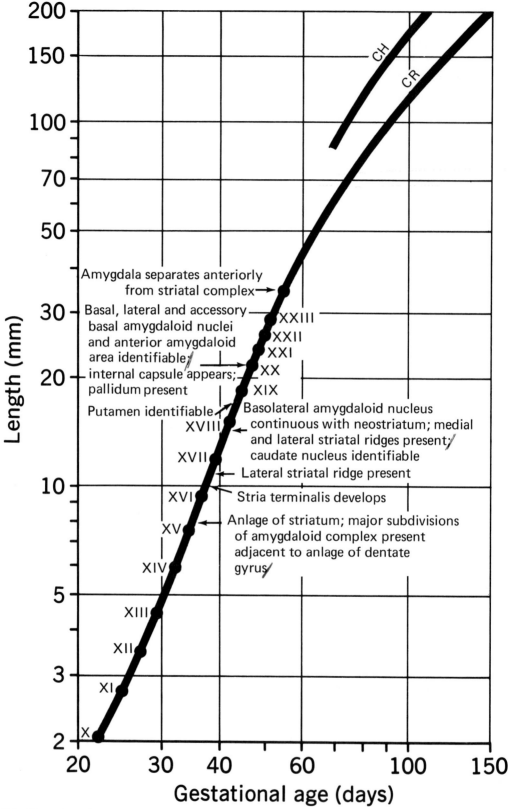

FIG. 12–8. Development of the striatal complex correlated with CR length and gestational age.

STRIATAL COMPLEX

The development of the striatal complex (Fig. 12–8) has been unusually poorly defined. Sharp[60] mentions a primitive corpus striatum in the ventrocaudal wall of the interventricular foramen at stage XV (8-mm CR), but Humphrey[31] identifies this as the primordial amygdala (archistriatum). Hewitt[28, 29] reports the basal ganglia to be represented by a single swelling in the wall of the lateral ventricle at 7.5-mm CR length, but he does not further identify the components. Very soon after the appearance of the primordial amygdala, the primitive neostriatum[31] appears deep to the primitive piriform cortex. Shortly afterwards, at stage XVIII (15-mm CR) at a time when the major subdivisions of the amygdaloid complex are already present, the primitive neostriatum is just becoming well delineated.

Before stage XVII (13-mm CR) only one striatal ridge is present, but soon thereafter two striatal ridges may be identified (at 15-mm,[28, 29] 18-mm[34] and 22-mm CR[31] length). Hewitt[29] identifies the first ridge to appear as the medial striatal ridge, but Humphrey[30, 31] identifies the first to appear as the lateral striatal ridge. The major source of neuroblasts for the amygdala is the lateral striatal ridge, but the medial striatal ridge contributes some neuroblasts until the internal capsule intervenes.[31] Between the two ridges is the striocaudate sulcus,[34] or interstriatal sulcus.[31] Hewitt[30, 31] describes a third striatal ridge as the source of the larger part of the head of the caudate nucleus, but other observers do not comment on its presence.

The striatal ridges represent large collections of germinal cells comprising the subependymal germinal matrix. A common error in several standard embryology texts is the identification of the striatal ridge or germinal matrix as the caudate nucleus, whereas the caudate nucleus is actually a much smaller structure, much deeper beneath the germinal matrix or striatal ridge. It is now generally agreed that during the first half of gestation the germinal matrix gives rise to neuroblasts migrating to various deep cerebral nuclei and to the cerebral cortex, and later in gestation it gives rise to glioblasts migrating especially to the developing cerebral white matter. The precise time at which migration

of the neuroblasts from each striatal ridge ceases is unclear and, except in the case of the amygdala, the destination of the neuroblasts arising in each striatal ridge is also poorly defined.

The appearance of the internal capsule aids in demarcating the subdivisions of the striatal complex. The internal capsule forms by the crossing of fibers between the diencephalon and telencephalon, just lateral to the lamina affixa. Present at stage XX (22-mm CR), it is distinct at stage XXII (27-mm CR) and forms the cerebral peduncle at 37-mm CR length. The caudate nucleus is the earliest identifiable part of the striatal complex, appearing at 15-mm[11] or 18-mm CR lengths.[34] The putamen has been identified at 18-mm CR length[30] and the globus pallidus at 22-mm[30] and 26-mm CR lengths.[34] The rapid growth of the internal capsule between 34- and 42-mm CR length separates the amygdala from the rest of the striatal complex, and it is now clearly possible also to speak of a caudate nucleus and a lentiform nucleus.

The differentiation of the two components of the lentiform nucleus still presents a major problem. Humphrey[31] maintains that the globus pallidus is already detectable with the first appearance of the internal capsule (22-mm CR length), but Cooper,[11] who identifies a lentiform nucleus at 22-mm CR length, does not mention all three major components of the striatal complex before 70-mm CR length. Somewhat similarly, Hewitt[11] finds the globus pallidus still indistinct at 70-mm CR length and not clearly defined until 135-mm CR length. To compound the problem, Kuhlenbeck and Haymaker[37] present the view that the globus pallidus is really a derivative of the hypothalamus, the neuroblasts migrating laterally as the internal capsule forms. An examination of actual sections of early fetuses clearly shows the difficulty in determining the boundaries of this junctional region to be much greater than one would imagine from an examination of adult tissue. In any event, the individual segments of the pallidum appear to develop at a relatively late date; Humphrey[31] notes them to be clearly delineated at 24.5 weeks.

Both Macchi[43] and Johnston[34] comment on the early close relationships of the striatal ridges rostral to the nucleus accumbens septi and of this nucleus to the anterior olfactory nucleus. The nucleus accumbens septi arises at the same time as the bed of the stria terminalis and the striatal complex (28-mm CR length[43]) and is considered a secondary olfactory center[34] (see Chapter 14).

RED NUCLEUS AND SUBSTANTIA NIGRA

According to Cooper,[11] the developments of the somatic efferent column, red nucleus and substantia nigra (Fig. 12–9) coincide with those of three related fiber pathways: 1) the posterior longitudinal bundle, 2) the brachium conjunctivum and 3) the cerebral peduncle, respectively.

During stage XV (7- to 9-mm CR) the basal lamina of the midbrain is larger than the alar lamina. At stage XVI (8- to 11-mm CR) the somatic efferent column is present, and in the midventral region of the basal plate neuroblasts are collecting between the two somatic efferent columns to form the midventral proliferation. Since Cooper[11] identified the pontine and medullary continuation of the midventral proliferation as the origin of the nuclei pontis and inferior olivary nucleus, it will be interesting to see if autoradiographic studies, comparable to those of Ellenberger et al.[19] with reference to the inferior olive, will identify the alar plate as the major source of the earlier cells migrating into the midventral proliferation. Be that as it may, by stage XVIII (11- to 14-mm CR) the midventral proliferation is well formed, and by stage XX (19- mm CR) fibers of the brachium conjunctivum are invading it. At that time some of the lateral cells of the midventral proliferation are displaced laterally to form the red nucleus, which thus arises concurrently with the arrival of the cerebellar fibers and creates, together with the somatic efferent column, the tegmentum of the midbrain. Slightly later, in stages XX–XXI (22- to 24-mm CR), the basal lamina thickens, and the fasciculus retroflexus may be seen passing through the medial part of the red nucleus. By stages XXI–XXII the mammillotegmental tract is present. At stage XXIII (27- to 31-mm CR) the dentate nucleus becomes identifiable, being separate from the neuroblasts that have already contributed to the brachium conjunctivum, and clusters of large cells

(pars magnocellularis) appear in the red nucleus. By 40-mm CR length the capsule of the red nucleus is well defined by the brachium conjunctivum, and by 90-mm CR length both large and small neurons are recognizable in the red nucleus. The brachium conjunctivum is finely myelinated (by light microscopy) by 180-mm CR length and heavily myelinated by the eighth month, but the red nucleus does not reach its full size until the fifth year of life.

The first evidence of the substantia nigra is seen during stages XX and XXI, when cells spread from the ventrolateral angle of the midventral proliferation and form a crescentic mass as the fibers of the descending cerebral peduncle reach the midbrain superficially. Other cells from the midventral proliferation form the nuclei of the basis pontis, their continuity with the nigral cells being established by stage XXIII. Beginning at 60-mm CR length two zones or strata of cells, the corpus and the cauda, can be distinguished in the substantia nigra. First to appear is the corpus, subdivided first into medial and lateral columns of cells and later with intermediate groups of cells appearing. Cooper[11] considers the corpus to be analogous to the pars compacta and to constitute the paleonigrum. The second stratum to appear is the cauda, corresponding to the pars reticulata and lying superficially. With formation of its major components, the substantia nigra becomes pyramidal shaped (90-mm CR length), its apex ventrolateral to the subthalamic nucleus and its base at the pontomesencephalic junction. At 190-mm CR length a third stratum, the caput, is formed; this lies at the junction of the basis pedunculi and tegmentum.

By the eighth fetal month (about 300-mm CR) myelinated fibers extend from the substantia nigra to the subthalamic nucleus and to the contralateral substantia nigra, as well as into the medial lemniscus, descending cerebrospinal fibers and temporopontine pathway.

Minute brown granules appear at the periphery of some nigral neurons at midterm (190-mm CR length) and increase gradually in number, but the pigmentation is not grossly visible until about five years and does not reach its adult characteristic until puberty.

caput

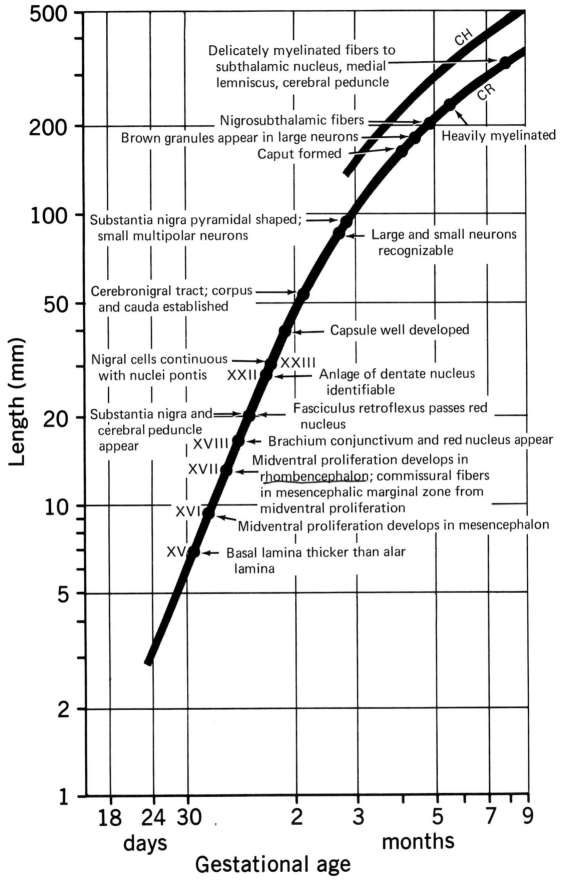

FIG. 12–9. Development of the red nucleus (to the right of the line) and substantia nigra (to the left of the line) correlated with CR length and gestational age.

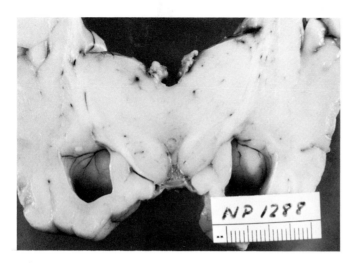
FIG. 12–10

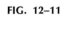

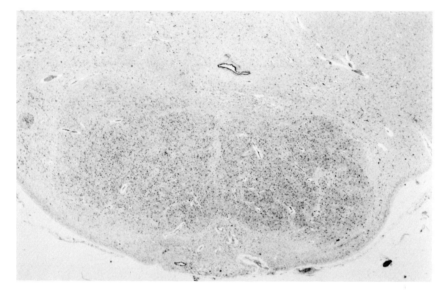
FIG. 12–11

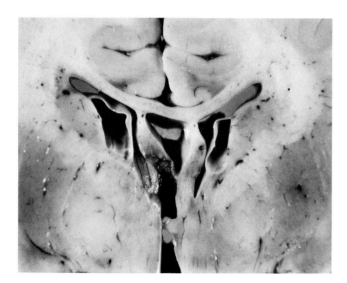
FIG. 12–12

◀ FIG. 12–10. Coronal section of a brain with the Arnold–Chiari malformation showing marked hydrocephalus and fusion of the thalami through a markedly enlarged massa intermedia. (#Np 1288)

◀ FIG. 12–11. Photomicrograph showing fusion of the mammillary bodies from a 16-month-old girl with Hurler syndrome, agenesis of the corpus callosum (see Fig. 16–6) and other malformations. (#Np 813)

◀ FIG. 12–12. Coronal section of the brain from a 5-month-old boy showing bilateral subependymal cysts and an incidental cavum septi pellucidi. Diffuse calcifications in the frontal white matter and retardation in development suggested a viral infection *in utero*. (#Np 1130)

ABNORMAL DEVELOPMENT

Developmental malformations of the deep cerebral nuclei are rare, and most commonly associated with malformations of other areas of the CNS. De Morsier[17] records one case of agenesis of the corpus callosum in which certain diencephalic structures, including the posterior commissure, epiphysis and optic chiasm were absent, and another case in which the floor of the third ventricle, including the mammillary bodies, was absent.

In cases of holoprosencephaly the caudate nucleus and putamen commonly form a single striatal bulge, the caudate nuclei may be fused,[16] the globus pallidus may be hyperplastic,[16] the globus pallidus and thalamus malformed (case 5[67]), the thalami fused[41] and the hypothalamus malformed.[67] The lamination of the lateral geniculate bodies was not apparent in other examples of holoprosencephaly,[47, 68] and both geniculate bodies were absent in another case.[6]

Fusion of the thalami has also been de-

FIG. 12–13. Prevalence of subependymal hemorrhages (±1 S.D. with the number of cases studied at each interval) in 278 premature infants weighing 500–1849 g at birth and dying with idiopathic respiratory distress syndrome, and in 19 stillborn infants of similar weight. (From Leech and Kohnen, 1974)

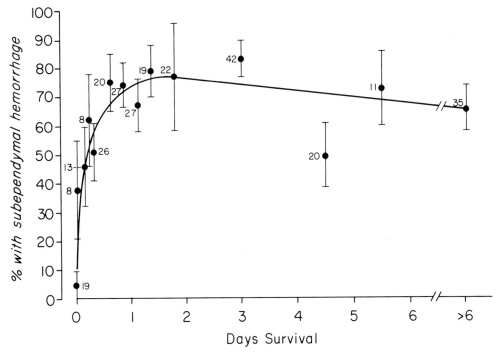

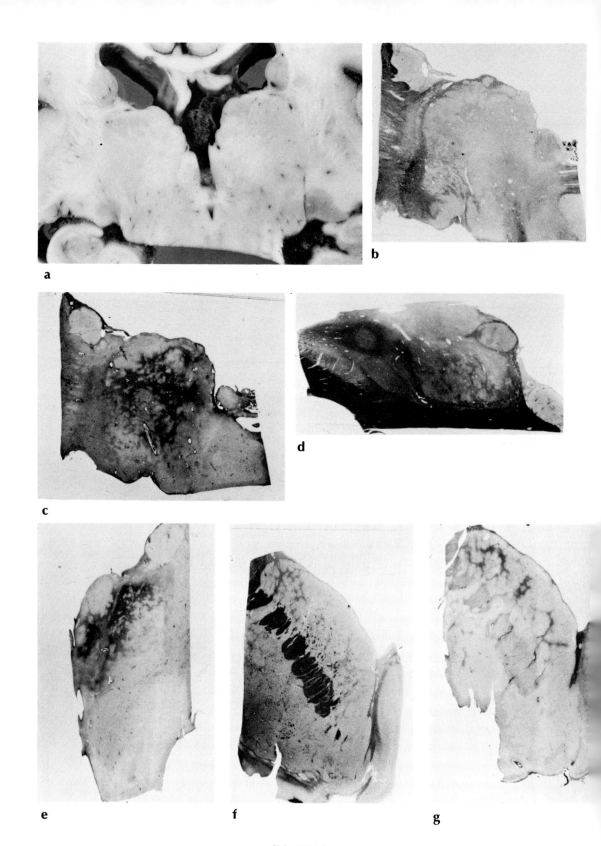

FIG. 12–14

FIG. 12–14. **a.** Status marmoratus involving posterior thalamus bilaterally in a 19-year-old boy with microcephaly (940 g) and sclerotic microgyria. He had started having epileptic seizures on the day of his birth (which had required forceps after a prolonged labor), and these continued throughout his life. He was mentally retarded, spastic and unable to speak. **b** and **c.** Low magnification photomicrographs showing hypomyelination of the gliotic regions shown in **a.** **d** and **e.** Dissociation between degrees of myelination and gliosis in medial and lateral thalamus. **f** and **g.** Congruence of myelination and gliosis in the striatum. (#Np 421)

scribed in agenesis of the corpus callosum[42] and is almost regularly observed in the Arnold–Chiari malformation (Fig. 12–10). The mammillary bodies may also be fused (Fig. 12–11).

OTHER ABNORMALITIES OF THE DEVELOPING DEEP CEREBRAL NUCLEI

Diseases of the deep cerebral nuclei, the basal ganglia and thalamus of classic terminology, are common in adult life, as Wilson originally recognized when he created the concept of diseases of the basal ganglia. They are also common in the immature, especially near the time of birth, when a selective vulnerability is readily evident in many acquired lesions, such as subependymal cysts and hemorrhages, status marmoratus, neonatal anoxic encephalopathy and Kernicterus.

SUBEPENDYMAL CYSTS

Gruenwald[24] described cystic disintegration of the subependymal regions of the corpora striata and thalamus, as well as in the cerebellum, in human embryos of 15-mm CR length and larger. From similar observations in malformed parts of the nervous systems of chick embryos where such disintegration was not expected, he raised, but could not resolve, the question of whether such lesions were related to the genesis of malformations. More recently, Shaw and Alvord[61, 62] have related such subependymal cysts overlying the medioventral aspect of the head of the caudate nucleus (Fig. 12–12) in the human to intrauterine viral infections. Such involvement of the telencephalic germinal matrix often results in imperfect development of the cerebral white matter and is considered the probable cause for the mental retardation which was present in practically all of the patients who survived long enough to be tested clinically.

SUBEPENDYMAL HEMORRHAGES

Remarkably little is known concerning the sequelae of subependymal hemorrhage (SEH), even though this is the most common gross lesion seen in premature infants coming to autopsy. It seems likely, however, that the destruction of the germinal matrix could cause further failure of development of the cerebral white matter specifically and that intraventricular extension of the hemorrhage (as occurs in 80% of the cases of SEH) could cause hydrocephalus by blockage of the aqueduct or in the subarachnoid spaces. Leech and Kohnen[39, 40] have investigated the situations in which these subependymal hemorrhages occur (Table 12–1). They practically do not occur in stillborns of any gestational age or in full term infants, but they are very commonly seen in premature infants (especially those under 1900 g birth weight). Such hemorrhages appear within one hour after birth and reach a peak incidence of about 80% at and after about 10 hours (Fig. 12–13). It is of some considerable importance pathogenetically that practically all the cases of SEH die with clinicopathologic evidences of severe infantile respiratory diseases, suggesting that hypoxia-acidosis may well be involved.

STATUS MARMORATUS

Status marmoratus is characterized by the presence of myelinated fibers in aggregations of a density abnormal for a given site.[50] Typically such aggregations are associated with abnormal collections of glial fibers, such that alternate sections stained for myelin and glia show the same patterns of fibers (Fig. 12–14). Rare examples fail to show gliosis, and occasionally a case with a grossly marbled appearance will not have increased numbers of myelinated fibers, showing only increased density of glial fibers (Fig. 12–14d, e).

Status marmoratus typically involves the

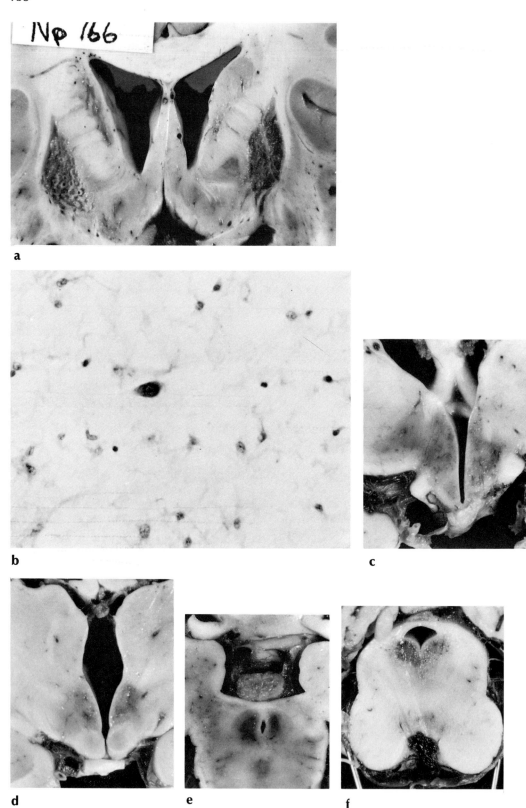

FIG. 12–15

◀ FIG. 12–15. **a.** Marked destruction of the putamen bilaterally due to subacute necrotizing encephalopathy in a 13-year-old boy, who was first noted to have dysarthria, dysphagia, and drooling at age 4½ years. Progressive stepwise deterioration in neurologic functions occurred with mask-like facies, rigidity and athetosis. Two siblings died of the same disease. **b.** High magnification photomicrograph of an isolated neuron persisting in the midst of spongy glial tissue. (#Np 766) **c,d,e** and **f.** Bilateral destruction of the hypothalamus and periaqueductal gray matter, sparing the mammillary bodies, in a 15-year-old girl who was mentally and physically retarded since birth with spastic quadriplegia and ataxia but without worsening of her neurologic status until shortly before death. (#Np 1003)

striatum and thalamus, usually equally in our experience, and occasionally other sites, such as the globus pallidus, red nucleus and cerebral cortex. Neuronal loss in the hippocampus was present in 4 of the 10 cases in our files not associated with other cortical damage, and 3 of these cases also showed diffuse gliosis of the brain stem reticular formation. Ulegyria (see Chapter 15) was associated with status marmoratus in 4 additional cases, and because of the association status marmoratus has also been attributed to hypoxia at birth, especially related to the drainage of the internal cerebral veins or vein of Galen. Indeed, status marmoratus associated with ulegyria has been demonstrated in a perinatally damaged monkey by Myers.[49]

Bignami and Ralston[4] demonstrated myelination of astrocytic processes during the late stages of Wallerian degeneration and suggested that such an occurrence might explain the concurrence of gliosis and hypermyelination in status marmoratus. More recent electron microscopic examination of such areas by Borit and Herndon[5] has confirmed the presence of myelinated fibrillary astrocytic processes. Thus, status marmoratus seems to represent an unusual response of sublethally damaged immature oligodendrocytes that wrap around the available astrocytic fibers at sites where axons have been at least partially destroyed. It seems equally possible that axons are also myelin-

ated, producing a haphazard pattern as would be expected with subsequent proliferation resembling an amputation neuroma, so commonly seen in peripheral nerves traumatized at any age but requiring special circumstances to be seen in the CNS.

Although status marmoratus is usually associated with the althetoid form of cerebral palsy,[44] review of our cases emphasizes that no single typical clinical picture emerges. Profound mental retardation, spasticity and epileptic seizures are common and, occasionally, opisthotonus. The mental retardation is of interest in view of the intact cortex present in many cases and as noted by Norman.[50] Although status marmoratus occurred in 4 of our 7 cases of ulegyria (see Chapter 15), an additional 10 cases did not have associated cortical lesions.

SUBACUTE NECROTIZING ENCEPHALOPATHY

Subacute necrotizing encephalomyelopathy (Leigh syndrome) is characterized by multifocal, bilateral, relatively symmetrical and sharply delineated areas of subtotal necrosis in the brain stem tegmentum, deep cerebral nuclei (especially subthalamus and putamen), cerebellum (especially the dentate nucleus) and even to some extent the spinal cord (Fig. 12–15). Vascular proliferation and spongiform gliosis are striking, especially in view of the preservation of at least some neurons in the center of the lesion. Such lesions may also involve the white matter, especially the posterior columns, corticospinal tracts, optic nerves, superior cerebellar peduncles and others. Histologically the lesions resemble Wernicke's disease due to thiamine deficiency, but the mammillary bodies are typically spared.[38,53,55] The condition commonly presents in infancy with feeding difficulties, psychomotor retardation, ophthalmoplegia, ataxia and weakness. Although originally considered a childhood disease exclusively, cases in juveniles[25,38,53]

TABLE 12–1. PREVALENCE OF CASES WITH SUBEPENDYMAL HEMORRHAGE

Birth Weight (g)	IRDS*	Still-born	Other†	Totals
500–1,899	181/273	1/20	8/28	190/321
1,900–2,499	9/23	1/8	1/8	11/39
2,500–	0/15	0/13	0/29	0/57
TOTALS	190/311	2/41	9/65	201/417

* Idiopathic respiratory distress syndrome.
† Pneumonia, sepsis, meningitis, enterocolitis, congenital heart disease.

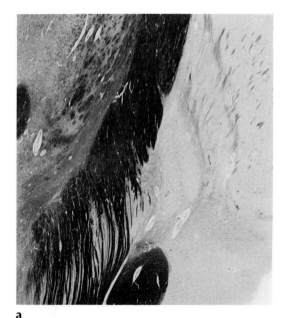

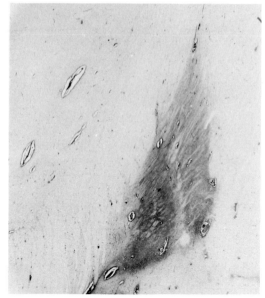

a   b

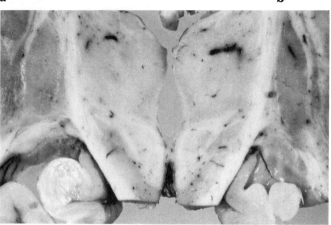

c

FIG. 12–16. **a** and **b.** Low magnification photomicrographs showing demyelination and gliosis of the globus pallidus in an 8-year-old girl who had had neonatal jaundice due to Rh incompatibility which was treated by multiple blood transfusions. She remained bedridden and spastic until her death from aspiration pneumonia. The subthalamic nuclei were similarly atrophic and gliotic. (#Np 183) **c.** Grossly visible atrophy of the globus pallidus of a 14-month-old boy with a similar history due to AB incompatibility: total bilirubin at 5 days of age was 29.6 mg %, which was reduced below 18.4 mg % by exchange transfusions.

and adults[20] are now well documented. Recent studies have shown that patients with Leigh encephalopathy exhibit an inhibition of the cerebral enzyme, adenosine triphosphate-thiamine pyrophosphate phosphotransferase.[13, 48] Thus, rather than representing an example of an enzyme deficiency, Leigh encephalopathy appears to represent an example of a recessively inherited disorder associated with an enzyme inhibitor.

NEUROAXONAL DYSTROPHY AND HALLERVORDEN–SPATZ DISEASE

Infantile neuroaxonal dystrophy (INAD) is a familial and progressive neurologic disease characterized pathologically by the appearance of axonal swellings or spheroids in the CNS.[27, 35] The axonal swellings characteristically appear in the posterior gray horns of the spinal cord, the inferior cerebellar peduncles and tegmentum of the brain stem,[26, 27, 57] but may be present throughout the CNS and even in the myenteric plexus and peripheral nerves.[35] Cerebellar cortical atrophy is present in many cases and viseral lipid storage may also be found. The disease presents commonly in infancy or later childhood with hypotonia, dementia, blindness and sometimes spasticity and ataxia.

Like INAD, Hallervorden-Spatz disease is characterized by the appearance of swollen axons, typically in the pallidum and substantia nigra. These nuclei also show a rusty discoloration which was originally considered to be the hallmark of the disease. The swollen axons may be present throughout the brain. Neuronal loss may be evident in the cerebral and cerebellar cortex, brain stem and spinal cord. Hallervorden–Spatz disease is a progressive degenerative disease which may present in the first decade or as late as the fourth decade with rigidity, intellectual deterioration, choreo-athetoid or dystonic movements, hyperreflexia, spasticity and epilepsy.[33, 57]

The relationship of INAD to Hallervorden–Spatz disease is unresolved, although a number of reported examples of INAD may be cases of so-called nonpigmented Hallervorden–Spatz disease.[32, 33, 65] The exact nature of Hallervorden–Spatz disease is further confused by the reported association with other diseases, including gargoylism and amaurotic idiocy. The question of the specificity of the pallidonigral pigmentation is unresolved.[18, 69]

The cardinal feature of both INAD and Hallervorden–Spatz disease is the axonal swellings. Such alterations in the axons may be seen as the result of toxic nitriles,[57] vitamin E deficiency,[52] autosomal recessive inheritance in the deer mouse[66] and in association with such conditions as mucoviscidosis and biliary atresia.[57] These findings have suggested that the human disease(s) is a hereditary metabolic disorder primarily involving the axon, but the specific defect is unknown.

KERNICTERUS

Kernicterus is an acute toxic bilirubin encephalopathy of the newborn infant resulting in bilirubin staining of certain nuclei of the brain. Characteristic structures involved include the subthalamus, globus pallidus, hypothalamus, hippocampus, flocculus of the cerebellum, and the nuclei about the aqueduct and in the floor of the fourth ventricle.[10, 70, 71] Histologically the involved neurons usually, but not always, show evidence of necrosis.

In patients who survive a long time, the affected nuclei usually show a marked loss of neurons with secondary gliosis, although the inferior olive is an exception. The classic syndrome of status dysmyelinisatus (with demyelination, gliosis and loss of neurons in the globus pallidus and subthalamus especially) is now generally accepted as one of the sequelae of kernicterus (Fig. 12–16).

As indicated by Zuelzer,[70] there may be considerable variability in the extent and intensity of the nuclear jaundice at autopsy. Review of twenty cases occurring during the past 3-1/2 years in this laboratory confirms such a variability. The thalamus was the single most common site of staining and was the only involved structure in one-fourth of the cases; indeed, unilateral staining may reflect the variability of the clinical sequelae, which may include mental retardation, spasticity, athetosis, sensorineural hearing loss, paresis of upward gaze and autonomic dysfunction.[14]

Kernicterus is typically associated with high levels of unconjugated bilirubin characteristic of hemolytic disease of the newborn. The effects of the bilirubin are potentiated by hypoxia, acidosis, prematurity and certain drugs, so that kernicterus may occur in premature infants and critically ill infants at surprisingly low bilirubin levels.[1, 14, 21] Kernicterus, not associated with hemolytic disease of the newborn, may become increasingly significant, for, as Odell et al[51] have emphasized, hyperbilirubinemia may be associated with a continuum of morbidity of which classic neonatal kernicterus is only one end of a spectrum of cerebral damage. Thus, as in so many forms of cerebral damage in the newborn, the severe forms are being readily recognized, but much remains in the elucidation of the milder forms of cerebral disease and their residua.

HAMARTOMA OF THE HYPOTHALAMUS

Hamartomas of the hypothalamus are rare tumors which arise from the tuber cinereum

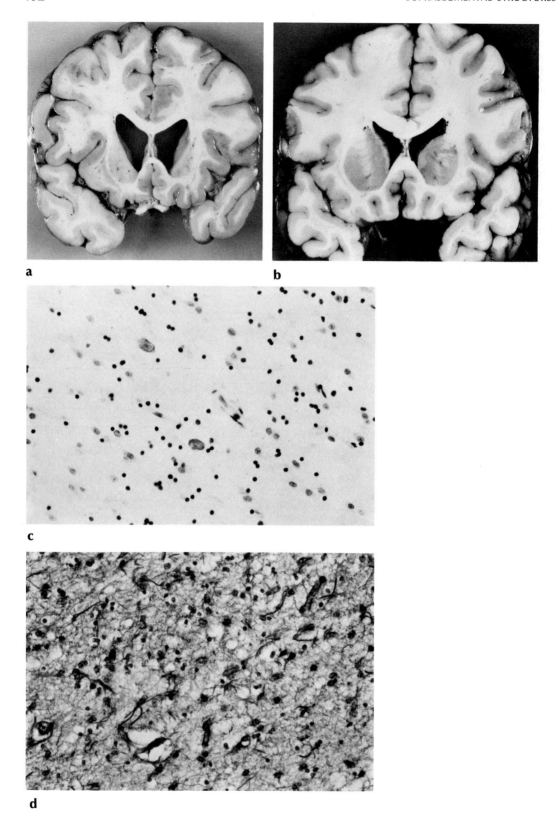

FIG. 12–17

◀ FIG. 12–17. **a.** Atrophy of the striatum due to Huntington's chorea in a 17-year-old boy, whose father, paternal uncle and paternal grandfather had died at relatively young ages of a similar disease with uncontrollable silly behavior, weakness and failing but large firm muscles, rigidity, ataxia and abnormal posturing. (#Np 913). **b.** Similar level of a normal control for comparison with **a. c** and **d.** High magnification photomicrographs showing paucity of neurons and gliosis of striatum illustrated in **a.**

and are frequently associated with precocious puberty. They are thought to represent hyperplastic nodules of displaced hypothalamic cells which occur while the chorda dorsalis and prechordal plate are withdrawing from the neural tube.[59] Histologically they consist of small and/or large nerve cells similar to those found in the tuber cinereum and adjacent hypothalamic structures.[3, 54, 59] They typically arise from the mammillary bodies, and only rarely from other regions of the hypothalamus. When the connections with the hypothalamus are lost,[3] precocious puberty does not develop, supposedly because of loss of the fiber connections with the tuberal nuclei.

In contrast to the hamartomas which usually present in the basal cisterns, intrinsic tumors of the third ventricle are usually gliomas[64] and, when they involve the anterior third ventricle, give rise to an entirely different clinical picture, Russell's diencephalic syndrome of early childhood.[58] Such infants typically present with subcutaneous wasting, euphoria and hyperactivity.[8, 9, 58] However, not all third ventricle tumors give rise to such a syndrome.

HUNTINGTON'S CHOREA

Huntington's chorea is a familial, inexorably progressive disorder characterized clinically by an abnormal movement disorder and mental deterioration. It is transmitted as an autosomal dominant with an incidence of about 5/100,000 population. It typically appears between the ages of 30–50 years, but about 10% of the cases may begin under the

age of 20 years, and 1–6% below 10 years of age and even before the age of 5 years.[7, 23, 45] Juvenile cases with Huntington's chorea differ in several respects from adults, especially with rigidity and akinesis rather than with the expected choreiform movements. Approximately one-third to one-half of the juvenile cases appear initially as this rigid-akinetic form with slow voluntary movements and loss of facial expression and associated movements.[6] There is a greater frequency of seizures, found in up to 50% of childhood cases,[45] as compared to the frequency of 2 to 7% in adult cases.[6] Cerebellar signs (incoordination, ataxia and intention tremor) and dementia are even more marked than in the adult.

Pathologically, Huntington's chorea is characterized by striking atrophy and gliosis of the striatum and less striking atrophy of the cerebral cortex (Fig. 12–17). There may be more widespread involvement of the CNS.[46] In children, severe alterations in the cerebellum correlate well with the clinical signs.[7, 45]

HYPOPIGMENTATION OF THE SUBSTANTIA NIGRA AND LOCUS CAERULEUS

The accumulation of melanin pigment in the cells of the brain stem, especially in the substantia nigra and locus caeruleus, appears to be delayed by many chronic diseases in children.[63] Once these cells become pigmented, about the time of puberty, they seem to be quite stable, since they disintegrate very slightly with normal aging, but quite extensively in Parkinsonism.[2]

REFERENCES

1. Ackerman BD, Dyer GY, Leydorf MM: Hyperbilirubinemia and kernicterus in small premature infants. Pediatrics 45:918–925, 1970

2. Alvord EC Jr, Forno LS, Kusske JA, Kauffman RJ, Rhodes JS, Goetowski CR: The pathology of Parkinsonism: A comparison of degenerations in cerebral cortex and brain stem. Adv Neurol 5:175–193, 1974

3. Bedwell SF, Lindenberg R: A hypothalamic hamartoma with dendritic proliferation and other neuronal changes associated with "blastomatoid" reaction of astrocytes. J Neuropathol Exp Neurol 20:219–236, 1961

4. Bignami A, Ralston HJ III: Myelination of fibrillary astroglial processes in long term Wallerian degeneration. The possible relationship to

status "marmoratus." Brain Res 11:710–713, 1968

5. Borit A, Herndon RM: The fine structure of plaques fibromyéliniques in ulegyria and in status marmoratus. Acta Neuropathol (Berl) 14:304–311, 1970

6. Bruyn GW: Huntington's chorea. Historical, clinical and laboratory synopsis. Handbook of Clinical Neurology, vol. 6. Diseases of the Basal Ganglia. Edited by PJ Vinken and GW Bruyn. North Holland Publishing Co., Amsterdam, 1968

7. Byers RK, Dodge JA: Huntington's chorea in children. Neurology (Minneap) 17:587–596, 1967

8. Carlson C, Kaplan S, Conte F, Lavetter A: Metabolic abnormalities in the diencephalic syndrome of infancy. Trans Am Neurol Assoc 91: 112–115, 1966

9. Chynn K, Sharkey R: Diencephalic syndrome of emaciation. Am J Roentgenol Radium Ther Nucl Med 95:917–920, 1965

10. Claireaux A: Haemolytic disease of the newborn. Part I. A clinical-pathological study of 157 cases. Arch Dis Child 25:61–80, 1950

11. Cooper ERA: The development of the human red nucleus and corpus striatum. Brain 69:34–44, 1946

12. Cooper ERA: The development of the thalamus. Acta Anat 9:201–226, 1950

13. Cooper JR, Pincus JH, Itokawa Y, Piros K: Experience with phosphoryl transferase inhibition in subacute necrotizing encephalomyelopathy. N Engl J Med 283:793–795, 1970

14. Crichton JV, Dunn HG, McBurney AK, Robertson A, Tredger E: Long-term effects of neonatal jaundice on brain function in children of low birth weight. Pediatrics 49:656–670, 1972

15. Dekaban A: Human thalamus: An anatomical, developmental, and pathological study. II. Development of the human thalamic nuclei. J Comp Neurol 100:63–97, 1954

16. De Lange C: Two cases of congenital anomalies of the brain. Am J Dis Child 53:429–444, 1937

17. De Morsier G: Median cranioencephalic dysraphia and olfactogenital dysplasia. World Neurol 3:485–504, 1962

18. DeMyer W, Harter DH, Zeman W: Familial spasticity, hyperkinesia and dementia. Acta Neuropathol 4:28–45, 1964

19. Ellenberger C Jr, Hanaway J, Netsky MG: Embryogenesis of the inferior olivary nucleus in the rat: A radioautographic study and a re-evaluation of the rhombic lip. J Comp Neurol 137: 71–88, 1969

20. Feigin I, Goebel H-H: "Infantile" subacute necrotizing encephalopathy in the adult. Neurology (Minneap) 19:749–759, 1969

21. Gartner LM, Snyder RN, Chabon RS, Berstein J: Kernicterus: high incidence in premature infants with low serum bilirubin concentrations. Pediatrics 45:906–917, 1970

22. Gilbert MS: The early development of the human diencephalon. J Comp Neurol 62:81–116, 1935

23. Goodman RM, Hall CL, Terango L, Perrine GA, Roberts PL: Huntington's chorea. Arch Neurol 15:345–355, 1966

24. Gruenwald P: Studies on developmental pathology. III. Disintegration in the nervous system of normal and maldeveloped embryos. J Neuropathol Exp Neurol 4:178–188, 1945

25. Hardman JM, Allen LW, Baughman FA Jr, Waterman DF: Subacute necrotizing encephalopathy in late adolescence. Arch Neurol 18: 478–486, 1968

26. Hedley-Whyte ET, Gilles FH, Uzman BG: Infantile neuroaxonal dystrophy. Neurology (Minneap) 18:891–906, 1968

27. Herman MM, Huttenlocher PR, Bensch KG: Electron microscopic observations in infantile neuroaxonal dystrophy. Arch Neurol 20:19–34, 1969

28. Hewitt W: The development of the human caudate and amygdaloid nucleus. J Anat 92:377–382, 1958

29. Hewitt W: The development of the human internal capsule and lentiform nucleus. J Anat 95:191–199, 1961

30. Humphrey T: The development of the human amygdala during early embryonic life. J Comp Neurol 132:135–166, 1968

31. Humphrey T: The development of the human amygdaloid complex. The Neurobiology of the Amygdala. Edited by BE Eleftheriou. New York–London, Plenum Press, 1972, pp. 21–77

32. Huttenlocher PR, Gilles FH: Infantile dystrophy. Neurology (Minneap) 17:1174–1184, 1967

33. Indravasu S, Dexter RA: Infantile neuroaxonal dystrophy and its relationship to Hallervorden–Spatz disease. Neurol 18:693–698, 1968

34. Johnston JB: Further contributions to the study of the evolution of the forebrain. J Comp Neurol 35:337–481, 1923

35. Kamoshita S, Neustein HB, Landing BH: Infantile neuroaxonal dystrophy with neonatal onset. J Neuropathol Exp Neurol 27:300–323, 1968

36. Kuhlenbeck H: The derivatives of the thalamus ventralis in the human brain and their relation to the so-called subthalamus. Milit Surg 102: 433–447, 1948

37. Kuhlenbeck H, Haymaker W: The derivatives of the hypothalamus in the human brain; their relation to the extrapyramidal and autonomic systems. Milit Surg 105:26–52, 1949

38. Lakke JPWF, Ebels EJ, Tenthye OJ: Infantile necrotizing encephalomyelopathy (Leigh). Arch Neurol 16:227–231, 1967

39. Leech RW, Kohnen P: Subependymal hemorrhages in the newborn infant (abstracted). J Neuropathol Exp Neurol 33:195, 1974

40. Leech RW, Kohnen P: Subependymal and in-

traventricular hemorrhages in the newborn. Am J Pathol 77:465–476, 1975

41. Lichtenstein BW, Maloney JE: Malformations of the forebrain. J Neuropathol Exp Neurol 13: 117–128, 1954

42. Loeser JD, Alvord EC Jr: Clinicopathological correlations in agenesis of the corpus callosum. Neurology (Minneap) 18:745–756, 1968

43. Macchi G: The ontogenetic development of the olfactory telencephalon in man. J Comp Neurol 95:245–305, 1951

44. Malamud N: Status marmoratus: A form of cerebral palsy following either birth injury or inflammation of the central nervous system. J Pediatr 37:610–619, 1950

45. Markham CH, Knox JW: Observations on Huntington's chorea in children. J Pediatr 67:46–57, 1965

46. McCaughey WTE: The pathologic spectrum of Huntington's chorea. J Nerv Ment Dis 133:91–103, 1961

47. Mettler FA, Marburg O: The diencephalon and telencephalon in a human case of cyclopia and arhinia. J Neuropathol Exp Neurol 2:111–131, 1943

48. Murphey JV, Craig LJ, Glen RH: Leigh disease. Biochemical characteristics of the inhibitor. Arch Neurol 31:220–227, 1974

49. Myers RE: Atrophic cortical sclerosis associated with status marmoratus in a perinatally damaged monkey. Neurology (Minneap) 19:1177–1188, 1969

50. Norman RM: État marbré of the corpus striatum following birth injury. J Neurol Psychiatr 10: 12–25, 1947

51. Odell GB, Storey GN, Rosenburg LA: Studies in kernicterus. III. The saturation of serum proteins with bilirubin during neonatal life and its relationship to brain damage at five years. J Pediatr 76:12–21, 1970

52. Pentschew A, Schwarz K: Systemic axonal dystrophy in vitamin E deficient adult rats. Acta Neuropathol (Berl) 1:313–334, 1962

53. Peterson H DeC, Alvord EC Jr: Necrotizing encephalopathy with predilection for the brain stem. Trans Am Neurol Assoc 89:104–107, 1964

54. Richter RB: True hamartoma of the hypothalamus associated with pubertas praecox. J Neuropathol Exp Neurol 10:368–383, 1951

55. Robinson F, Solitaire GB, Lamarche JB, Levy LL: Necrotizing encephalomyelopathy of childhood. Neurology (Minneap) 17:472–484, 1967

56. Rosales RK, Lemay MJ, Yakovlev PI: The development and involution of massa intermedia with regard to age and sex. J Neuropathol Exp Neurol 27:166, 1968

57. Sacks OW, Brown WJ: The axonal dystrophies. Bull Los Angeles Neurol Soc 31:35–41, 1966

58. Salmon MA: Russell's diencephalic syndrome of early childhood. J Neurol Neurosurg Psychiatry 35:196–201, 1972

59. Schmidt E, Hallervorden J, Spatz H: Die Entstehung der Hamartome am Hypothalamus mit und ohne Pubertas praecox. Deutsche Zeitschrift für Nervenheilkunde 177:235–262, 1958

60. Sharp JA: The junctional region of cerebral hemispheres and third ventricle in mammalian embryos. J Anat 93:159–168, 1959

61. Shaw CM: Subependymal germinolysis. J Neuropathol Exp Neurol 32:153, 1973

62. Shaw CM, Alvord EC Jr: Subependymal germinolysis. Arch Neurol, 31:374–381, 1974

63. Spence AM, Gilles FH: Underpigmentation of the substantia nigra in chronic disease in children. Neurology (Minneap) 21:386–390, 1971

64. Stein BM, Fraser RAR, Tenner MS: Tumours of the third ventricle in children. J Neurol Neurosurg Psychiatry 35:776–788, 1972

65. Thibault J: Neuroaxonal dystrophy. A case of non-pigmented type and protracted course. Acta Neuropathol (Berl) 21:232–238, 1972

66. Vandermeer J, Barto E: Axonal dystrophy in a deer mouse (Peromysius Maniculatus) with an inherited ataxia and tremor. J Neuropathol Exp Neurol 28:257–266, 1969

67. Yakovlev PI: Pathoarchitectonic studies of cerebral malformations: III. Arhinencephalies (holotelencephalies). J Neuropathol Exp Neurol 18:22–55, 1959

68. Yakovlev PI, Wadsworth RC: Schizencephalies. A study of the congenital clefts in the cerebral mantle. II. Clefts with hydrocephalus and lips separated. J Neuropathol Exp Neurol 5:169–206, 1946

69. Zeman W, Scarpelli DG: The non-specific lesions of Hallervorden–Spatz disease. A histochemical study. J Neuropathol Exp Neurol 17: 622–630, 1958

70. Zuelzer WW: Bilirubin and mental retardation. Res Publ Assoc Res Nerv Ment Dis 34:183–195, 1962

71. Zuelzer WW, Mudgett RT: Kernicterus. Etiologic study based on analysis of 55 cases. Pediatrics 6:452–474, 1950

chapter 13

OPTIC SYSTEM

A protrusion of the diencephalon leads to the formation of the visual apparatus. The development of the visual system has been discussed by Cooper,[4] Barber,[2] Duke-Elder and Cook,[6] Mann[15] and most comprehensively by O'Rahilly.[17] The histology of the developing retina has been studied by Hollenberg and Spira.[10]

NORMAL DEVELOPMENT*

GENERAL DEVELOPMENT (FIGS. 13–1 AND 13–2)

During stage X (at 7–8 somites) a thickening and a shallow groove on the cephalic neural folds are the first indication of the developing eye. During stage XI (2.5- to 4.5-mm CR) this optic primordium progresses to become an optic evagination with a cavity called the optic ventricle. This evagination, the optic vesicle, during stage XII (3- to 5-mm CR) is surrounded by a sheath of mesenchyme. In stage XIII (4- to 6-mm CR) the optic vesicle establishes contact with the surface ectoderm, which then thickens to several cell layers at the site of contact. Late in stage XIII and early in stage XIV (5- to 7-mm CR), the retinal portion becomes morphologically distinguishable from the optic stalk, and invagination of the retinal disc forms a hollow optic cup containing an intraretinal space. The ventral portion of the optic cup is incomplete, the open space being known as the choroid or retinal fissure. The thickened surface ectoderm

* See Chapter 1 for background information on embryologic development and staging system.

(lens disc) also indents and closes completely to form the lens vesicle which marks the onset of stage XV (7- to 9-mm CR) together with the appearance of pigment in the external layer of the retina. The inner layer of the retina, still separated by the intraretinal space, soon begins to differentiate into sensory neural elements. The lens vesicle, no longer in contact with the surface ectoderm, shows some early differentiation of lens fibers but still contains a moderately large cavity. This cavity later reduces in size; it becomes slitlike in stage XVIII (13- to 17-mm CR) and closes in stage XX (18- to 22-mm CR). The choroid (retinal) fissure begins to close during stage XVI (8- to 11-mm CR), and, except for a small opening that persists as the hyaloid canal and permits blood vessels to enter the eye, it is completely closed in stage XVIII (13- to 17-mm CR).

During stage XVII (11- to 14-mm CR), a migration and alignment of cells in the inner layer of the retina defines its inner nuclear layer. This process starts in the area of the future macula lutea. The inner nuclear layer becomes more distinct during stage XVIII (13- to 17-mm CR) as the cellular migration is more widespread. Streeter[21] likens this migration to the early establishment of the mantle zone in the spinal cord.

Optic nerve fibers, arising from ganglion cells, form a network on the surface of the retina in stage XIX (16- to 18-mm CR). Some of these fibers go into the optic stalk but do not reach the brain until stage XX.[4] The cavity of the stalk itself is nearly closed in stage XIX and is completely closed in stage XX. The initial steps in the formation

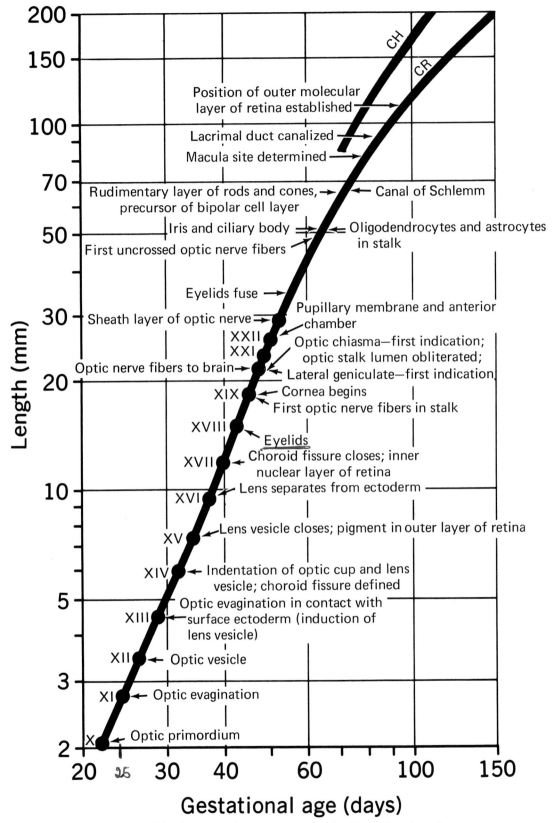

FIG. 13–1. Development of the human optic system correlated with CR length and gestational age.

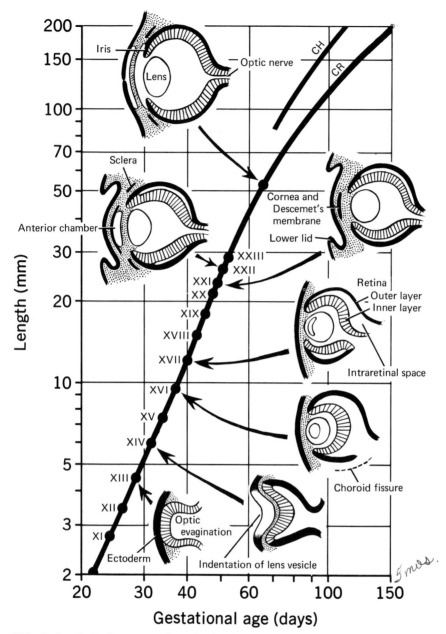

FIG. 13–2. Sagittal sections through the human eye during embryonic and early fetal periods.

of the future cornea take place in stage XIX as two layers of mesodermal cells are found between the surface ectoderm and the lens. In stage XX (18- to 22-mm CR) the retro-lental blood vessels are present, the optic disc is defined, the optic chiasm is formed and the first indication of the dorsal nucleus of the lateral geniculate body is found.[4] A

definitive cornea is present in stage XXI (22- to 24-mm CR), and Descemet's membrane is beginning to form in some embryos. Further mesodermal cells migrate over the surface of the lens as the pupillary membrane. The region between Descemet's membrane and the pupillary membrane develops into the anterior chamber. Around the remaining portion of the outer layer of the retina, mesoderm condenses to form the choroid (continuous with the pia mater) and sclera (continuous with the dura mater). In stage XXII (23- to 28-mm CR) an aggregation of nerve cells found at the entrance of the hyaloid artery into the vitreous cavity marks the site of Bergmeister's papilla. The previously mentioned hyaloid canal (the bulbar remnant of the choroid fissure), containing hyaloid vessels, is located in its final position in stage XXIII (27- to 31-mm CR). During this same period, a mesodermal sheath forms around the optic nerve.

By the end of the embryonic period, the eye has differentiated to a point where most of its features are identifiable. Like most other structures in the CNS, the eye still undergoes many important changes during fetal life. Sometime between 30- and 35-mm CR length the ventral nucleus of the lateral geniculate body appears.[4] It is not until from 40- to 50-mm CR length that uncrossed nerve fibers are found in the optic chiasm, glial differentiation occurs in the optic stalk, and the dorsal nucleus of the lateral geniculate body is continuous with the pulvinar of the thalamus. At 65-mm CR length the canal of Schlemm, the pupillary border of the iris and the rudimentary ciliary processes are differentiating. Primitive rods and cones are seen in the inner layer of retina, and the precursor layer of bipolar cells appears. The bipolar cells do not become well defined until 170-mm CR length, when lamination of the lateral geniculate body also occurs. The visual pathways are complete at 250-mm CR length, including differentiation of the macula and the retinal layers.

Canalization of the lacrimal duct is found at 90-mm CR length.

MUSCLES FOR EXTRAOCULAR MOVEMENT

Gilbert[8] has extensively studied the development of the muscles that control eye movements. The lateral rectus and superior oblique muscles arise from a mass of mesenchymal cells, termed the *maxillomandibular mesoderm*, which is first seen in stage XI (2.5- to 4.5-mm CR) and lies on the dorsocaudal surface of the optic vesicle in stage XII (3- to 5-mm CR). In stage XIII (4- to 6-mm CR) the primordium of the lateral rectus muscle appears as a condensation within the maxillomandibular mesoderm, and the primordium of the superior oblique muscle appears in stage XIV (5- to 7-mm CR) as a second condensation. The origin and insertion of the lateral rectus are defined by stage XX (18- to 22-mm CR), and a few muscle fibers are found in it at this time. The superior oblique forms a trochlear angle in stage XVII (11- to 14-mm CR), but the actual trochlea is not formed until stage XX.

The remaining muscles controlling extraocular movements are derived from another group of mesodermal cells termed the *premandibular condensation*. In stage XIV (5- to 7-mm CR) the primordium of the superior rectus appears, and in stage XVI (8- to 11-mm CR) the primordia of the medial rectus and the inferior rectus appear. The primordium of the inferior oblique is formed from the distal end of the inferior rectus in stage XVII (11- to 14-mm CR), and these two muscles retain intimate contact until the inferior oblique becomes attached to the eyeball in stage XX (18- to 22-mm CR). During stages XXII and XXIII (23- to 31-mm CR) the levator palpebrae superioris forms from the superior rectus and grows into the eyelid.

OPTIC AXIS

Because of the association of ocular hypo- and hypertelorism with many syndromes involving the CNS, the optic axis or angle is important. When the bilateral optic evaginations first arise in stage XI, this angle is nearly 180°. Throughout the remainder of embryonic and fetal life, this angle progressively decreases; by the time of birth it is nearly the same as that in an adult (70°), although there is some disagreement as to actual figures.[2, 15, 24]

INTEROCULAR DISTANCE

Of more practical use clinically is the determination of interocular distances, especially external measurements, such as the inner (inter-) canthal, interpupillary and outer orbital distances. Such measurements are available for the fetal period[24] and from birth to adulthood.[13] Virtually every aspect of the growth of the eye has been measured and tabulated.[12,18,19] The eye is about 17 mm in diameter at birth and from 23 to 24 mm in the adult.[23]

aphakia

ABNORMAL DEVELOPMENT

While writing his book on teratology, Ballantyne[1] stated that "a book might easily be written instead of part of a chapter, upon the structural anomalies of the eye and its appendages. The multiplicity of its malformations is fully explained by the complexity of the development of the eye." He then by footnote acknowledged such a work by Van Duyse, prepared in the same year, 1905. Two recent works[5,14] published in English on malformations of the eye comprehensively categorize and discuss the subject.

Although there are many malformations of clinical and scientific interest, only a few will be discussed in the present chapter. The following brief classification of eye anomalies is intended only to provide examples of the varieties of malformations that exist. Fortunately, the incidence of most of them individually is very low, but collectively they are encountered frequently enough that most clinicians dealing with children are exposed to malformed eyes several times and should have some understanding of them/

A. Anomalies of Induction and Initial Organogenesis
  1. Anophthalmia
  2. Congenital cystic eye
  3. Microthalmia with cysts
  4. Colobomata
  5. Aplasia of retina
  6. Primary aphakia
  7. Cyclopia
B. Anomalies of Differentiation
  1. Cornea
    a. Absence
    b. Megalo- and microcornea
    c. Shape
    d. Opacities
  2. Iris
    a. Aniridia
    b. Colobomata
    c. Congenital anisocoria
  3. Retina
    a. Outer layer
    b. Inner layer
    c. Cysts

  d. Macular aplasia, hypoplasia, degeneration
  4. Lens
    a. Secondary aphakia and microphakia
    b. Failure of separation
    c. Colobomata
    d. Ectopic
    e. Cataracts
  5. Optic Nerve (and disc)
    a. Aplasia, hypoplasia
    b. Position of disc
    c. Shape of disc
C. Anomalies of Supporting Structures
  1. Vasculature
    a. Persistence of hyaloid artery
    b. Absence of retinal vessels
    c. Aneurysms of retinal vessels
  2. Eyelids
    a. Cryptophthalmus
    b. Inner and epicanthus configuration
    c. Hypotrichosis
  3. Conjunctiva
    a. Absence
  4. Lacrimal Gland
    a. Absence
  5. Muscles
    a. External and internal ophthalmoplegia

ANOPHTHALMIA

Clinically, this diagnosis is applied to any case in which there appears to be complete absence of an eye, but in most cases there are microscopic remnants so that anophthalmia is actually an extreme form of microphthalmia. There are three types of anophthalmia: 1) primary, in which the optic primordium (stage X) fails to either form or evaginate; 2) secondary, which appears as a consequence of a lack of any forebrain differentiation; and 3) tertiary, in which optic evagination begins in stage XI but subsequently undergoes degeneration.[14] Anophthalmia has been produced experimentally in rodents with such teratogens as hypervitaminosis A, ionizing irradiation and triparanol;[11] in addition, anophthalmia may occur spontaneously, sometimes as a genetic mutant.

Bilateral anophthalmia is three times more frequent than unilateral. The bony orbit is small but formed correctly. The lids are also

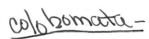

colobomata —

well formed but are sometimes adherent, diminishing the palpebral fissure. There may be abnormalities of the eyelashes in some cases. The lacrimal system, including the duct, is usually intact. Depending on which pathogenetic type is involved, the optic nerves and chiasm may be rudimentary or absent, and the optic foramen may be extremely small, allowing passage only of the ophthalmic artery. Many variations are found centrally, and neural connections to the lateral geniculate or superior colliculus may be either normal or abnormal. Cranial nerves III, IV and VI may also be absent. Encephalocele and the absence of either the corpus callosum or occipital lobes represent other CNS defects that have been associated with anophthalmia.[22]

Most human cases occur sporadically, but pedigrees have been published with several cases in one sibship or family. Both sexes are affected with equal frequency. Some cases have associated malformations of other systems, and anophthalmia can be a feature of such clearly established syndromes as trisomy 13.

MICROPHTHALMIA

Microphthalmia can occur either unilaterally or bilaterally. It affects either sex with equal frequency, occurs sporadically in most cases and can be associated with other CNS anomalies. There is a marked variability in the nature of the lesion, which in its severest form may be erroneously regarded as anophthalmia. It is sometimes found in association with colobomata and cataracts.

Microphthalmia is usually present in trisomy 13 and is frequently seen in children born with the congenital rubella syndrome, cytomegalic inclusion disease and toxoplasmosis, as described in Chapter 23. Microphthalmia has been reported with prenatal irradiation.[22]

MICROPHTHALMIA WITH CYSTS

Microphthalmia with cysts is one of several conditions arising from failure of the choroid (retinal) fissure to undergo correct formation in stage XV or closure in stage XVII (Fig. 13–3). The malformation may be unilateral or bilateral; the infant presents with bulging lower lids. In the usual case, severe microph-

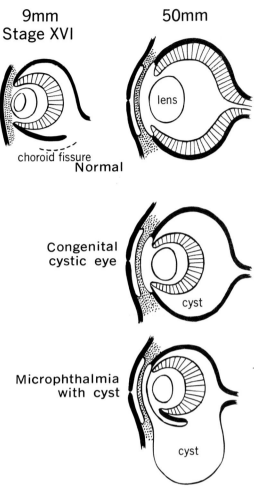

FIG. 13–3. Relationships between normal eyes at different times in development (above) and certain ocular anomalies (congenital cystic eye and microphthalmia with cyst). (Adapted from Mann, 1957)

thalmia accompanies this anomaly, but some infants can be born with normal-sized eyes associated with orbital cysts. There may be associated colobomata of the iris and retina, and occasionally more than one cyst may be present in the same eye. Histologically, the cyst contains anomalous retinal elements, glia and connective tissue.

CONGENITAL CYSTIC EYE

After the optic stalk evaginates from the telencephalon, it may fail to invaginate to form an optic cup. If the optic cup does not form (stage XIV), the prospective layers of the retina (inner and outer) remain separated, and a cystic cavity develops (Fig. 13–3). Depending on the size of the cyst, the newborn infant may have an eye that appears small, normal or large. Histologic examination of the anterior and posterior walls of the cyst reveals various retinal remnants. As with anophthalmia, there are varying degrees of associated abnormalities of the lids, orbit and optic nerve.

COLOBOMATA

The term *coloboma* denotes a hole or fissure in any ocular structure. The typical congenital coloboma arises as a defect in closure of the choroid fissure and, therefore, may involve the iris, choroid, retina and optic nerve (stalk). The sclera is usually thinned but intact. Since the choroid fissure begins to close in stage XVI and completes its closure during stage XVII, these defects must arise before the 44th day of gestation. Colobomata arising from faulty closure of the choroid fissure are located on the inferior-medial aspect of the eye. Those involving the iris appear as a black gap, whereas those involving the retina appear as a white area. If the extent of the retinal defect includes the optic disc, the macula is usually abnormal, and there is a reduction of visual acuity.

Although colobomata may be independent of other anomalies, they are frequently helpful in the clinical diagnosis of certain syndromes:[20] 1) coloboma of iris with anal atresia and small extra chromosome, 2) Goltz, 3) Reiger, 4) trisomy 13 and 5) 4p— syndrome. They are occasionally present in patients with basal cell nevus, Goldenhar, Marfan, Rubenstein–Taybi, Sturge–Weber, penta–X and trisomy 18 syndromes. Experimentally colobomata have been produced in mice with ionizing radiation and have sporadically occurred in association with otocephaly.[11]

CYCLOPIA

Cyclopia, as part of the holoprosencephaly spectrum, is discussed in Chapter 14. The optic nerves may be separate, partially fused, completely united or rudimentary. There may be one or two retinas, lenses or choroids. The medial rectus muscles are absent but the lateral recti present, while the superior and inferior recti are frequently duplicated. Four eyelids are usually present with varying degrees of fusion such that a quadrangular arrangement usually surrounds a single orbit and is usually incapable of closing.

ANOMALIES OF THE CORNEA

Absence of the Cornea

Absence of the cornea refers to the rare condition in which the cornea undergoes early metaplasia because of failure of the lids to form in stage XVIII. There is usually associated microphthalmia, and other anomalies are common.

Corneal Opacities

Corneal opacities are relatively uncommon. Feigin and Caplan[7] list four general categories in which opacities are found: 1) appearing at birth, 2) associated with systemic disease, 3) associated with infections and 4) hereditary corneal dystrophies.

There are few conditions in which there is a primary structural anomaly of the cornea based on faulty differentiation. Duke–Elder[6] and Mann[14] agree that in some cases, termed *congenital leukoma,* the failure of Descemet's membrane (and endothelium) to develop correctly in stage XXI may lead to corneal opacification. Feigin and Caplan[7] note that congenital glaucoma may produce corneal opacity because of increased intraocular pressure, and both conditions may be found in association with aniridia, possibly implicating another developmental anomaly. In addition, normal differentiation may be affected in some cases of congenital rubella, resulting in corneal opacity (*e.g.,* case 13 of Boniuk and Zimmermann[3]). There is inconclusive evidence that failure of the lens vesicle to separate from the surface ectoderm (stage XVI) causes opacification of the cornea.

After the cornea is formed, there are many situations that can lead to various types of opacities: maternal syphilis (acquired by the fetus *in utero*), gonorrhea and inclusion cell blenorrhea (acquired by the baby during delivery). Rupture of Descemet's membrane during a traumatic birth and congenital glaucoma from any cause are associated with opacities. Cloudy cornea is a frequent finding in several of the mucopolysaccharidoses (*e.g.*, Hurler, Morquio, Scheie and Maroteaux–Lamy).

Other corneal malformations, such as abnormal shapes (vertical and horizontal ovals) and size (megalo- and microcornea) are rare. Congenital megalocornea, usually transmitted as a sex-linked recessive, can be associated with discoloration of the lens and can be confused with congenital glaucoma. Unlike the latter, there is no increase in intraocular tension. Congenital microcornea may lead to an erroneous assumption of microphthalmia, but in at least one syndrome (oculodentodigital) it is associated with microphthalmia. In both megalo- and microcornea, appropriate measurements by an ophthalmologist provide correct diagnosis.

ANOMALIES OF THE IRIS

Aniridia

Absence of the iris, *aniridia* (a term applied whenever a major portion is missing), is easily diagnosed in the newborn. It is usually bilateral and frequently not associated with other abnormalities since the iris begins development comparatively late (50-mm CR length). In some cases it is associated with defects of the skeletal system or ears and is transmitted as either an autosomal dominant, or more rarely, as a recessive trait. There is equal incidence in males and females. Other ocular defects (*e.g.*, corneal or lenticular opacities, ectopic lens, cataracts and hypoplasia of the ciliary process) are commonly found. Mental retardation is often present. Probably the most significant association is that of aniridia with the subsequent finding of Wilm tumor, first reported by Miller *et al.*[16] Whereas the incidence of aniridia is 1/50,000 in the general population, it is 1/73 in patients with Wilm tumor, and at least 25 such cases have been reported.[9]

ANOMALIES OF THE RETINA

Aplasia

Aplasia of the retina includes several conditions in which the rods, cones or other neural elements fail to develop (or perhaps secondarily degenerate) in the embryologically inner layer of the retina. However, the retina is present.

Chorioretinitis

As previously mentioned, the optic vesicle is composed of an outer layer, an inner layer and an intraretinal space situated between them. The outer layer becomes the pigment layer and in conjunction with the choroid pigment undergoes degeneration following a variety of infections, some of which may be congenital, including toxoplasmosis, cytomegalovirus, rubella virus and syphilis.

Pigmentation

In albinism, an autosomal recessive condition, there is lack of pigmentation of the retina as well as of other parts of the body. Because of the absence of the enzyme tyrosinase, melanin production cannot occur. In contrast, congenital melanosis of the retina is characterized by hyperplasia of the retinal pigment cells, causing dark areas on ophthalmoscopic examination of the retina. Hyperpigmentation can also be found in the inner layer of the retina, usually as small black dots in one sector. In this situation, the term *congenital pigmentation of the retina* is applied.[14] Retinal hyperpigmentation is found in association with several syndromes, *e.g.*, Cockayne, Chédiak–Higashi, Hurler, Laurence–Moon–Biedl and Werner,[20] and may be of some diagnostic help to the clinician.

Rosettes and Retinal Folds

The inner layer of the optic vesicle may undergo several changes, such as forming rosettes and retinal folds, both considered embryonic proliferative phenomena; usually these changes arise after closure of the choroid fissure in stage XVII. They can, however, also be found in association with colobomata, in which case an earlier onset is suggested.

Primary Congenital Detachment

We are unable to find a study that determines when the intraretinal space is normally obliterated by fusion of the inner and outer retinal layers. In some tissue sections they appear to be approximated by stage XXIII, and in other sections they are still separated at that time. Undoubtedly, fixation artifact makes this difficult to determine. When these retinal layers fail to fuse, primary congenital detachment results. This condition is commonly associated with a microphthalmic eye and may be complete or partial. Secondary detachments can also occur.

Macular Cyst

The macula is the point that eventually has the highest capacity for visual discrimination. Its site, lateral to the optic disc, is determined at about 85-mm CR length, but differentiation continues through several postnatal months. Anomalies of position and size (including aplasia), as well as various degenerations, have been reported. Although any part of the retina may contain a cyst, the macular region is one of the most common sites. The pathogenesis of these cysts is not entirely clear, but they may arise in retinal folds.

ANOMALIES OF THE LENS

Absence of the lens (aphakia) may be *primary* (*e.g.*, Mann,[14] Figs. 226, 227, from a

sectioned 13-mm CR length human embryo, in which the inner and outer retinal layers of a well-formed optic cup were present, but the lens was completely absent). However, aphakia is usually *secondary, i.e.*, the lens forms and subsequently undergoes either rupture of its capsule or degeneration. The pathogenesis of primary aphakia is unknown, but it may be due to either interruption of the initial vascularity or intrauterine infection, and it is usually associated with microphthalmia or colobomata. Microphakia, an abnormally small lens, is rare but has been described in Marfan syndrome.

Colobomata of the lens (see Colobomata) appear as notches in the margin and are usually secondary to anomalies of the suspensory ligament. Irregularities or notches of the border of the lens are also seen in ectopia lentis (dislocation of the lens), which is found in homocystinuria and Marfan syndrome and is therefore a physical finding of some help in differential diagnosis.

Opacity of the lens (*cataract*) can occur either pre- or postnatally. Since the lens never undergoes a phase in which it is not transparent, cataracts cannot be caused from an arrest in development. Smith[20] lists 24 different syndromes in which they occur, perhaps the best known being that of congenital rubella embryopathy (see Chapter 23).

REFERENCES

1. Ballantyne JW: The Embryo, Manual of Antenatal Pathology and Hygiene. Vol. II. New York, William Wood, 1905, pp. 406–420

2. Barber AN: Embryology of the Human Eye. St. Louis, CV Mosby, 1955

3. Boniuk M, Zimmermann LE: Ocular pathology in the rubella syndrome. Arch Ophthalmol 77: 455–473, 1967

4. Cooper ERA: The development of the human lateral geniculate body. Brain 68:222–239, 1945

5. Duke-Elder S: Normal and abnormal development, congenital deformities. System of Ophthalmology, vol III, pt 2. London, Henry Kimpton, 1964

6. Duke-Elder S, Cook C: Normal and abnormal development, embryology. System of Ophthalmology, vol III, pt 1. London, Henry Kimpton, 1964

7. Feigin RD, Caplan DB: Corneal opacities in infancy and childhood. J Pediatr 69:383–392, 1966

8. Gilbert PW: The origin and development of the human extrinsic ocular muscles. Contrib Embryol 36:61–78, 1959

9. Haicken BN, Miller DR: Simultaneous occurrence of congenital aniridia, hamartoma and Wilm's tumor. J Pediatr 78:497–502, 1971

10. Hollenberg MJ, Spira AW: Early development of the human retina. Can J Ophthalmol 7:472–491, 1972

11. Kalter H: Teratology of the Central Nervous System. Chicago, Univ Chicago Press, 1968

12. Keyes JEL: Observations of four thousand optic foramina in human skulls. Arch Ophthalmol 13: 538–568, 1935

13. Laestadius ND, Aase JM, Smith DW: Normal inner canthal and outer orbital dimensions. J Pediatr 74:465–468, 1969

14. Mann, I: Developmental Abnormalities of the Eye, ed 2. Philadelphia, JB Lippincott, 1957

15. Mann I: The Development of the Human Eye, ed 3. New York, Grune & Stratton, 1964

16. Miller RW, Fraumeni JF, Manning MD: Association of Wilm's tumor with aniridia, hemihypertrophy and other congenital malformations. N Engl J Med 270:922–927, 1964

17. O'Rahilly R: The early development of the eye in staged human embryos. Contrib Embryol 38:1–42, 1966

18. Scammon RE, Hesdorffer MB: Growth in mass and volume of the human lens in postnatal life. Arch Ophthalmol 17:104–112, 1937

19. Scammon RE, Wilmer HA: Growth of the components of the human eyeball. II. Comparison of the calculated volumes of the eyes of the newborn and of adults, and their components. Arch Ophthalmol 43:620–637, 1950

20. Smith DW: Recognizable Patterns of Human Malformation. Philadelphia, WB Saunders, 1970

21. Streeter GL: Developmental Horizons in Human Embryos. Embryology reprint, vol II. Washington DC, Carnegie Inst Wash, 1951

22. Warkany J: Congenital Malformations. Chicago, Year Book Med Publ, 1971

23. Wilmer HA, Scammon RE: Growth of the components of the human eyeball. I. Diagrams, calculations, computations and reference tables. Arch Ophthalmol 43:599–619, 1950

24. Zimmermann AA, Armstrong EL, Scammon RE: The change in position of the eyeballs during fetal life. Anat Rec 59:109–134, 1934

Rd. 4/12/88

chapter 14

OLFACTORY AND LIMBIC SYSTEMS

NORMAL DEVELOPMENT*

ANATOMY—DEFINITIONS

The contents of the *rhinencephalon* (the classic term for what should be the anatomic substrate of the olfactory system) have varied over the years as physiologic information has accumulated.[59, 60] At the present time, it would appear that the major components of the classic rhinencephalon should be separated off as the *limbic lobe* since it is not essential for olfactory discrimination. Thus, only a very small part of the CNS—the primary olfactory nerves, olfactory bulbs, olfactory tracts and basal olfactory cortex (including the tuberculum olfactorium, diagonal band of Broca, piriform and prepiriform cortex)—is necessary for olfaction. The amygdala, septal nuclei, hippocampus, fornix, mammillary bodies, anterior thalamus, cingulate gyrus, cingulum, parahippocampus and dentate gyrus comprise the bulk of the limbic system, to which the nervus terminalis and vomeronasal nerves can be included for this discussion. Much more is known about the phylogenetic development of these structures, which form a limbus or belt about the foramen of Monro,[60] than is known about their ontogenetic development in man. Most notable in this area are the studies of Humphrey,[24-32] but even she has covered only the earliest stages.

* See Chapter 1 for background information on embryologic development and staging system.

OLFACTORY NERVE AND BULB, VOMERONASAL NERVE AND NERVUS TERMINALIS (FIG. 14–1)

At the beginning of the fourth week of gestation, the anterior neuropore is still open, and the olfactory areas are not yet differentiated. After completion of the lamina terminalis and closure of the anterior neuropore (stage XI), the olfactory placode appears in stage XIII.[3] The first bipolar cells resembling olfactory nerves appear in the olfactory placode in stage XVI (8- to 11-mm CR)[50] and by 14-mm CR (stage XVIII) the nerve fibers are well defined, passing obliquely upward and forward. They begin to enter the brain shortly thereafter (16-mm CR; stage XVIII), and the olfactory nerve is defined by 17-mm CR (stage XIX).

There is no evidence of an olfactory bulb when the nerve fibers are first attached to the brain, but soon afterwards the olfactory bulb begins as a slight bulge (17-mm CR; stage XIX), and by 22-mm CR (stage XX) it consists of a slight protrusion directed downward and slightly backward. At this time, the primitive anterior olfactory nucleus is present,[28] and the lateral olfactory tract fibers are approaching the prepiriform cortex. By stage XXII (23- to 28-mm CR) all layers of the bulb are represented. The mitral cells are present, and the fila olfactoria appear as the bulb constricts at its base (29-mm CR; stage XXIII). With further evagination of the bulb, the fissura prima of His appears at 32-mm CR length.[34] As the neopallium begins its great growth, the ol-

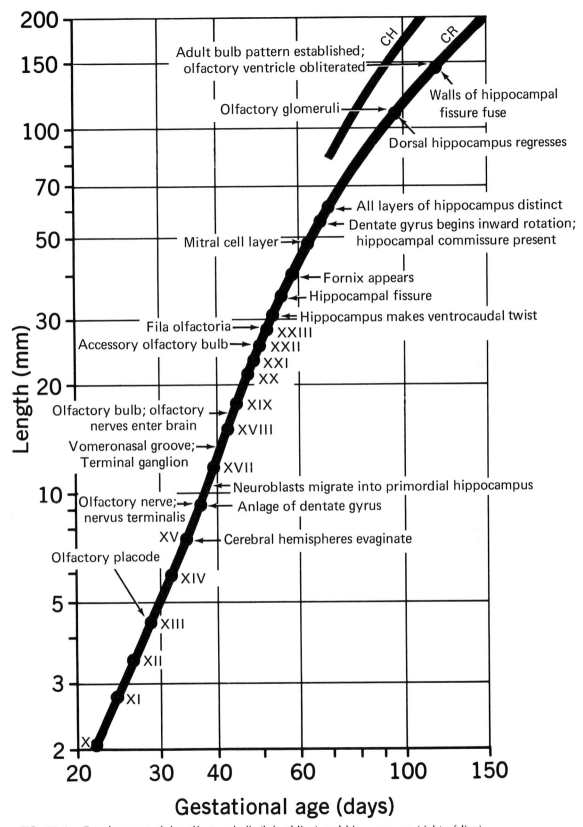

FIG. 14–1. Development of the olfactory bulb (left of line) and hippocampus (right of line) correlated with CR length and gestational age.

factory bulb begins to rotate forward (44-mm CR length). At 49-mm CR length the mitral cells are arranged into sectors as in the adult. The mitral olfactory connections with the entering fila olfactoria are being made by the end of the 3rd month (100-mm CR length). The olfactory glomeruli (representing the synapses of the entering olfactory fila on the mitral cell dendrites) appear at 112-mm CR length, and the adult pattern on the bulb is established by 145-mm CR length. The olfactory ventricle begins to close during the 14th week (115-mm CR length) and is no longer present at 145-mm CR length (the end of the 4th month).

The vomeronasal organ, a pocket lying in the nasal septum and lined by a specialized epithelium, is not found in the adult but can be demonstrated in human embryos. It first appears as a groove in the nasal septum at stage XVIII (13- to 17-mm CR).[24] Nerve fibers from the region of this organ may be traced into the vomeronasal nerve, the nervus terminalis and the nasopalatine branch of the trigeminal nerve. The vomeronasal nerve arises from cells found in the medial border of the olfactory placode and is difficult to separate from elements of the nervus terminalis, which also arises in the same area at about the same time.[49] The fibers of the vomeronasal nerve pass dorsomedially along the developing olfactory bulb to enter a special part, the accessory olfactory formation. At first this formation is distinguishable only on the basis of the entering nerves, but by stage XXII (26-mm CR) sufficient changes have occurred to separate the two bulbs. The accessory olfactory bulb appears as an eminence on the surface of the developing olfactory bulb and moves from a medial (during stage XVIII; 14-mm CR) to a dorsolateral position by 160-mm CR length.[4] The change in position occurs with the anterior rotation of the olfactory bulb. The accessory olfactory bulb begins to regress at 61-mm CR length and is vestigial by the time the olfactory ventricle is obliterated (145-mm CR length). The development of the vomeronasal nerve and accessory olfactory bulb parallels the development and regression of the vomeronasal organ (Jacobson's organ) in the human embryo.

The nervus terminalis is an independent nerve probably subserving both sensory and autonomic functions to the nasal septum. It is characterized by ganglion cells along its course and has been reported in human adults.[8] The anlage of the nerve is present in embryos from stage XVI to stage XVII (9- to 14-mm CR) and develops from cells lying in the medial aspect of the olfactory placode. The nervus terminalis is closely associated with the vomeronasal nerve. In stage XVII (14-mm CR), the cells of the terminal ganglion form irregular masses along the medial side of the olfactory nerve.[49] Initially the ganglion is intimately associated with the olfactory nerve and adjacent forebrain, but by stage XXI (23-mm CR) it is separate, and by 38-mm CR length it is a fairly compact mass. The nervus terminalis maintains its relationship with the olfactory nerve, with fibers coursing over the surface of the olfactory nerve to enter the telenecphalon caudal to the base of the olfactory bulb. In 47-mm CR length embryos, although the olfactory bulb has grown much larger, the nervus terminalis and its ganglion have not increased in size; by 78-mm CR length the nerve forms a single bundle lying on the medial surface of the olfactory bulb. On entering the brain, the fibers end in the septal nuclei, in that part of the olfactory system corresponding to the anterior perforated substance in adults, in the precommissural region and in the anterior portion of the supraoptic nucleus.[42]

HIPPOCAMPAL FORMATION (FIGS. 14–1 AND 14–2)

The cerebral hemispheres begin to evaginate in stage XV, the hippocampal formation (hippocampus and dentate gyrus) being the first cortex to differentiate. During its development, the hippocampal formation undergoes a complex sequence of alterations as it extends in a crescentic fashion beginning from its anterior end at the medial side of the olfactory evagination, proceeding back to the posterior end of the cerebral hemisphere before the temporal lobe forms, and continuing anteroventrally to the temporal tip. During this sequence one part of the hippocampal formation regresses as another appears. Humphrey[28] notes that differentiation in the dentate gyrus generally follows developmental changes in the olfactory bulbs, whereas the differentiation of the hippo-

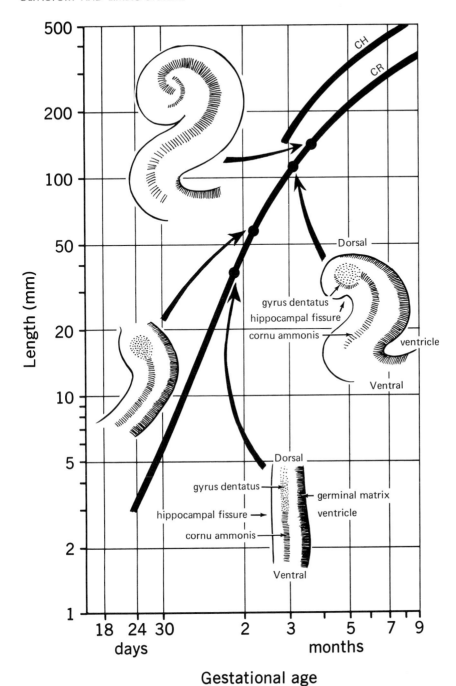

FIG. 14–2. Stages of development of the hippocampus and hippocampal fissure correlated with CR length and gestational age.

campus (cornu ammonis) generally precedes the development of the olfactory bulbs.

The first appearance of the hippocampal formation is in the dorsomedial wall of the cerebral hemisphere adjacent to the lamina terminalis at stage XVI (9-mm CR). The primordium of the dentate gyrus appears as a cell-free marginal zone (marginal velum of Hines), representing the site into which cells will later migrate to form the dentate gyrus.[25, 26, 28] This zone was identified as the primordium hippocampi by Hines.[22] By stage XVII (11-mm CR), the earliest migration of neuroblasts from the ependymal surface takes place to form the primordial hippocampus. By 33-mm CR length, a primitive pyramidal cell layer is formed within the hippocampus. The differentiation of the pallium into its three subdivisions (archi- paleo- and neocortex) has thus begun. The hippocampal formation makes a ventrocaudal curve posteriorly. Initially the best-developed part of the hippocampus is anterior; by 44-mm CR length, the best-developed part has shifted posteriorly to lie dorsolateral to the diencephalon. All subdivisions of the hippocampal formation are identifiable by 70-mm CR length. The primordium of the fornix is identifiable at 40-mm CR length in the precommissural area; the psalterium hippocampi and hippocampal commissure are identifiable at between 55- and 60-mm CR length.[51]

According to Humphrey,[29] the hippocampal fissure is first identifiable at 37-mm CR length but does not appear well formed until the cells of the dentate gyrus form a ball-like mass in its fimbrial end (56-mm CR). At the time of its intermediate stage of development, the dentate gyrus rotates toward the hippocampus to the fissure. The fissure identified by Humphrey is not, therefore, the one that Hines[22] identified in stage XX (19-mm CR). As the dentate gyrus continues to rotate inward, its relationship with the hippocampus changes from a dorsoventral orientation to a medio–lateral one. The dentate gyrus comes to lie lateral to the hippocampal fissure and the hippocampus still further laterally beneath the ventricular surface. Although it may be detected earlier, the fimbriodentate fissure is present at 110-mm CR length, by which time all layers of the hippocampus are represented and the

fibers of the alveus are collecting along the ependymal layer. At between 79- and 85-mm CR length, all layers and subdivisions of both dentate gyrus and hippocampus are represented.[37]

The groove or indentation of the hippocampal fissure is defined by the position of the granular layer of the dentate gyrus. As the hippocampal formation develops, the groove deepens, rotates and eventually is partly obliterated, leaving a microscopically visible fibrovascular scar between the dentate gyrus and H1. The hippocampal fissure appears first at 37-mm CR length and is located along the posterolateral surface of the diencephalon. With migration of the hippocampus into the developing temporal lobe ventrolaterally, by 112-mm CR length the best-developed part of the hippocampal fissure is actually in the temporal lobe. As the fissure deepens, the cortical walls come in contact and begin to fuse (144-mm CR length), and the leptomeninges are resorbed so that only a superficial fissure remains at 275-mm CR length. The perforant bundle or the direct temporoammonic tract of Cajal may be seen by 150-mm CR length. Most fibers of the perforant bundle pass through the compressed zone at the depth of the fissure rather than through the area of fusion, although a few fibers may be seen crossing the region of fusion at from 20 to 25 weeks gestation.

At 144-mm CR length, the best-developed region of the hippocampal formation is seen in the temporal lobe rather than over the diencephalon. Shortly before this time, at 110-mm CR length and coincident with the development of the corpus callosum, the dorsal (supracallosal) hippocampus begins to show regressive changes. This regression is firmly established by 160-mm CR length. With continued rolling in of the dentate gyrus, the interlocking of the hippocampus and dentate gyrus on the temporal lobe takes place at from 112- to 143-mm CR length, thus establishing the adult relationships. The growth of the corpus callosum dorsally and the retreat of the hippocampus into the developing temporal lobe are completed at the same time. Remnants of the early development of the dorsal hippocampus include the striae Lancisii (induseum griseum) above the corpus callosum and the septohippocampal nucleus below it.

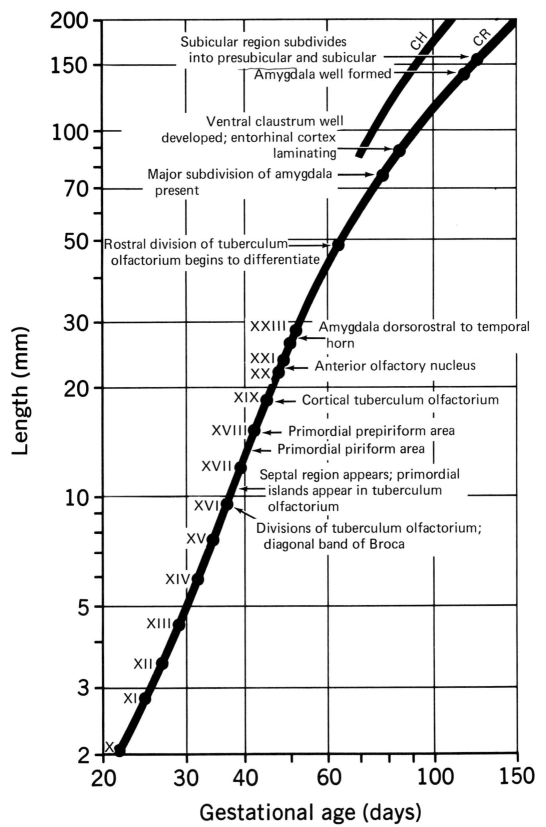

FIG. 14–3. Development of the olfactory-related areas correlated with CR length and gestational age.

RELATED AREAS (FIG. 14–3)

Anterior Olfactory Nucleus

The anterior olfactory nucleus forms a discontinuous ring of scattered neurons about the olfactory ventricle, anteriorly becoming continuous with the internal granular layer of the olfactory bulb and posteriorly extending into the olfactory trigone. Behind the olfactory stalk, the anterior olfactory nucleus extends laterally to become continuous with the prepiriform cortex, posteriorly toward the parolfactory area, dorsally toward the neopallium and dorsomedially toward the anterior part of the hippocampus.

The anterior olfactory nucleus is present in embryos at stage XXI (22-mm CR),[25] and by the time the bulb is elongating (32-mm CR length) the nucleus completely surrounds the ventricle. The various parts of the nucleus develop in a fashion consistent with the development of the other areas with which they come in contact. Thus, the medial part remains small until the anterior portion of the hippocampus begins to enlarge at 45-mm CR length, but the close association of the medial anterior olfactory nucleus with the hippocampus is lost in adults. With the appearance of the tuberculum olfactorium, the ventral part differentiates into three subdivisions that also become indistinct with time. The lateral part develops early and rapidly, as does the adjacent piriform cortex.

Anterior Perforated Substance

The anterior perforated substance, or tuberculum olfactorium, is relatively quite small and inconspicuous in the adult, but in the embryo it forms a significant part of the basal region and is central, both figuratively and anatomically, to the rhinencephalon. Anteriorly the anterior perforated substance is continuous with the ventral part of the anterior olfactory nucleus. Posteriorly it is bordered by the diagonal band of Broca, laterally by the prepiriform cortex (anteriorly) and the piriform cortex (posteriorly) and medially by the septal region and subcallosal gyrus. Humphrey[30] divides it into three zones anteroposteriorly, as well as into three longitudinal zones and three cortical layers. Within the cellular layers are the islands of Calleja, the medial island being the most prominent in the adult.

Before any olfactory fibers penetrate the brain, the caudal, middle and rostral subdivisions of the tuberculum olfactorium can be identified (stage XVI; 8- to 11-mm CR) with the primitive diagonal band of Broca. The caudal regions of the tuberculum olfactorium show the earliest development. With the development of the mitral cell layer in the olfactory bulb (49-mm CR length), the rostral subdivision begins to differentiate so that a distinct caudorostral sequence of development is apparent.

The relations of the borders of the tuberculum olfactorium change with increasing age because of the growth and differentiation of contiguous structures. The posterior boundary, initially formed by the diagonal band, does not change. From stage XX (22-mm CR) on, with the growth and development of the olfactory bulb and tract, the ventral part of the anterior olfactory nucleus is the anterior boundary. The tuberculum olfactorium is initially bordered laterally by the primordial piriform region and medially by undifferentiated neuroepithelium. In stage XVII (at about 11-mm CR), the septal region appears posteromedially and the primordial hippocampus anteromedially, with undifferentiated neuroepithelium accounting for most of the border. As the medial and lateral septal nuclei appear, the septal region further encroaches on the tuberculum, and by the end of embryonic development (31-mm CR), the medial border is formed by the medial part of the anterior olfactory nucleus, a small continuation of the hippocampal formation and the septal nuclei. With further rapid growth, the hippocampal formation comes to form a large part of the medial border. However, with the subsequent appearance of the corpus callosum and growth of the neopallium, all connections are reduced to the rudimentary status of the adult, and the larger role of the hippocampus in the medial boundary of the tuberculum olfactorium is lost.

Prepiriform and Piriform Cortex

Laterally, during stages XVII–XVIII (13- to 15-mm CR), the primordial prepiriform cortex constitutes most of the boundary, and only posterolaterally is the piriform cortex present. The lateral olfactory tract separates the lateral zone of the tuberculum from the prepiriform cortex. With the growth of the anterior olfactory nucleus, its lateral part separates the prepiriform cortex from the tuberculum olfactorium anteriorly in stage XXII (27-mm CR), but the prepiriform cortex grows rapidly and constitutes the entire lateral border by 40-mm CR length. Only later with the further growth of the piriform cortex does the lateral border approach that of the adult.

As the gross boundaries of the tuberculum are changing, there are cyclic alterations in its histology. Primordial islands develop in stage XVI (8- to 11-mm CR); soon thereafter the major anteroposterior subdivisions appear. These islands reach a peak and then disappear between stages XVIII and XX (13- to 18-mm CR). Secondary islands then appear but become diffuse by 40-mm CR length. Their later development is not known, but Humphrey[30] suggests that they probably disappear and are replaced at a still later time by the islands of Calleja typical of the adult.

The parolfactory area of Broca, or the precommissural septum, is poorly divided into the medial and lateral septal nuclei, mentioned above, and is continuous with the scattered gray of the septum pellucidum, nucleus accumbens septi and septohippocampal nucleus. The nucleus accumbens septi is first identified when the mitral cell layers of the olfactory bulb are differentiating at the end of stage XXIII. Initially ventral, it assumes its medial position after 90-mm CR length as the olfactory bulb elongates. Although the continuity of the septal region with the hippocampal formation is still well defined at 80-mm CR length, by 160-mm CR length that contact is lost, and the relationship of the hippocampus with the corpus callosum is firmly established.

Septal Region

The primordial septal region appears in stage XVI (11-mm CR),[30] begins to rapidly increase in size during stage XX (18- to 21-mm CR) and by from 32- to 35-mm CR length appears as a discrete but small bulge lying medial to and between the developing paleostriatum and olfactory bulb.[4] By the middle of the third month, the septal nuclei have grown rapidly, but less rapidly than the striate body, and have extended forward to lie next to the midline below the corpus callosum and septum pellucidum; with increasing age the nuclei are markedly reduced in size, especially relative to the massive neopallium.

The prepiriform cortex in the adult is a small band of gray matter adjacent to the lateral olfactory striae. It appears in the primordial piriform area relatively early (14- to 18-mm CR; stages XVIII to XIX) and is quite large by 40-mm CR length. At this stage the anterior commissure with its anterior and posterior divisions is well developed. At 100-mm CR length, the prepiriform cortex is a conspicuous part of the base of the brain.[4] By 160-mm CR length there is a clear polymorphic cell layer. By 250-mm CR length the outer granular layer arises, but the cortex is reduced to a narrow strip passing from the olfactory trigone to the base of the insula near the uncus.

The piriform lobe is located basally, and with the developing amygdaloid complex it forms a large part of the primitive temporal lobe. The ventral claustrum is clearly visible by 87-mm CR length, when the entorhinal cortex begins to laminate. By from 110- to 120-mm CR length, the entorhinal cortex surpasses the prepiriform cortex in extent and in complexity is nearer that of the neopallium.

By 160-mm CR length, the piriform cortex has assumed a medial position, appearing on the inner aspect of the temporal lobe. At this time the piriform lobe (including entorhinal cortex, subiculum, periamygdaloid cortex and ventral claustrum) and the postcallosal hippocampal formation form two-thirds of the olfactory telencephalon. The subicular area is subdivided into a presubicular and subicular region by 160-mm CR length.

Amygdala (Figure 14–4)

Constituting the subcortical gray of the piriform lobe, or the traditional secondary olfactory projection field, the amygdaloid complex is considered here although we recognize that concepts of the function of this area are changing rapidly.[17, 40]

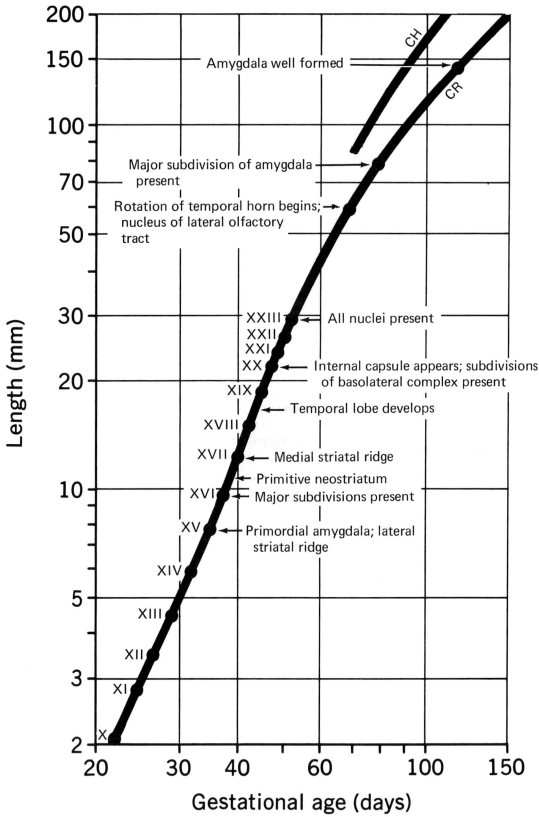

FIG. 14–4. Development of the amygdaloid complex and contiguous structures correlated with CR length and gestational age. (See also Fig. 12–8)

The amygdaloid complex, or archistriatum, is the first portion and, morphologically, the most complicated part of the human striatal complex to appear. The amygdaloid complex is overlaid by the periamygdaloid cortex of the hippocampal gyrus and is fused with the tail of the caudate nucleus and the ventral claustrum. At least a portion of it, the cortical medial division, is associated during development with other olfactory regions, including the tuberculum olfactorium, the nucleus of the lateral olfactory tract and the diagonal band of Broca.

The three major subdivisions include: 1) the corticomedial complex (cortical, medial and central nuclei); 2) the basolateral group (lateral, basal and accessory basal); and 3) an undifferentiated anterior region, the anterior amygdaloid area.[31,32,36] The following account of its development will follow the studies of Humphrey.[31,32]

The primordial amygdala is recognized as a thickening in the ventrocaudal wall of the interventricular foramen as soon as the cerebral hemisphere has evaginated (6- to 9.5-mm CR; stages XIV–XVI). The amygdala appears adjacent to the primordial hippocampal formation. The migrating neuroblasts which give rise to the amygdaloid complex originate from a slight elevation of the ventricular wall which constitutes the lateral striatal elevation. The major subdivisions of the complex are recognized very soon after the appearance of the primordial amygdaloid region develops, i.e., at stage XVI (10-mm CR). The primitive neostriatum appears anteriorly in the lateral striatal ridge slightly later, as does the primordial piriform cortex. In stage XVII (13-mm CR), the medial striatal ridge is present.

Almost as soon as the primordial amygdala can be recognized, the divisions of the corticomedial complex develop, particularly the medial nucleus that is adjacent to the anlage of the dentate gyrus and the cortical nucleus that is lateral to it and continuous with the piriform cortex. The subdivisions of the basolateral complex differentiate later, in stage XX (20- to 21-mm CR), but rapidly outstrip the corticomedial complex. The central nucleus appears in embryos of stages XX–XXI (22-mm CR), by which time the basolateral complex has separated from the common caudate–putamen primordium. All amygdaloid nuclei are present by stages XXI–XXII, except for the nucleus of the lateral olfactory tract, which does not appear until 48- to 60-mm CR length and is not well developed until 114-mm CR length. Macchi[45] found all major subdivisions present by 80-mm CR length, and Johnston[35] notes that the complex was well developed by 145-mm CR length.

The gross relationships are continuously changing. At stage XVII (13.5-mm CR), the amygdaloid complex is directly posterior to the lateral ventricle, whereas by stage XXII (24.5-mm CR), with the development of the temporal horn, the complex has been carried forward; it comes to lie anterior and lateral to the ventricle by stage XXIII (27.4-mm CR length). From 34- to 42-mm CR length, the relations to the internal capsule become important as it separates the amygdaloid complex from the caudate nucleus, putamen and globus pallidus. During the same period the temporal horn grows farther forward, medial to the complex. From 48- to 60.5-mm CR length, there is additional growth of the inferior horn, and a medial rotation of the temporal pole begins. At the same time, the basolateral complex increases markedly in size and by 114-mm CR length has grown forward. The transitional zone from amygdaloid complex to piriform cortex becomes larger and more distinct while that with the hippocampal region is poorly represented.

By 216-mm CR length, there has been additional growth of the temporal lobe such that the amygdaloid complex almost overlaps the lateral part of the tuberculum olfactorium. There has also been further medial rotation such that those nuclei that were lateral in earlier stages are now basal or ventral in position. By this late stage the corticomedial complex is less extensive, whereas the basolateral complex has increased further in size. Some slight rotation remains to be accomplished between this period (216-mm CR length) and birth.

ABNORMAL DEVELOPMENT

HOLOPROSENCEPHALY (ARHINENCEPHALY)

Nosology

Kundrat coined the term arhinencephaly in 1832 to describe the cardinal feature of a highly complex malformation that includes facial abnormalities, absence of the olfactory bulbs and tracts and failure of cleavage of the forebrain with the resultant production of a telencephalic holosphere. Yakovlev[61] correctly pointed out that the term is a misnomer, implying agenesis of the rhinencephalon, and showed that, although the olfactory bulbs fail to develop, the primary defect is the failure of evagination of the secondary telencephalic vesicles. For that reason he termed the malformation holotelencephaly.

De Myer and Zeman[14] introduced the term holoprosencephaly to emphasize the general arrest of prosencephalic cleavage and tectogenesis. De Myer and Zeman[14] further subdivided the malformation into a spectrum of related anatomic disorders. "Alobar holoprosencephaly" was used to describe the most severe form of the malformation, whereas "lobar holoprosencephaly" was used for the least severely affected cases demonstrating absence of the olfactory bulbs and tracts as the most common abnormality. "Semilobar holoprosencephaly" was reserved for a number of cases with characteristics falling in between the alobar and lobar forms. The term holoprosencephaly is more appropriate for the most severe cases, since it implies a tendency for the prosencephalon to remain a whole or single incompletely cleft bulb with severe malformations of both telencephalon and diencephalon. However, in less severe forms the diencephalon largely escapes, so that the term holotelencephaly would be more appropriate. The older term arhinencephaly is well established, but it should be modified to indicate mild, moderate or severe forms depending on how much more than the olfactory bulbs and tracts are missing or malformed.

Anatomy

According to Cohen et al.,[7] the holoprosencephalies comprise a spectrum of related disorders in which failure of midline cleavage of the embryonic forebrain is the basic feature. The absence of the olfactory bulbs and tracts is characteristic of even the mildest forms of the disorder. The most severe forms are characterized by the production of a telencephalon in the form of a holosphere with a single ventricular cavity.

Many different authors have given the impression that the anatomy of this complex

malformation is well known; clearly that is not the case. There are very few adequate histologic studies of the many cases said to fall in this category on gross inspection alone. Furthermore, the entire complex is inextricably mixed with considerations of the facial abnormalities said to occur so frequently with this disorder.

In the typical and most severe form of holoprosencephaly, the brain consists of a holosphere composed of relatively large, simply convoluted gyri (Figs. 14–5 through 14–7). The sphere may be compressed anteriorly, opening posteriorly into a large bulging cavity, the covering membrane of which represents the roofing membrane of the telencephalon medium. This membrane (Fig. 14–7) is attached to a ridgelike thickening that is shaped like a horseshoe and is seen histologically to be the hippocampal formation. Successive architectonic fields[61] include the periprepiriform cortex, limbic region, gigantopyramidal (motor) area and homotypical eulaminate cortex. The prepiriform, periprepiriform and insular regions are located more ventrally. The olfactory bulbs and tracts are absent, as are the prefrontal granular areas of the frontal lobes.

Such cases, representing the alobar form of De Myer and Zeman,[14] have been reported by Bishop et al.,[6] DeLange,[12] De Myer and Zeman (case 3),[14] De Myer et al.,[15] Fatt,[18] Haworth et al.,[21] Lichtenstein and Maloney (case 2),[43] Marburg and Warner,[46] Yakovlev[61] and Zellweger (case 3).[62] Cases probably belonging in this group include those reported by Barber and Muelling[2] and Landau et al.[41]

The mildest form of this complex is the case with a simple absence of only the olfactory bulbs and tracts, which may be unilateral but is more commonly bilateral, and therefore most appropriately termed arhinencephaly. Such a group is best exemplified by the case of Stewart,[56] histologically shown to demonstrate absence of the olfactory trigone, area olfactoria, diagonal band of Broca and a hypoplastic dentate gyrus. Simple aplasia of the olfactory bulb and tracts may be associated with other distinct malformations, including agenesis of the corpus callosum,[13] agenesis of the septum pellucidum and hypoplasia of the hippocampal formation and corpus callosum.[10] Other relatively pure forms include those reported by

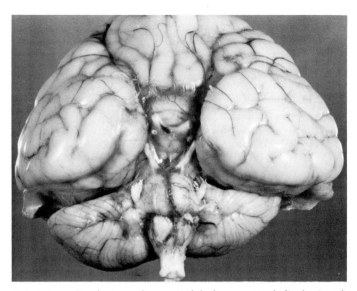

FIG. 14–5. Basal view of a typical holoprosencephalic brain of a 4-month-old boy with progressive hydrocephalus and a depressed nasal bridge. There is absence of both olfactory bulbs, fusion of the frontal lobes and marked shortening of the temporal and occipital lobes. (#Np 103).

FIG. 14–6. **a.** Anteroposterior view of a ventriculogram showing air in the single holosphere similar to that in Fig. 14–5. (UWH #18-26-25). **b.** Coronal section of the holoprosencephalic brain shown in Fig. 14–5 to be compared with the ventriculogram shown in Fig. 14–6a. Note the single ventricular cavity and fusion of the thalami behind the paired striatum. (#Np 103)

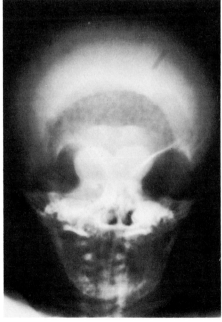

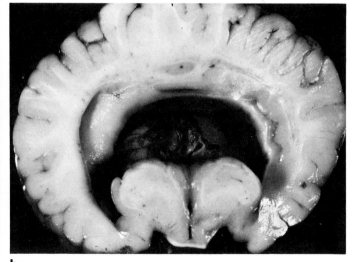

a   b

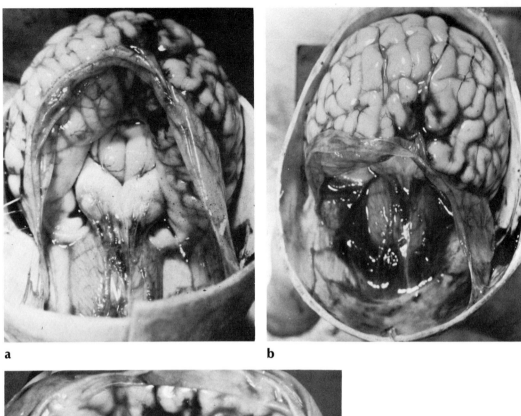

a   b

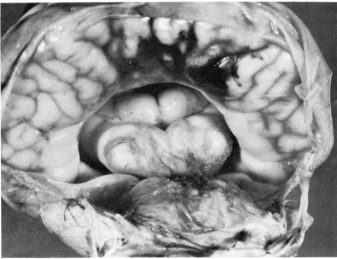

c

FIG. 14–7.   **a.** Dorsoposterior view of the holoprosencephalic brain shown in Figs. 14–5 and 14–6**b.** The roofing membrane of the telencephalon medium has been opened to reveal the deep cerebral nuclei in the floor. (#Np 103) **b.** Dorsal view of the same brain, better showing the extent of the cerebral defect in relation to the cranial cavity. **c.** Posterior view of the same brain (after removal from the skull) revealing the fused deep cerebral nuclei in the floor of the single holosphere.

hamartoma

TABLE 14–1. FACIAL FEATURES IN HOLOPROSENCEPHALY

Facial Type*	Main Facial Features†	Usual Cerebral Malformation
Cyclopia	Median monophthalmia, synophthalmia or anophthalmia; proboscis may be single, double or absent; hypognathia in some cases	Alobar holoprosencephaly‡
Ethmocephaly	Ocular hypotelorism; proboscis may be single, double or absent	Alobar holoprosencephaly‡
Premaxillary agenesis	Ocular hypotelorism, flat nose and median cleft lip	Usually alobar holoprosencephaly‡
Cebocephaly	Ocular hypotelorism and single nostril nose	Usually alobar holoprosencephaly‡
Less-severe facial dysmorphia	Variable features including ocular hypotelorism or hypertelorism, flat nose, unilateral or bilateral cleft lip, iris coloboma or other anomalies; slight or no facial dysmorphia in some cases	Usually semilobar (moderate) or lobar (mild) holotelencephaly

* Transitional facial forms are known to occur.

† Only the main distinguishing features are listed here. Features such as microcephaly, other eye anomalies, ear anomalies and other defects also occur.

‡ Severe arhinencephaly or typical holoprosencephaly.

Biemond[5] and Issajew,[33] whereas an example associated with several other malformations, including a midline hamartoma and meningeal angiomatosis, is reported by Gitlin and Behar.[20]

There are a few cases which can be accepted as forming a bridge between the severe cases of holoprosencephaly and the mild cases of arhinencephaly: case 10 of Yakovlev,[61] case 1 of DeLange[11] and that of Bannwarth.[1] Such cases demonstrate, in addition to the aplasia of the olfactory bulbs and tracts, varying degrees of hypoplasia of the cerebral mantle, over well-formed lateral ventricles or over a single ventricle, with varying degrees of fusion of the basal ganglia and/or thalami.

Other cases that have been confused with and sometimes presented as examples of holoprosencephaly without arhinencephaly include examples of agenesis of the corpus callosum or agenesis of the septum pellucidum. Such malformations have what may appear to be a single ventricle and may be associated with abnormalities of gyral formation. Included here are case 1 of Lichtenstein and Maloney,[43] which shows simple agenesis of the septum pellucidum; the cases of Kautzky,[37] which show agenesis of the septum pellucidum, hypoplastic corpus callosum and fusion of the frontal lobes (heterotopias) across the midline; the case of Gaustaut and De Wulf,[19] which shows

agenesis of the septum pellucidum and partial agenesis of the corpus callosum with heterotopic gray matter in the midline; and the case of Ortiz de Zarate,[48] which shows agenesis of the septum pellucidum and absence of the posterior corpus callosum with fusion of the cortical gyri posteriorly. In all of these cases, the olfactory bulbs are either present, hypoplastic or not mentioned.

Facial Dysmorphia and Holoprosencephaly

The association of certain characteristic facial malformations with holoprosencephaly has been so striking that they have been considered virtually pathognomonic of holoprosencephaly.[7,15] They are included here (Table 14–1) because any understanding of the etiology and pathogenesis of holoprosencephaly must include consideration of the facial abnormalities, but it must be noted that the association is not invariable.

CYCLOPIA. The most severe of these facial malformations is cyclopia, characterized by the presence of a single eye located in the area normally occupied by the root of the nose. Various degrees of doubling of intrinsic structures occur, and the optic nerves may be single, double or absent.[55] There is usually a single proboscislike appendage located above the eye, but there may be more than one proboscis or none. Numerous facial bones are usually absent, including the ethmoids, nasal bones, turbinates, vomer, middle of the body of the sphenoid, lacrimal, premaxilla and zygomatic portions of the malar bones.

ETHMOCEPHALY.   In ethmocephaly the orbits are separate but closer than normal, and there may be one or more proboscides or none. Several bones may be absent, including the nasal bones, premaxilla, septum of the ethmoid and turbinates; others may be fused, including the lacrimal and palatine bones.

CEBOCEPHALY.   Cebocephaly is characterized by hypotelorism and a flat rudimentary nose, which is present in its usual position. The optic foramina lie close together and the nasal septum and premaxilla are absent. There may be a median cleft lip.[7]

PREMAXILLARY AGENESIS.   Premaxillary agenesis is characterized by ocular hypotelorism, a flat nose and a median cleft lip in which the premaxillary bone is absent, but the hard palate is intact.[7,14]

LESS-SEVERE FACIAL DYSMORPHIA.   Among this group of facial abnormalities are children[7,14] with less-severe anomalies, including unilateral or bilateral cleft lip with preservation of the philtrum–premaxilla anlage, hypotelorism and a flat nose.

As with the brain, so with the face; in many transitional cases the above terms must be considered as identifying only the most common forms. Unfortunately, all authors have not used these terms in the same way.[18] Also, although holoprosencephaly is frequently associated with these facial anomalies, such is not always the case,[7] and there is no correlation of mild facial anomalies with mild cerebral anomalies. Indeed, the less-severe forms of holoprosencephaly usually have no facial anomalies.[11,18,56]

Other Associated Anomalies

In addition to the facial and cerebral abnormalities already discussed above, other anomalies are quite common. Within the CNS, microcephaly is typically present. The anterior commissure has been absent in some cases,[2,13] but serial sections[61] may be necessary to detect small ones. The pyramidal tracts are usually poorly formed, but other anomalies of the brainstem are uncommon. Vascular abnormalities have been noted in the CNS in several cases, usually at the base of the brain.[11,20,46] The presence of hydranencephaly or anencephaly has been mentioned,[7,55] but one must be careful in examining such cases to be certain whether the olfactory bulbs and tracts have been merely destroyed. If anencephaly results from failure of closure of the anterior neuropore, one would expect the olfactory ventricles to share in the subsequent malformation.

The hypophysis is absent in many cases, particularly in cyclopia, and is associated with other endocrine abnormalities.[7,16,21,23,52,55] Although Rogers[52] found the hypophysis to be present in one-half of his cases, Sedano and Gorlin[55] found it present in only about 15% of the cases reviewed. Among other endocrine abnormalities one should note that hypogonadism and anosmia are transmitted as an X-linked recessive trait in the Kallman syndrome.

Polydactyly and syndactyly are frequently present, as are visceral anomalies, such as congenital heart disease, situs inversus viscerum and anomalies of the genitourinary system.[7,23,41,55,61] Occasional cases show no extracranial abnormalities.

Cytogenetics

Chromosomal aberrations associated with syndromes of congenital malformations have excited considerable comment in recent years.[58,59] Cohen et al.[7] have reviewed this aspect in great detail. Of the many chromosomal syndromes that have been associated with holoprosencephaly, the most common are trisomy 13, 18p− and Dq−, but cases have been reported with no chromosomal abnormalities,[6,41] especially those cases with the less severe forms of arhinencephaly.

Pathogenesis

From the foregoing discussion it is clear that arhinencephaly and holoprosencephaly must be considered part of a symptom–complex that is probably etiologically heterogeneous. Cohen et al.[7] postulate that the basic defect relates to a faulty embryonic interaction be-

anosmia.-

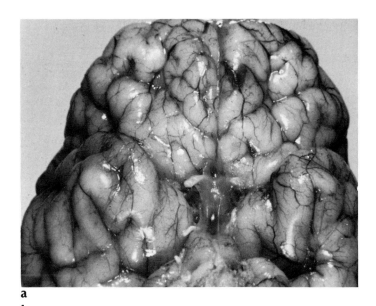

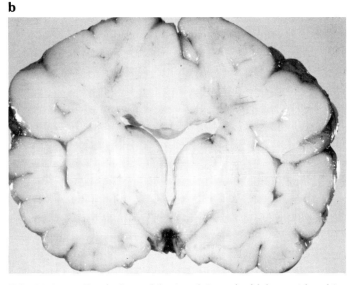

FIG. 14–8. **a.** Basal view of brain of 2-week-old boy with arhinencephaly but with relatively well-formed frontal and temporal lobes. There were multiple anomalies of skeletal, cardiac and renal systems. **b.** Coronal section of the brain reveals a T-shaped ventricular system with a large mass of gray and white matter blending with the corpus callosum and obliterating most of the superior longitudinal fissure. (#Np 417)

tween the notochordal plate, the neuroectoderm of the brain plate and the oral plate. Thus, when the notochordal plate terminates further caudally than normal, there is an inhibition of the neuroectoderm, and the optic anlagen fail to migrate laterally, producing various degrees of hypotelorism, synophthalmia or cyclopia.

Any faulty interaction of the olfactory placodes and the rostral end of the brain may result in a displacement of the placodes. Mesenchymal proliferation around the placodes may result in proboscis formation. Faulty interaction of the olfactory placodes with the oral plate may result in malformations of the primary oral plate with lack of fusion of the maxillary primordia and production of a median pseudocleft. Faulty

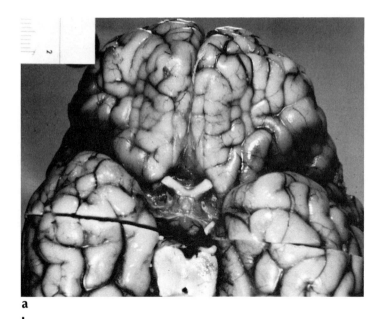

a

b

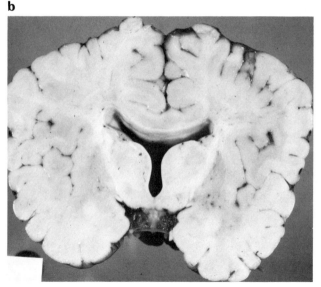

FIG. 14–9. **a.** Basal view of the brain of a 3-month-old girl with multiple congenital malformations of skeletal, cardiac and genitourinary systems but with well-preserved olfactory
tracts. **b.** Coronal section of the brain reveals a T-shaped ventricular system with a thick
layer of cortex covering the corpus callosum. (#Np 647)

interaction of the notochord, prochordal
plate and surface ectoderm may result in
failure of the oral plate to develop with an
abnormal or absent Rathke's pouch and its
derivatives.

Cohen et al.[7] regard notochordal length as
a polygenic trait, thus accounting for the variety of chromosomal abnormalities encountered. Rogers[53,54] has produced cyclopia by
both chemical and traumatic techniques,
suggesting that the stimuli act either on the
prechordal substrate or on the neural tissue
of the telencephalon and diencephalon.
Krafka[38] suggests a vascular basis for the
malformation, but it is more likely that the
vascular abnormalities he found, and those
cited previously, are either a result or a part
of the entire complex.

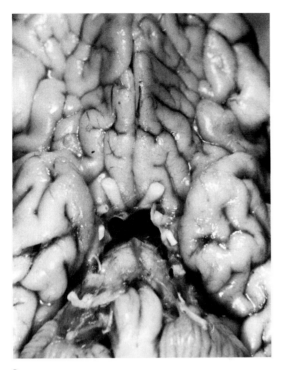

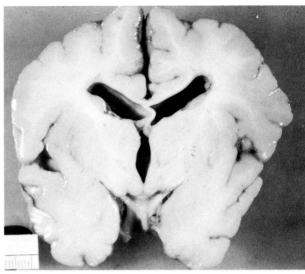

b

a

FIG. 14–10. **a.** Basal view of the brain of an 8-month-old boy with multiple skeletal anomalies and arhinencephaly. Thick neuronal and glial heterotopias were noted microscopically, filling the leptomeninges under the anterior perforated space, evidence perhaps of abnormal involution of the olfactory tracts. **b.** Coronal section of the brain reveals slightly hydrocephalic but normally shaped ventricles. The corpus callosum is thin and covered with a thin layer of gray matter. (#Np 835)

ABNORMALITIES OF THE HIPPOCAMPAL FORMATION

The hippocampal formation is a readily recognized histoanatomic structure. Characteristically, its hippocampus and dentate gyrus are in the form of interlocking C's. As noted previously, the early ventral-to-dorsal arrangement of the dentate gyrus and hippocampus changes by rotating medially (dentate gyrus) to laterally (hippocampus). Because of its characteristic appearance, abnormalities in the hippocampal formation are readily recognized and have been described in a variety of CNS malformations.

In typical holoprosencephaly, as noted already, the hippocampal formation forms an undivided horseshoe-shaped transverse gyrus about the dorsal border of the holosphere.[61] In less-severe forms, other abnormalities may be seen, such as hypoplasia of the dentate gyrus in a case of aplasia of the olfactory nerves and bulbs.[56]

Hypoplastic and malrotated hippocampal formations may also be seen in cases of agenesis of the septum pellucidum,[10,43,47] agenesis of the corpus callosum[44] and trisomy 18 syndrome.[57] The temporal lobes may also be quite small[10] or abnormal.[44] In the case of Nathan and Smith,[47] both the hippocampus and dentate gyrus lay on the surface with no hippocampal fissure being identified. The alveus was poorly developed, and the fornix could not be identified. An additional abnormality was the presence of heterotopias occupying much of the corpus callosum.

PERSONAL STUDIES

From the above review of the "spectrum" of previously reported abnormalities of the brain, face and other organs in association with absence of the olfactory bulbs and tracts, it is obvious that much further work must be done to synthesize a completely satisfactory picture since there are still insufficient numbers of cases which have been studied adequately both anatomically and clinically. Our own studies are unfortunately

TABLE 14–2. SOME FEATURES OF CASES WITH ARHINENCEPHALY AND/OR RELATED MALFORMATIONS

| | Arhinencephaly | | | | Olfactory Tracts Normal | |
| | Bilateral | | | Unilateral | Agenesis of Septum Pellucidum | Agenesis of Corpus Callosum |
	Single Spherical Ventricle	Single T-shaped Ventricle	Normal Ventricles	Normal Ventricles	Single T-shaped Ventricle	
Total no. of cases	13	6	24	12	5	18
Macrocephaly or hydrocephaly	6/13	2/6	2/24	1/12	3/5	4/18
Corpus callosum:						
Absent	13/13	3/6	1/24	1/12	0/4	13/18
Normal	0/13	0/6	20/24	9/12	4/4	0/18
With gray matter	0/13	3/6	0/24	0/12	1/4	0/18
Hypoplastic	0/13	0/6	3/24	2/12	0/4	5/18
Single diencephalic mass	13/13	0/6	0/23	0/12	0/5	0/18
Bilateral but fused thalami	0/13	0/6	0/24	1/12	3/5	1/18
Other CNS anomalies:						
Forebrain	—	4/6	14/24	8/12	4/5	8/18
Cerebellum	1/13	5/6	10/24	3/12	1/5	5/18
Other	3/13	1/3	1/24	2/12	2/5	7/18
Facial abnormalities:[1]						
Severe	5/13	0/6	0/24	0/12	0/5	0/18
Moderate	2/13	2/6	8/24	3/12	3/5	1/18
Mild	2/13	1/6	6/24	1/12	0/5	3/18
None	4/13	3/6	10/24	8/12	2/5	14/18
Other organ abnormalities[2]	10/13	3/6	16/24	8/12	3/5	7/18
Chromosomal abnormalities proven:						
Trisomy D = 13–15	1/3	—	6/9	1/3	—	—
Trisomy E = 18	—	1/2	—	—	—	1/3
Trisomy G = 21	—	—	—	1/3	—	1/3
Other						
Minor abnormalities of 21–22	—	—	1/9	—	—	—
Normal	2/3	1/2	2/9	1/3	2/2	1/3
Chromosomal abnormalities suspected:	—	—	3			
Down syndrome (clinical)	—	—	—	(2)		
Other diseases:						
Congenital Rubella	—	—	—	(1)		
Subependymal germinolysis	1	—	—	2		
Encephalocele	—	1	—	—		
Arnold–Chiari	—	—	2	—		
Kallman	—	—	2			

[1] *Severe:* absence of nose or eyes, cyclopia, severe microphthalmia, in association with cleft lip and/or palate.
   Moderate: cleft lip and/or palate alone or with mild microphthalmia, coloboma.
   Mild: deformed ears, skin tags, micrognathia.
   None: "suspicious-looking facies" or no abnormalities recognized.
[2] *Cardiac:* interventricular or interatrial septal defect, dextroposition of the heart, hypoplastic ventricle or atrium, tetralogy of Fallot, bicuspid aortic valve.
   Skeletal: clubbing of hands or feet, fusions of vetrebrae, hemivertebrae, partial agenesis of clavicle, rocker bottom feet, polydactyly.
   Genitourinary: horseshoe kidney, polycystic kidney, hypoplastic kidney, hypospadias, cryptorchidism, bicornuate uterus, double ureter.
   Gastrointestinal: Meckel diverticulum, accessory spleen, accessory lobe of liver, esophageal atresia, malrotation of the intestine.

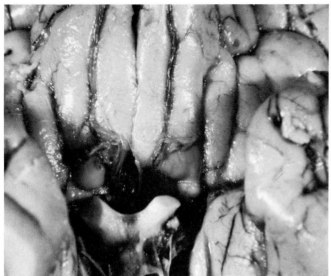

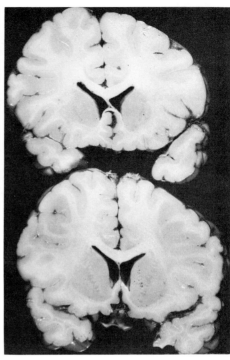

a

FIG. 14–11. **a.** Basal view of the brain of a 46-year-old, mildly mentally retarded man with undescended testes, aspermatogenesis and minor anomalies. No other members of his family were affected. Arhinencephaly was proven microscopically even though the olfactory sulci are well-formed. **b.** Coronal sections of the brain reveal it to be well-formed otherwise. (#Np 302)

b

also still incomplete, but Table 14–2 summarizes our preliminary examinations of 78 cases, 55 with arhinencephaly (Shaw, unpublished data) and 23 without arhinencephaly but with agenesis of the septum pellucidum or corpus callosum (many of these having been reviewed by Loeser and Alvord[44]).

It would appear that there is only one relatively homogeneous group, the 13 cases of bilateral arhinencephaly with a single spherical forebrain ventricle (Figs. 14–5 through 14–7). These cases can be considered as typical holoprosencephaly, in which failure to develop a midline cleft extends to involve most of the diencephalon as well as the telencephalon. Only the eyes typically escape, but even these may be affected in cyclopia, the most severe form of holoprosencephaly.

The "spectrum" breaks at this point, however, in that all the other groups appear to be relatively heterogeneous, with the other congenital malformations occurring either in isolation or in association with one another,

even with or without arhinencephaly. Some of these could be considered examples of "holotelencephaly," the diencephalon generally being spared. A single T-shaped ventricle, for example, results from absence of the septum pellucidum and can be seen equally frequently in cases with (Fig. 14–8) or without (Fig. 14–9) agenesis of the olfactory bulbs and tracts. In those with arhinencephaly the corpus callosum is absent where there is a cerebral cleavage, which may be either complete or focal posteriorly. In those without arhinencephaly the corpus callosum is usually normal. Cases in each group may show incomplete midline separation of the telencephalon with cortical gray matter covering the corpus callosum (Fig. 14–10). Whether the corpus callosum is absent—or hidden, undifferentiated—in cases without a cerebral cleavage is difficult to prove, and one should be careful to note that "absence" of the corpus callosum in Table 14–2 is not meant to imply real similarity between the typical holoprosencephalic cases and those with typical agenesis of the corpus callosum. "Incomplete midline separation" of the diencephalon, *i.e.*, fusion of the thalami (which

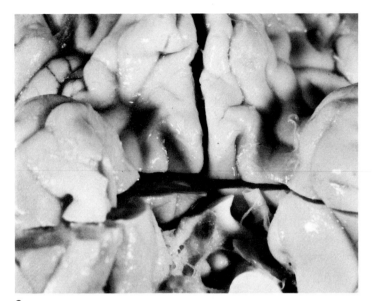

a

b

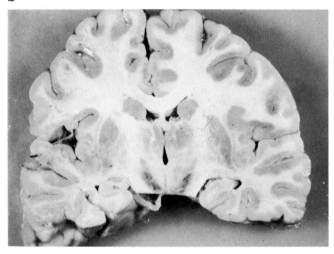

FIG. 14–12.   **a.** Basal view of the brain of a 30-year-old man with X-linked anosmia, hypo-gonadism and epilepsy (Kallmann's syndrome). Note the poorly formed olfactory sulci. Microscopic sections reveal gliosis extending into the leptomeninges beneath the olfactory area. **b.** Coronal section of the brain reveals it to be well-formed, but microscopically there was diffuse gliosis about the lateral and third ventricles. (#Np 2624)

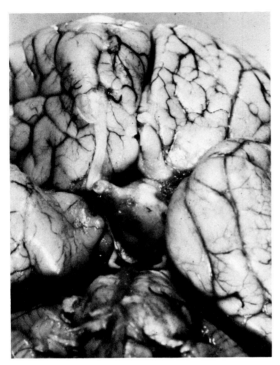

FIG. 14–13. Basal view of the brain of a 13-month-old boy with agenesis of the left olfactory tract and corpus callosum, and with contralateral hydrocephalus (see Fig 7–11). (#Np 541)

may well represent increased fusion of the diencephalon through excessive formation of the massa intermedia or "third ventricular adhesion"), occurs surprisingly only in those cases without arhinencephaly—and not in all of those. Rarely is it seen in cases of unilateral absence of the olfactory bulb and tract or of agenesis of the corpus callosum, and more commonly but in milder degree in cases with the Arnold–Chiari malformation. Other anomalies of the forebrain, not seen in holoprosencephaly, occur frequently in all the groups of cases, and include polymicrogyria, subcortical or subependymal heterotopias, hypoplastic or malrotated hippocampus or dentate gyrus.

Even in the most homogeneous group, those with holoprosencephaly, there is some heterogeneity in the CNS and even greater heterogeneity outside the CNS. Thus, enlargement of the head may or may not be present and anomalies of the subtentorial parts of the CNS are rather infrequent. Severe facial abnormalities (cebocephaly, cyclopia, absence of the nose or eyes, severe microphthalmia—frequently associated with cleft lip and/or palate) occur only in association with holoprosencephaly, but the converse is not true; many cases with holoprosencephaly have normal or nearly normal facies. Various degrees of anomalies of other organs involving the skeletal system, genitourinary system, gastrointestinal system and cardiovascular system are frequent in all groups, but their severity does not necessarily correlate with the severity of the CNS malformations.

So, when one looks at the various other groups, already heterogeneous with respect to associations of the major malformations, it is not surprising that they are heterogeneous with respect to other anomalies in the brain or elsewhere. The one thing that can be said is that these cases do not show the single diencephalic mass characteristic of, or the severe facial anomalies frequently seen in, holoprosencephaly. But all the other anomalies are frequently seen in each group—except for facial anomalies with agenesis of the corpus callosum—leading to the suspicions that no one anomaly is primary and that various causative factors must be considered. Indeed, trisomy D was frequently suspected clinically because of the multiplicity of anomalies, but unfortunately it was frequently either not sought or not present.

Of special interest are two groups of cases, one with mental retardation and the other with unilateral absence of one olfactory bulb and tract. Mental retardation may be associated with arhinencephaly (Fig. 14–11), especially in cases of Kallman syndrome, which consists of mental retardation with anosmia (arhinencephaly) and hypogonadism transmitted as an X-linked recessive (Fig. 14–12). Unilateral arhinencephaly (Figs. 7–11, 14–13 and 14–14) suggests that a secondary destruction rather than a primary malformation was at work. Severe hypoplasia (or atrophy) of one or both olfactory tracts was frequently found microscopically in cases of gross arhinencephaly with an otherwise relatively well-developed forebrain. The same variation in other associated anomalies, even chromosomal, appears to occur in this group. If a destructive agent, viral or other, is likely to be the cause of the unilateral arhinencephaly, is it also likely to be the cause of other anomalies? We suspect so.

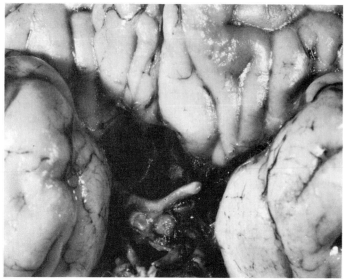

a

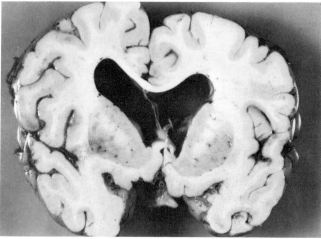

b

FIG. 14–14.   **a.** Basal view of the brain of a 47-year-old man, blind and mentally retarded since early infancy, with unilateral arhinencephaly. **b.** Coronal section of the brain reveals moderate hydrocephalus secondary to aqueductal gliosis and stenosis. There is also diffuse gliosis of the cerebral, cerebellar and brain stem white matter. (#Np 2180)

REFERENCES

1. Bannwarth A: Gehirnmissbildung und Epilepsi. Nervenarzt 13:97–103, 1940

2. Barber AN, Muelling RJ: Cyclopia with complete separation of the neural and mesodermal elements of the eye. Arch Opthalmol 43:989–1003, 1950

3. Bartelmez GW, Dekaban AS: The early development of the human brain. Contrib Embryol 37:13–32, 1962

4. Baxter JS: Frazier's Manual of Embryology, ed 3. London, Bailliere, Tindall & Cox, 1953

5. Biemond A: Ueber einen Fall von Kernaplasie (Moebius), kombiniert mit Arhinencephalie. Acta Psychiatr Neurol Scand 11:48–62, 1936

6. Bishop K, Connolly JM, Carter CH, Carpenter DG: Holoprosencephaly. J Pediatr 65:406–414, 1964

7. Cohen MM Jr, Jirásek JE, Guzman RT, Gorlin RJ, Peterson MQ: Holoprosencephaly and facial dysmorphia: nosology, etiology and pathogenesis. Birth Defects 7:125–135, 1971

8. Crosby EC, Humphrey T: Studies of the verte-

brate telencephalon. II. The nuclear pattern of the anterior olfactory nucleus, tuberculum olfactorium and the amygdaloid complex in adult man. J Comp Neurol 74:309–352, 1941

9. Currarino G, Silverman FN: Orbital hypotelorism, arhinencephaly, and trigonocephaly. Radiology 74:206–217, 1960

10. Dekaban A: Arhinencephaly in an infant born to a diabetic mother. J Neuropathol Exp Neurol 18:620–626, 1959

11. De Lange C: Two cases of congenital anomalies of the brain. Am J Dis Child 53:429–444, 1937

12. De Lange C: Cebocephalia minor. Acta Psychiatr Neurol Scand 15:299–336, 1940

13. De Morsier G: Etudes sur les dysraphies cranioencephaliques. Schweiz Arch Neurol Neurochir Psychiatr 74:309–361, 1955

14. De Myer W, Zeman W: Alobar holoprosencephaly (arhinencephaly) with median cleft lip and palate: clinical, electroencephalographic and nosologic considerations. Confin Neurol 23:1–36, 1963

15. De Myer W, Zeman W, Palmer CG: The face predicts the brain: diagnostic significance of median facial anomalies for holoprosencephaly (arhinencephaly). Pediatrics 34:256–263, 1964

16. Edmonds HW: Pituitary, adrenal and thyroid in cyclopia. Arch Pathol 50:727–735, 1950

17. Eleftheriou BE: Introductory remarks. The Neurobiology of the Amygdala. New York–London, Plenum Press, 1972

18. Fatt CY: Cebocephaly: a report of five postmortem cases and a review of literature. Aust Paediatr J 8:52–56, 1972

19. Gaustaut H, De Wulf: Etude de deux cas d'une dysgénésie cérébrale exceptionnelle: la synraphie des fissures cérébrale, et des anomalies anatomiques et cliniques qu'elle entraine. Rev Neurol (Paris) 79:591–601, 1947

20. Gitlin G, Behar AJ: Meningeal angiomatosis, arhinencephaly, agenesis of the corpus callosum and large hamartoma of the brain, with neoplasia, in an infant having bilateral nasal proboscis. Acta Anat (Basel) 41:56–79, 1960

21. Haworth JC, Medovy H, Lewis AJ: Cebocephaly with endocrine dysgenesis. J Pediatr 59:726–733, 1961

22. Hines M: Studies in the growth and differentiation of the telecephalon in man. The fissura hippocampi. J Comp Neurol 34:73–171, 1922

23. Hintz KL, Menking M, Sotos JF: Familial holoprosencephaly with endocrine dysgenesis. J Pediatr 72:81–87, 1968

24. Humphrey T: The development of the olfactory and the accessory olfactory formations in human embryos and fetuses. J Comp Neurol 73:431–468, 1940

25. Humphrey T: The development of the anterior olfactory nucleus of human fetuses. Prog Brain Res 3:170–190, 1963

26. Humphrey T: Some observations on the development of the human hippocampal formation. Trans Am Neurol Assoc 82:207–209, 1964

27. Humphrey T: The development of the human hippocampal formation correlated with some aspects of its phylogenetic history. Evolution of the Forebrain. Edited by R Hassler and H Stephen. Stuttgart, Georg Thieme Verlag, 1966, pp. 104–116

28. Humphrey T: Correlations between the development of the hippocampal formation and the differentiation of the olfactory bulbs. Ala J Med Sci 3:235–269, 1966

29. Humphrey T: The development of the human hippocampal fissure. J Anat 101:655–676, 1967

30. Humphrey T: The development of the human tuberculum olfactorium during the first three months of embryonic life. J Hirnforsch 9:437–469, 1967

31. Humphrey T: The development of the human amygdala during early embryonic life. J Comp Neurol 132:135–166, 1968

32. Humphrey T: The development of the human amygdaloid complex. The Neurobiology of the Amygdala. Edited by BE Eleftheriou. New York–London, Plenum Press, 1972, pp. 21–77

33. Issajew PO: Ein Fall der Abwesenheit des N. olfactorius. Anat Anz 74:398–400, 1932

34. Johnston JB: Nervus terminalis in reptiles and mammals. J Comp Neurol 23:97–120, 1913

35. Johnston JB: The morphology of the septum, hippocampus, and pallial commissures in reptiles and mammals. J Comp Neurol 23:371–478, 1913

36. Johnston JB: Further contribution to the study of the evolution of the forebrain. J Comp Neurol 35:337–481, 1923

37. Kautzky R: Uber einen Fall von Missbildung im Gebiete des Endhirnes. Z Anat Entwicklungsgesch 106:447–461, 1937

38. Krafka J: Cyclopia and arhinia. Arch Ophthalmol 33:128–136, 1945

39. Kuhlenbeck H: General discussion on the terminology of the rhinencephalon. Prog Brain Res 3:243–244, 1963

40. Lammers HJ: The neural connections of the amygdaloid complex in mammals. The Neurobiology of the Amygdala. Edited by BE Eleftherion. New York–London, Plenum Press, 1972, pp. 123–144

41. Landau JW, Barry JM, Koch R: Arhinencephaly. J Pediatr 62:895–900, 1963

42. Larsell O: The nervus terminalis. Ann Otol Rhinol Laryngol 59:414–438, 1950

43. Lichtenstein BW, Maloney JE: Malformation of the forebrain. J Neuropathol Exp Neurol 13:117–128, 1954

44. Loeser JD, Alvord EC Jr: Agenesis of the corpus callosum. Brain 91:553–570, 1968

45. Macchi G: The ontogenetic development of the olfactory telencephalon in man. J Comp Neurol 95:245–305, 1951

46. Marburg V, Warner FJ: The brain in a case of human cyclopia. J Nerv Ment Dis 103:319–330, 1946

47. Nathan PW, Smith MC: Normal mentality associated with a maldeveloped "rhinencephalon." J Neurol Neurosurg Psychiatry 13:191–197, 1950

48. Ortiz de Zarate JC: Partial holoprosencephaly. Psychiatr Neurol (Basel) 154: 311–318, 1967

49. Pearson AA: The development of the nervus terminalis in man. J Comp Neurol 75:39–66, 1941

50. Pearson AA: The development of the olfactory nerve in man. J Comp Neurol 75:199–217, 1941

51. Rakic P, Yakovlev PI: Development of the corpus callosum and cavum septi in man. J Comp Neurol 132:45–72, 1968

52. Rogers, KT: Presence of the pituitary in perfect cyclopia. Anat Rec 128:213–218, 1957

53. Rogers KT: Experimental production of perfect cyclopia in the chick by means of LiCl, with a survey of the literature on cyclopia produced experimentally by various means. Dev Biol 8: 129–150, 1963

54. Rogers KT: Experimental production of perfect cyclopia by removal of the telencephalon and reversal of bilateralization in somite-stage chicks. Am J Anat 115:487–508, 1964

55. Sedano HO, Gorlin RI: The oral manifestation of cyclopia. Oral Surg 16:823–838, 1963

56. Stewart RM: Arhinencephaly. J Neurol Neurosurg Psychiatry 2:303–312, 1939

57. Sumi SM: Brain malformations in the trisomy 18 syndrome. Brain 93:821–830, 1970

58. Warkany J: Congenital Malformations. Chicago, Year Book Med Publ, 1971, pp. 201–210

59. Warkany J, Passarge E, Smith LB: Congenital malformations in autosomal trisomy syndromes. Am J Dis Child 112:502–517, 1966

60. White LE: A morphologic concept of the limbic lobe. Int Rev Neurobiol 8:1–34, 1965

61. Yakovlev PI: Pathoarchitectonic studies of cerebral malformations. III. Arhinencephalies (Holotelencephalies). J Neuropathol Exp Neurol 18:22–55, 1959

62. Zellweger VH: Kasuistischer Beitrag zum Problem der Cyclencephalie und des congenital single lateral ventricle. Helv Paediatr Acta 7: 98–104, 1952

Rd. 4/18/88

chapter 15

FOREBRAIN CORTEX

NORMAL DEVELOPMENT*

EARLY GENERAL DIFFERENTIATION[6, 46, 73]

The bilateral cerebral vesicles first appear in stage XV (7- to 9-mm CR) as outpocketings of the telencephalon from the region of the foramina of Monro (Fig. 15–1). At this time, the walls of the vesicles are of uniform thickness and are connected in the midline by the lamina terminalis. During stage XVI (8- to 11-mm CR), the cerebral vesicles expand (rostrally, caudally and ventrally), and their walls begin to differentiate in two places: 1) dorsally as the primordium of the hippocampus and 2) ventrally as the primordium of the corpus striatum. The lamina terminalis does not grow and now forms a keel for the bilateral expansion.

In stage XVII (11- to 14-mm CR), there is dorsal expansion such that the top portions of the cerebral vesicles lie slightly above the level of the lamina terminalis. This expansion provides the first indication of the sites of the superior longitudinal fissure and the interventricular foramina of Monro. The areas that will become the frontal and parietal lobes can now be identified, but as yet they have no resemblance to their final form. Increased vascularity on the dorsal–medial wall of each vesicle marks the primordia of the choroid plexuses of the lateral ventricles. Later, in stage XIX (16- to 18-mm CR), the wall indents at this position to form the choroidal fissure. On the ventral aspect of the cerebral vesicle the corpus striatum is

---

* See Chapter 1 for background information on embryologic development and staging system.

---

thickening, and some fibers can be found between it and the thalamus. During stage XIX the occipital pole forms, and in stage XXIII (27- to 31-mm CR) the primoridium of the temporal pole is present.

TELENCEPHALON MEDIUM

By the end of stage XVII (14-mm CR), the region of the lamina terminalis connecting the two cerebral vesicles in the midline is properly termed the *telencephalon medium,* i.e., the structures demarcated by the preoptic recess rostrally and the velum transversum caudally.[46] Early in stage XVIII (13- to 17-mm CR), the telencephalon medium has two subdivisions: 1) rostrally the lamina terminalis and 2) caudally the area choroidea. Each of these can be further subdivided, the lamina terminalis into a thick *pars crassa* and a thin *pars tenuis,* and the area choroidea into the *tela choroidea telencephali medii* and the *paraphyseal arch.* In stage XIX (16- to 18-mm CR), a sharp midline angle, the *angulus terminalis,* forms between the lamina terminalis and the area choroidea. At this time the major components of the telencephalon medium are present. As noted by Hines[46] these are:

Preoptic recess
Lamina terminalis
  Pars crassa
  Pars tenuis
Angulus terminalis
Area choroidea
  Tela choroidea
  Paraphyseal arch
Velum transversum

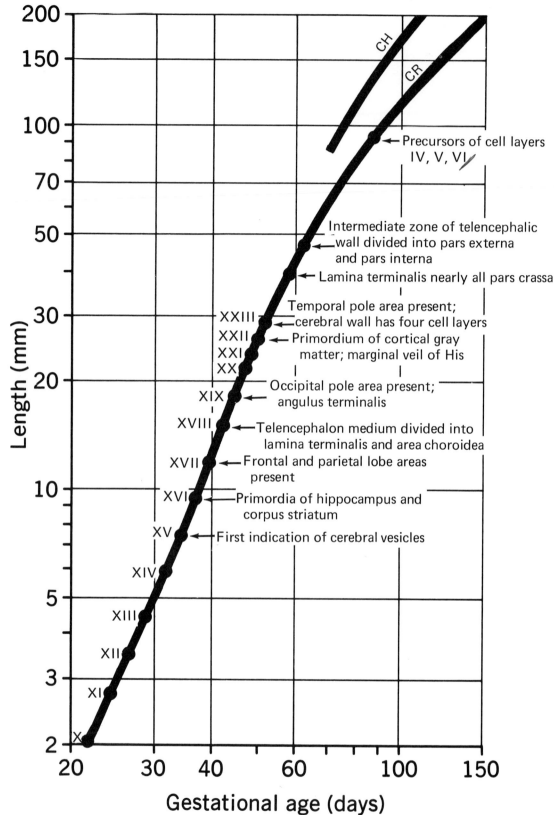

FIG. 15–1. Development of the cerebral cortex correlated with CR length and gestational age

The medial wall of the hemisphere along the area choroidea undergoes further changes. A portion designated as the area intercalata lies opposite the tela choroidea, but neither participates in the formation of the choroid plexus. Instead, just caudal, the paraphyseal arch forms a midline bridge for the lamina epithelialis, which very soon invaginates into the ventricle to begin formation of the choroid plexuses during stage XIX (16- to 18-mm CR). This mechanism forms the choroidal fissure. This fissure differs from the nearby hippocampal fissure (fissura hippocampi), which lies dorsally, by being more extensive and later to develop.[47] By stages XXII and XXIII (23- to 31-mm CR), more changes in the lamina terminalis are apparent.[6, 46] The pars tenuis of the lamina terminalis thickens as the pars crassa encroaches upon it, and the angulus terminalis becomes more obtuse. Ventral to the lamina terminalis, the primordium of the optic chiasm now contains some decussating fibers, and the primordia of the anterior and hippocampal commissures are defined. In an early fetus (40-mm CR length), the lamina terminalis is nearly all pars crassa, while the relationships of the area choroidea are approximately the same as before. The angulus terminalis between these two midline areas becomes less distinct as growth proceeds.

CORPUS STRIATUM

As described in Chapter 12, the primordium of the corpus striatum appears in stage XVI (8- to 11-mm CR) as a thickening of the inferior–lateral wall of the cerebral vesicle. Between it and the developing thalamus is a depression marking the future stria terminalis.[14] The corpus striatum rapidly thickens, and in stage XVII (11- to 14-mm CR) fibers are found between it and the ventral thalamus. During stages XXI and XXII (22- to 28-mm CR), descending fibers of the internal capsule divide the corpus striatum into medial and lateral components. The medial part becomes the caudate nucleus, and the lateral part forms the lentiform nucleus.[44]

The lentiform nucleus subdivides into the globus pallidus, which is derived from a medial lamina of cells (possibly from the hypothalamus, as discussed in Chapter 12), and the putamen, derived from a lateral lamina. These lamina are present by stage XVIII (13- to 17-mm CR), but the identification of the nuclei themselves takes place later—the putamen in stage XXII (23- to 28-mm CR) and the globus pallidus between 70- and 135-mm CR length.[45]

DIFFERENTIATION OF THE CORTICAL SURFACE

The external surface of the postnatal cerebral cortex is marked by numerous grooves (sulci and fissures) bordering the gyri. These grooves develop in a pattern that can serve as an indicator of developmental age (Figs. 15–2 through 15–4).

The formation of sulci and fissures is associated with an increase in the surface area of the cerebrum. Hesdorffer and Scammon[43] measured both total (including the portions buried in the sulci and fissures) and free (visible) surface area in 20 brains ranging in age from the 4th gestational month to the 50th postnatal year. They did not have any cases between the 2nd and 26th year after birth, and there was a marked variability among some cases of comparable ages. Figure 15–5 utilizes some of their points to show quantitatively the difference between the externally visible and buried cerebral surfaces.

CYTOARCHITECTURE

From the time that the bilateral cerebral vesicles first appear in stage XV (7- to 9-mm CR) until stage XVIII (13- to 17-mm CR), the main changes in the cerebral wall are an increase in the thickness of the ependymal zone and a differentiation of the hippocampus and striatal regions. Beginning in stage XVIII (13- to 17-mm CR), the wall begins to differentiate; the ependymal zone can then be subdivided into an inner dense layer of cells and an outer sparse layer, regarded as the mantle layer. Additionally, a small marginal zone is present around the periphery. In stage XXII (25-mm CR), a layer of neuroblasts that has migrated from the ependymal zone into the marginal zone forms the primordium of the cortical gray. This layer, regarded as mainly comprising pyramidal cells, is still bordered externally by a relatively acellular area, now known as the marginal veil of His. By stage XXIII (27- to 31-mm CR) the cerebral wall has four defined layers. From without inward there

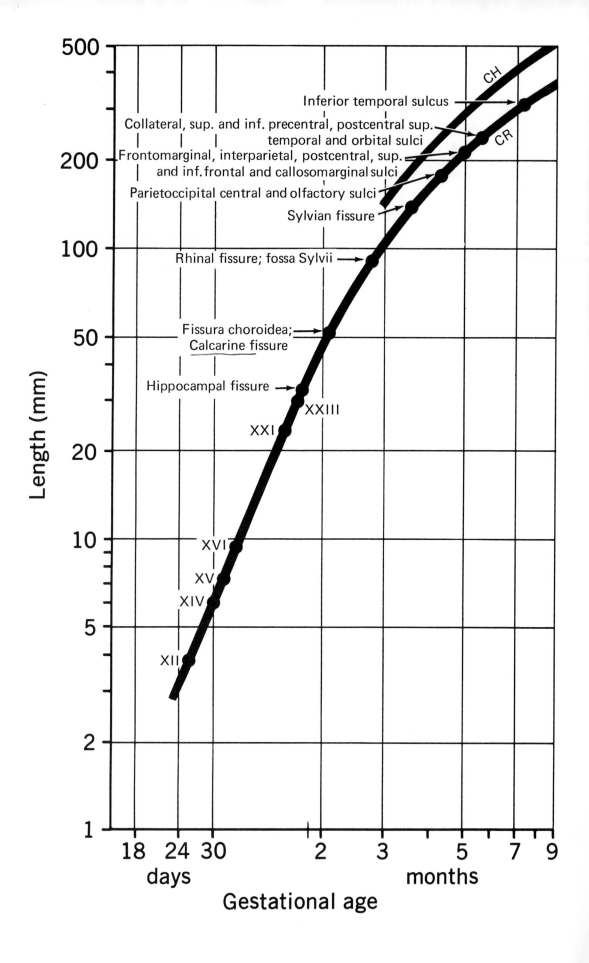

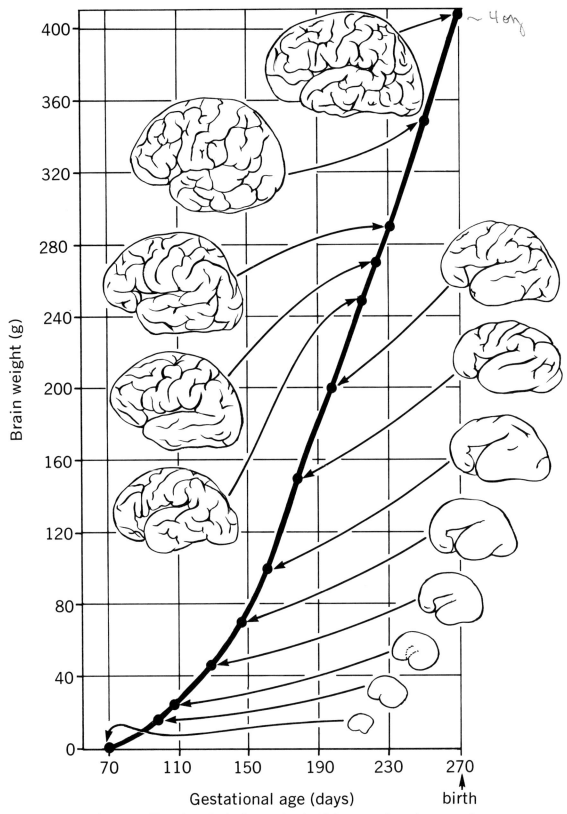

~ 4 on

FIG. 15–3. Development of lateral cerebral sulci correlated with brain weight and gestational age. (Adapted from Larroche, 1966)

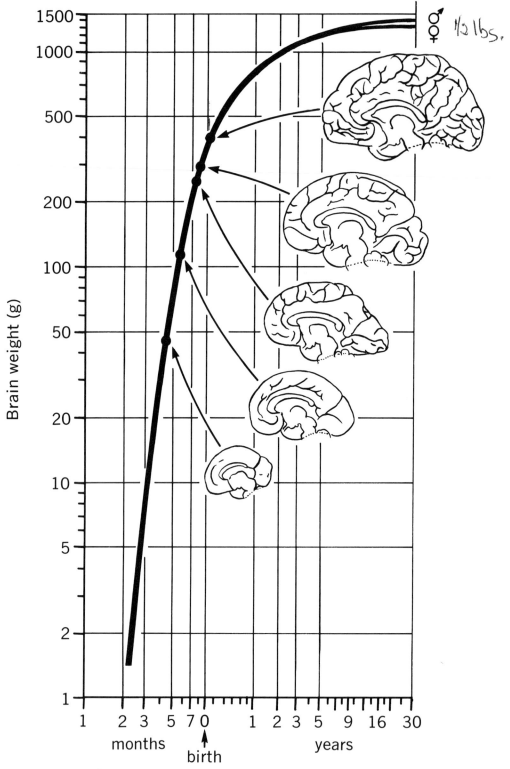

FIG. 15-4. Development of medial cerebral sulci correlated with brain weight and gestational age. (Adapted from Larroche, 1966)

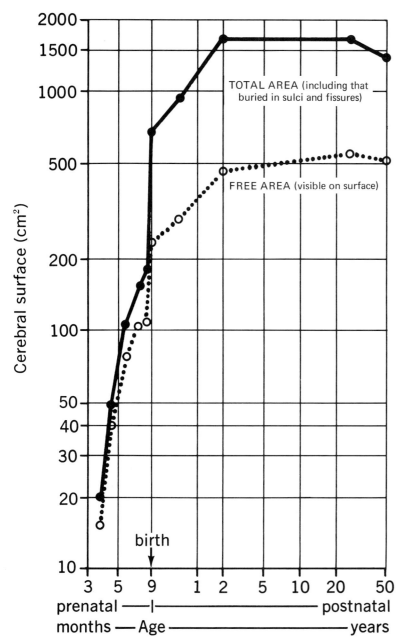

FIG. 15–5. Total surface area of cerebral cortex contrasted with externally visible surface area. After birth, the area buried in sulci and fissures is approximately twice the visible area. (Adapted from Hesdorffer and Scammon, 1935)

is: 1) the marginal veil of His, 2) the layer of cells that has migrated to form the primordium of the cortical cellular layer, 3) an intermediate zone (the mantle layer, which is now gradually widening and has a sparser cellular population) and 4) the innermost ependymal layer from which the cells are continuing to proliferate. By 46-mm CR length the intermediate zone has become quite broad and is subdivided into two layers: 1) the outer, intermediate layer (the pars externa, which consists of fibers from the internal capsule and a few nuclei) and 2) an inner, nuclear portion (the pars in-

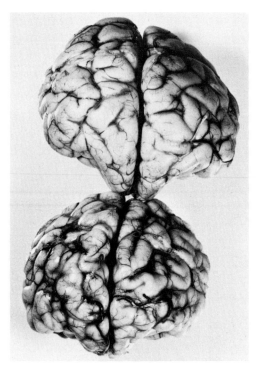

FIG. 15–6.   Mild degree of pachygyria, most prominent in upper portion of specimen. (#TCH-A-59-13)

FIG. 15–7.   Severe degree of diffuse pachygyria with a large central area of agyria from a 7-year-old boy with atonic diplegia and massive spasms. (#D-249) (From Druckman *et al.*, 1959)

terna, which has spongioblasts and neuroblasts)*

When the fetus reaches 80-mm CR length, the cortical layer begins to show signs of differentiation in its deeper portion, close to the pars externa of the intermediate zone* The nature of this change is better characterized at 95-mm CR length, when three layers are noted that are probably the precursors of layers IV, V and VI.[34] Differentiation beyond this time is extremely complex and varies in the different regions of the brain* Streeter[73] states that during the sixth or seventh month of intrauterine life the cells become grouped into the six layers corresponding to those found in the adult cortex. Other studies that expand on the histogenesis of the cerebral cortex during specific periods are those by Streeter,[72] Mellus,[58] Bolton and Moyes,[8] Kershman,[50] Brun,[10] Poliakov,[69] Rabinowicz,[70] Duckett and Pearse[33] and Conel[13]

According to Brun,[10] a subpial layer of granule cells "appears first in the basal allocortex, especially the paleocortex, in the 12th to 13th "foetal week" (*i.e.*, menstrual age, about 70–80 days gestation, corresponding to the 60- to 80-mm CR length, Ed.) by radial migration from the wide periventricular matrix in the telencephalon medium. From the paleocortex it spreads over the cerebral hemispheres, apparently by tangential migration beneath the pial membrane, though it was not possible to rule out spread also by radial migration from the periventricular matrix through the isocortical plate" into the lamina zonalis* This layer of granule cells

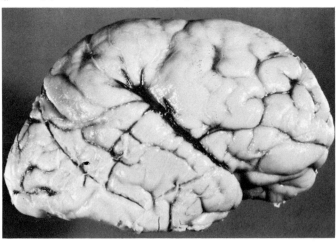

hydramnios –

reaches its maximal width at 22 fetal weeks (menstrual age about 20 weeks gestation, or 200-mm CR length) and then resolves by inward migration of its cells, just as in the development of the cerebellar cortex (see Chapter 10). The resolution largely parallels "the regional maturation of the isocortical plate, as expressed by its cytoarchitectonic differentiation and later by its myelination."

ABNORMAL DEVELOPMENT

PACHYGYRIA AND AGYRIA (LISSENCEPHALY)

Pachygyria refers to a condition in which one or more gyri are abnormally broad (Fig. 15–6). The more extensive the disorder, the fewer the gyri that can be found, until complete agyria results. The associated sulci are wide and shallow and have an abnormal pattern. The usual specimen has pachygyria in some areas and agyria in other areas (Figs. 15–6 to 15–9). Microcephaly is commonly found with pachygyria, but only a small percentage (1.5%) of microcephalic brains have pachygyria.[22] Seizures and mental retardation are frequent.

Histologically, the cortex is thickened, but the volume remains about normal, so that the ratio of gray to white matter is increased.[22, 41] An absolute decrease in the amount of white matter, coupled with the decreased cortical folding, accounts for the shift in this ratio. The claustrum and capsula extrema are usually absent, and there is a diminution (and distortion) of the cellular layers in the cortex (Fig. 15–10). Other changes are common. The substantia nigra has decreased pigmentation. In the cerebellum, which is also small, there is cellular distortion, and the Purkinje and basket cells are sometimes absent, while the molecular layer may have increased cellularity. In the cerebellar white matter there are usually ectopic nodules of cerebellar cortex. The medulla usually has nodules of ectopic inferior olive, and the inferior olivary nucleus itself is small and incomplete. Fibrous gliosis is present in both the brain stem and spinal cord.

Crome[22] believes that the difference between agyria (lissencephaly) and pachygyria is only one of degree since the gray matter is arranged in four layers and the

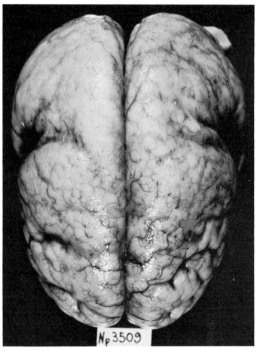

FIG. 15–8. Dorsal view of the brain of a 9-month-old boy who died suddenly, with severe pachygyria and agyria. (#Np 3509)

gray to white ratio increases in both conditions. The four layers are: "1) marginal, containing a slight excess of nerve fibers, 2) superficial cellular, 3) sparsely cellular, containing a large number of tangential and some radial nerve fibers, and 4) deep cellular, formed by nerve cells without definite orientation and a lattice-like network of nerve fibers." It is worth noting that the same four layers generally exist in microgyric cortex. Although the four-layered cortex resembles one of the stages seen in the early fetus, the nature of the layers is slightly different. In general, however, it has been postulated that pachygyria is the result of a failure in the migration of cells that would become the layers of superficial cortex.[41]

Lissencephaly refers to a relatively complete "agyria" in which most of the surface of the brain appears smooth. The pregnancy is frequently complicated by hydramnios, and microcephaly is usually present at birth. Dieker et al.[30] suggest that a characteristic phenotype of dysmorphic facial features permits consideration of a "lissencephaly syndrome," i.e., that the CNS anomaly can be

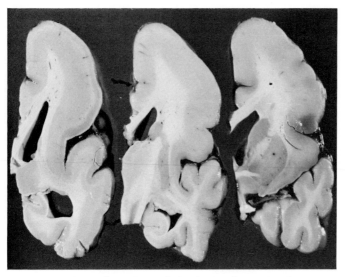

FIG. 15–9. Coronal sections of the brain shown in Fig. 15–7. Note thick agyric central cortex and transition from normal to pachygyric temporal cortex. (From Druckman *et al.*, 1959)

FIG. 15–10. Photomicrograph of the superficial half of the central agyric cortex (lissencephaly) showing a general diminution of cells on the right and an arrangement in vertical columns only in the middle layer. The deep layer of diffuse cells remained the same throughout the unphotographed, deeper half of the agyric cortex. A normal control (full thickness) is on the left. (From Druckman *et al.*, 1959)

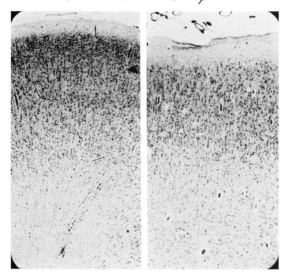

predicted. Autosomal recessive inheritance is suggested in some cases. Most patients with lissencephaly show a marked failure to thrive; there is a high incidence of serious congenital defects of the heart, kidney and eye, and most patients die within the first year. Severe psychomotor retardation is present, and seizures are common. EEG frequently reveals hypsarhythmia.[32]

Wesenberg *et al.*[77] suggest that the following radiographic findings may be helpful in the diagnosis: 1) a small (3-mm) midline

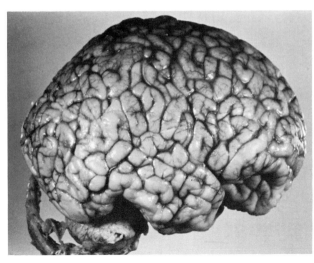

FIG. 15–11.   Lateral view of a brain with generalized mild polymicrogyria, as typically seen in cases with the Arnold–Chiari malformation. (#Np 431)

calcification, thought to lie in the roof of the third ventricle (this was present in Wesenberg's two cases and also in two of four cases reported by Dieker *et al.*[30]); 2) ventricular dilatation most prominently posteriorly, sometimes known as colpocephaly; 3) nodularity in the ventricular walls secondary to heterotopic neurons; 4) cavum septi pellucidi; and 5) arteriographic evidence of a "shallow indentation of the middle cerebral artery at the site of the Sylvian fissure and absence of the Sylvian fissure and absence of the Sylvian point" in addition to other arterial changes.[77]

Neuropathologic examination[27,30,32,37,49,59][74] frequently reveals the presence of a few sulci and fissures, especially at the poles and inferiorly (Sylvian, calcarine, parietooccipital) with the central frontoparietal area of the brain being smooth. The temporal lobe enlarges posteriorly, so that the Sylvian fissure rises at a 45° angle. Overall brain weight may be reduced, but not necessarily.

On coronal sections the affected cortex appears very thick, there is markedly decreased white matter, and the gray–white junction is blurred. The ventricles may be enlarged, and the walls are frequently studded with heterotopic gray matter nodules. A cavum septi pellucidi is common. The corpus callosum may be normal, thin or absent. Myelination may be decreased in all areas. The usual case has very thick cortex,

in four layers as noted above; in many cases there is no definite cortical lamination, while in others (*e.g.*, Miller[59]) some stratification, although abnormal, exists. Walker[74] found a definite increase in the number of blood vessels in the cortex. Druckman *et al.*[32] found increased numbers of oligodendroglia in groups between bundles of myelinated fibers. There may be a lack of development of a subarachnoid space, with a thickened arachnoid being fused with a mass of glia.

The medulla lacks the olivary and pyramidal prominences, and the corticospinal and corticobulbar tracts may show decreased myelination, but the cross-sectional area of the pyramids may be normal.[32] Most striking is the aberrant pattern of the inferior olivary nucleus, which is incomplete, malformed and heterotopic.

The surface of the cerebellum may appear normal, or it may have anomalous folial patterns. The vermis may be normal or dysplastic. The dentate nucleus is usually abnormal, and there is usually a loss of Purkinje cells. Numerous foci of heterotopic cerebellar gray are common.

MICROGYRIA

In microgyria there is a reduction in the size and an increase in the number of the gyri (Figs. 15–11 and 15–12). Some have frontoparietal-temporal gyri in the concentric

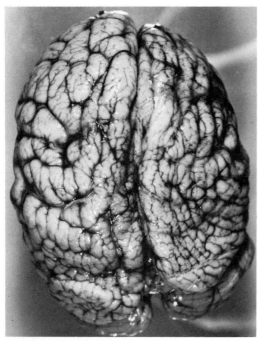

a

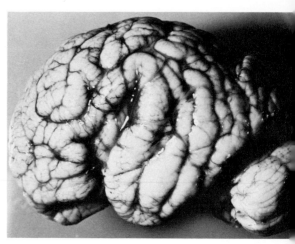

b

FIG. 15–12. **a.** Dorsal view of the brain of a 9-year-old boy with severe microcephaly (700 g) and polymicrogyria. Note the regional differences with the parietooccipital regions being severely involved and a gradation to a more normal pattern frontally (especially on the larger hemisphere). (#Np 2267) **b** and **c.** *Lateral views.* Note the concentric patterns of gyri about the lateral fissures with **b**, general pachygyria of the left hemisphere and **c**, general microgyria of the right hemisphere.

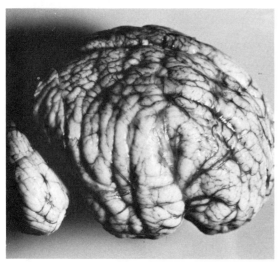

c

horseshoe-shaped pattern characteristic of the cetacean brain (Fig. 15–12 b, c). At least two types must be differentiated. One is a dysplastic malformation without obvious cause, and the other is encephaloclastic, a partial continuation of the growth of obviously damaged cortex; the latter is usually known as sclerotic microgyria or ulegyria (see below). Although there is some variability, the typical microgyric cortex has four

layers.[21] The first layer corresponds to the marginal layer; the second layer is broad and has small round nerve cells in its superficial region, while deeper there are multipolar or pyramidal cells; the third layer is mainly composed of myelinated fibers with sparse cells; the fourth layer has pyramidal and round cells. This histologic pattern of microgyric cortex can also be seen in areas where the gross pattern is not microgyric. Gliosis is frequently found in the subpial area and around the ventricles. There is usually decreased white matter, sometimes containing heterotopic ganglion cells.[75] An alteration in the ganglioside pattern has been reported in microgyric cortex.[38]

In individual brains that do not have generalized microgyria, one or more gyri may be distinctly small. Such is frequently the case of the superior temporal gyrus in Down syndrome (Fig. 15–13).

MISCELLANEOUS GYRAL PATTERNS

In some brains the gyral patterns are abnormal but do not fit the true picture of either pachygyria or microgyria (Fig. 15–14).

BRAIN WARTS

Grcevic and Robert [36] provide an extensive description of the gross and microscopic characteristics of brain warts (also known as *verrucose dysplasia*). These consist of round nodules (up to 5 mm diameter) on the cortical surface that are usually outlined by a groove containing a small blood vessel (Fig. 15–15). The surface of a brain wart is smooth and has the same consistency and color as the surrounding cortex. The overlying pia mater is frequently adherent and thickened. Brain warts can be found associated with normal or microgyric cortex and may occur on the surface or in the depths of sulci.

Depending on the location of the brain wart, three histologic patterns are evident. The superficial nodules have an outer accumulation of ganglion cells of varying shapes. The molecular layer is frequently absent (or thin), and the second and third cellular layers appear to herniate through it. The nodule contains a bundle of aberrant myelinated nerve fibers that originates in the subcortical white, enters the stalk of the nodule where it forms a dense central core and then expands into a brushlike formation at the surface. Within the center of the myelinated nerve stalk is a blood vessel.

A similar but slightly different histologic picture is found in brain warts of an *intracortical* nature, *i.e.*, those that do not protrude beyond the surface. These are also found in normal or microgyric cortex and show a disorganization of cells of the second and third cortical layers. An accumulation of these cells extends to the surface where they are covered by a thin membrane of glia and fibroblasts. The central myelinated bundle is much smaller, and the blood vessel is usually lacking.

A third type of nodule can be found in areas with microgyric cortex. These contain loops of ganglion cells as well as areas lacking any organization. The central radial-oriented bundle of myelinated fibers described above is present in most of these nodules. Superficial cortical vessels are increased in number and size, and some pial vessels are imbedded in the cortex.

Crome[23] found brain warts in a microcephalic brain with ventricular dilatation and shrunken basal ganglia. Only a few central myelinated fibers were found, and the core of the wart consisted predominantly of neurons.

SCHIZENCEPHALY

Yakovlev and Wadsworth[79] contributed greatly to our understanding of diseases of the cerebral mantle (affecting both gray and white matter) when they distinguished between dysplastic and encephaloclastic forms of porencephaly (see below). To avoid confusion, they identified the dysplastic form as schizencephaly. This type appears to have a developmental origin with no evidence of destruction of tissue or gliosis and typically is bilaterally symmetric. The orientation of the cleftlike defect is along a fissure (Fig. 15–16), and the hallmark of schizencephaly is a "piaependymal seam." In two later articles, Yakovlev and Wadsworth[80, 81] further define the morphology of schizencephaly depending on whether or not the clefts have fused lips or separated lips. In cases with fused lips, the ventricular system may be slightly enlarged, with most of the enlargement occurring in the occipital horns of the lateral ventricles; this is not considered a true hydrocephalus, but rather colpocephaly, and is believed to result from an abnormal continuation of normal embryonic and fetal ventricular dilatation. In cases with separated lips, marked hydrocephalus is present.

Other CNS malformations associated with schizencephaly include heterotopic nodules of gray matter within the white matter, absence of the corpus callosum and septum pellucidum, enlargement of the corpus striatum and atrophy of the lateral geniculate bodies.

Unfortunately not all cases of schizencephaly have a piaependymal seam (*e.g.*, Cohn and Neumann[12]). The variability of these defects is further described in articles by Dekaban[28] and Norman *et al.*[63] and illustrated in Fig. 15–17.

OTHER ABNORMALITIES OF THE DEVELOPING CEREBRAL CORTEX

As we have illustrated throughout this book, not all abnormalities of the developing brain can be considered malformations. As evidence of destruction of previously formed

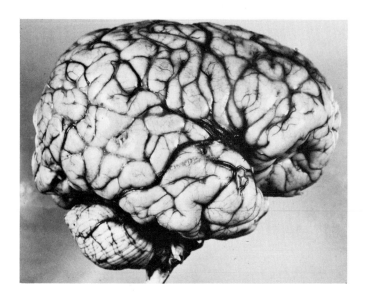

FIG. 15–13

FIG. 15–14

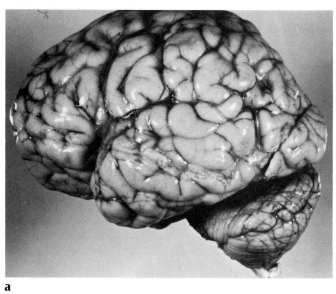

a

b

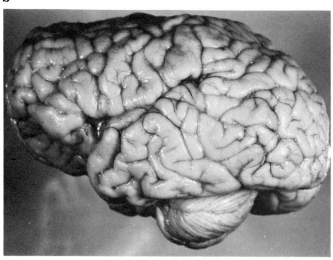

FIG. 15–13. Lateral view of the brain of a 10-year-old boy with Down's syndrome showing the typical small superior temporal gyrus. (#Np 779)

FIG. 15–14. **a.** Lateral view of the brain of a 7-year-old girl with normal mental development but with an abnormally simple gyral pattern. This is not truly pachygyria but resembles it in several areas. (#Np 387) **b.** Lateral view of the brain of an 8-month-old boy with multiple congenital anomalies including arhinencephaly and a somewhat jumbled abnormal gyral pattern. (#Np 835)

FIG. 15–15. **a.** Surface of the brain of a 4-year-old normally developed boy with multiple brain warts. One is present in the center of the photo (*arrow*). (#Np 856) **b.** Coronal section of the brain shown in 15–15**a** demonstrating a brain wart (*arrow*)

tissue and reactions of the surviving cellular elements is recognized in any particular case, one is justified in classifying that case as due to an acquired encephaloclastic process. Without such evidence we tend to classify the disease as a dysplastic process, but such a classification must contain at least some errors, since the distinction may be arbitrarily resting only on two temporal factors, *i.e.*, if a destructive process occurs before there are any astrocytes to react to form gliosis, and if sufficient time elapses for absorption of the debris before our examination of the specimen, we may be misled into believing that the etiologic agent was not acquired but was erroneously built into the planning of the "dysplastic" lesions discussed above.

Be that as it may, there are many cases in which the lesion was obviously acquired,

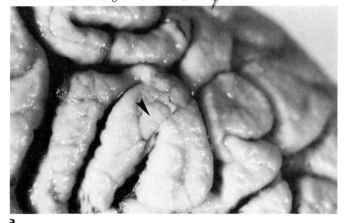

a

b

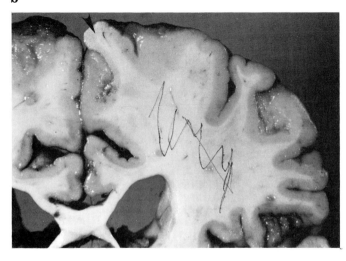

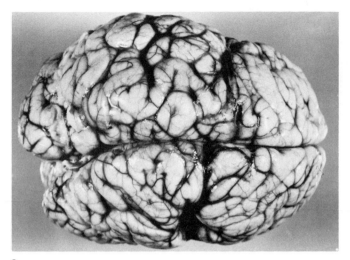

FIG. 15–16

a

b

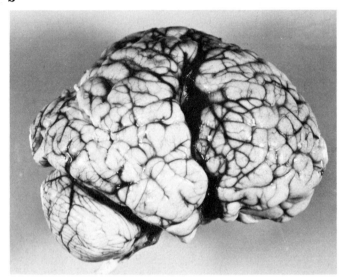

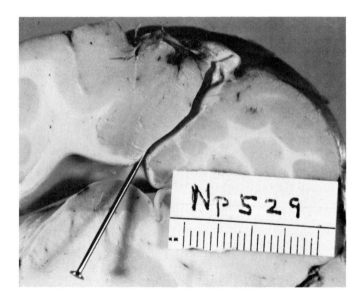

FIG. 15–17

FIG. 15–16. **a.** Dorsal view of the brain of a 10-month-old markedly retarded boy with bilateral but slightly asymmetric clefts, the wider one (right) communicating with the ventricle (as in porencephaly). The narrower one (left) resembles schizencephaly. (#Np 2210) **b.** Lateral view of the same brain with porencephaly or schizencephaly.

FIG. 15–17. A schizencephaly-like cleft with lips separated occurring within large subcortical heterotopias in a 2-year-old boy who developed hydrocephalus following neonatal Pseudomonas meningitis. He was severely retarded mentally and physically and died of acute hydrocephalus in spite of a ventriculoatrial shunt which had been inserted at age 5 months. The "pia-ependymal membrane" fusing with the molecular layer of the cortex and the cleft itself are unusual in being lined not by ependyma but by gliotic white matter continuous with the subependymal glia. On the opposite side were similar masses of heterotopic gray matter without a cleft (*i.e.*, schizencephaly with lips fused). (#Np 529)

encephaloclastic, with obvious secondary gliosis, but with varying degrees of continued growth of the partially damaged cells at the margin of the lesion. These lesions are heterogeneous but very significant because of their frequent association with mental retardation, epilepsy and "cerebral palsy." The lesions may range from focal cortical lesions, such as ulegyria, to the widespread cerebral damage characteristic of the walnut brain or of multiple cystic encephalomalacia. The perinatal encephaloclastic processes are as follows:

I. Focal cortical atrophy and scarring
      (ulegyria, atrophic sclerosis, sclerotic microgyria, nodular cortical sclerosis)
II. Diffuse cerebral cortical atrophy
      (walnut brain)
III. Multicystic encephalomalacia
      (pseudocystic brain, polyporencephaly, central porencephaly)
IV. Related disorders
      (porencephaly, hydranencephaly)
V. Associated lesions
      status marmoratus, état fibreux (see Chapter 12)

Most appear to be related to perinatal asphyxia, but the role of other factors—including impaired arterial circulation, impaired venous drainage, hypotension, brain swelling, or viral infections—has not been resolved.[15, 18, 19, 20, 56, 61] Some, such as porencephaly, may be related to infectious processes.[64, 65] Part of the problem of understanding the pathogenesis of these lesions results from the difficulty in establishing in retrospect 1) the exact nature of the insult (*e.g.*, hypoxia, hypotension, alone or combined, infection or other process), 2) the severity or degree of the insult, 3) the rapidity of onset of the insult, 4) the duration of the insult, and 5) the age of the infant at the time of the insult. Obviously, the permutations are great enough to provide theoretical explanations for the variety of lesions seen.

ULEGYRIA (SCLEROTIC MICROGYRIA)

The best example of these encephaloclastic processes is ulegyria (lobar sclerosis or sclerotic microgyria). According to Courville,[19] who has reviewed the entire category of brain damage secondary to birth injury in great detail, ulegyria is a restricted variety of cortical nodular sclerosis, which he defines as an irregular shrinkage or atrophy of limited portions of the cerebral cortex. Typically, most of the destruction of the cortex is buried in the depth of the sulci. The crests of the gyri are relatively spared, appearing as mushroom-like caps over the severely gliotic core of each gyrus (Fig. 15–18). Acute lesions of the same pattern may be seen in infants dying near term (Fig. 15–19).

Courville[19] restricts ulegyria to lesions involving the dorsolateral aspect of the frontal and/or parietooccipital cortex in a watershed distribution typical of hypoperfusion, but allows nodular cortical sclerosis to be focal, multifocal or generalized, unilateral or bilateral. We see no particular value in using such distinctions. Typical distributions also include the upper central area, as in Little disease, with spastic paraplegia, and a more extensive central lesion, often bilateral and symmetrical.

Generalized ulegyria can be found in progressive degeneration of the cerebral cortex, a lesion which appears to begin postnatally and progresses to a walnut brain (see below).[53]

As shown in Fig. 15–18, the postulated hypoxia may be less severe at sites not showing ulegyria, instead showing only an arrest of development recognized as hemiatrophy or hemihypoplasia. Without microscopic

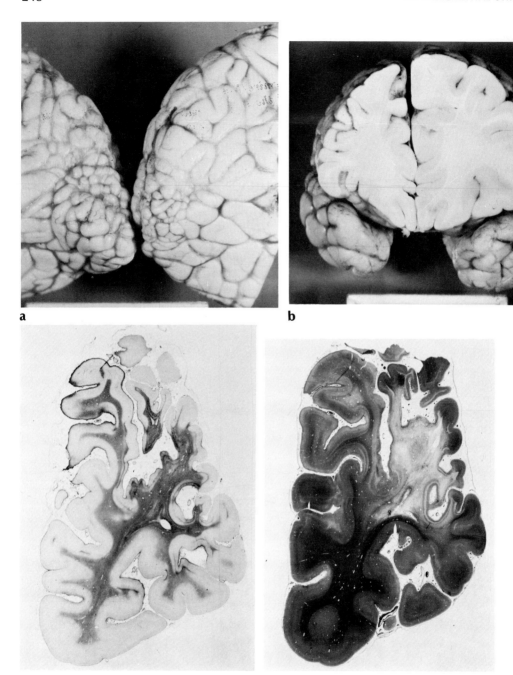

FIG. 15–18. **a.** Ulegyria (sclerotic microgyria) of both occipital lobes from a 10-year-old microcephalic boy with a 6-year history of epilepsy. **b.** The right cerebral hemisphere is smaller than the left (hemiatrophy), but the whole brain is smaller than normal, weighing only 870 g. **c** and **d.** Low-power photomicrographs of the ulegyric occipital lobe stained by Holzer and myelin sheath techniques. Note the severe destruction of the cerebral cortex at the depths of the sulci with relative preservation of the crests of the gyri which create the microgyria shown in **a. e** and **f.** Low-power photomicrographs of the right superior frontal region stained by Holzer and myelin sheath techniques. Note the similar pattern of the gliotic process accompanying a less severe destruction of the hemiatrophic cortex. (#D-218)

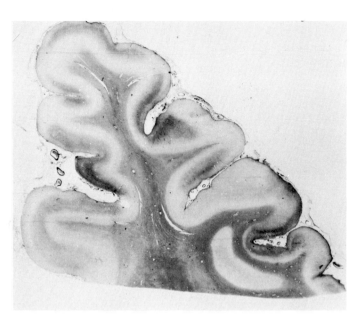

e

f

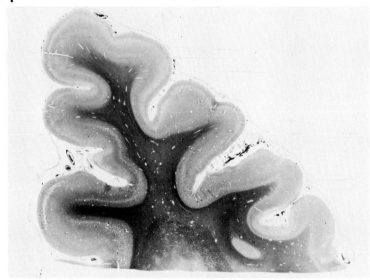

demonstration of the gliosis in the typical pattern, worse at the depths of sulci, one could erroneously regard this as a dysplastic process.

In brains with ulegyria there may be other subcortical lesions, such as status marmoratus,[9] which was present in 4 of 7 cases of ulegyria in our files and was not associated with ulegyria in an additional 10 cases (see Chapter 12).

WALNUT BRAIN AND ALPERS DISEASE

There are an increasing number of cases characterized by a uniform severe atrophy of the brain secondary to a diffuse neuronal necrosis of the cerebral cortex. Often necrosis occurs in a laminar pattern, and there may be striking gliosis, vascular proliferation and microcystic alterations. The basal ganglia frequently show similar changes, as do

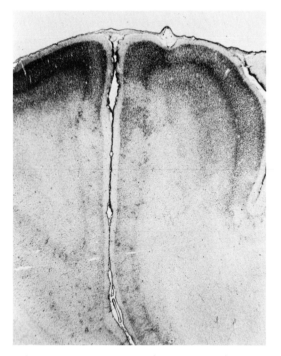

FIG. 15–19. Low-power photomicrograph of a Nissl-stained section of the occipital cortex from a neonate who survived only 44 hours. Note the acute selective neuronal necrosis in the same pattern as shown in Fig. 15–18. (#D-409)

the substantia nigra and occasionally, the cerebellum. Clinically, many cases have had onset during the first postnatal year, frequently near birth, with subsequent mental deterioration, spasticity, seizures, myoclonus, blindness and deafness. Characteristically the disease is progressive to death in months or a few years.

Such cases have been published under a variety of terms, including progressive cerebral degeneration of infancy (Alpers[3,4]), poliodystrophia cerebri progressiva (Christensen and Krabbe[11]), poliodysplasia cerebri (Kramer[51]), familial diffuse progressive encephalopathy (Liu and Sylvester[55]), Alpers disease (Blackwood *et al.*[7]), progressive poliodystrophy (Dreifuss and Netsky[31]) and walnut brain (Courville,[16] Laurence and Cavanagh[53]). The last term (Fig. 15–20) emphasizes the severe degree of cortical convolutional atrophy that can be obtained. Although grouped here for purposes of discussion, there is no agreement that the reported cases constitute a nosologic entity, and a variety of etiologic possibilities

exist, including especially a slow virus infection such as occurs in the histologially similar Jakob–Creutzfeldt disease, which is usually considered to occur only in adults/

Anoxia has been emphasized as a cause of walnut brain,[16] for cases with diffuse softening of the gray matter but with less severe cortical atrophy,[17] and for cases with even less striking cortical alterations.[2] However, there is frequently little clinical evidence for an asphyxial episode—and even in some considered anoxic in origin, other members of the family were involved.[2,16] Many are clearly familial[7,53,55] which suggests a possible metabolic disorder. Epileptic seizures have also been emphasized as a possible cause with concomitant hypoxia, but in some cases seizures were never present,[11] or developed only after the onset of the disease process.[53] Many cases represent sporadic occurrences[3,11,31,51] in which a common etiologic factor is difficult to discover/

FIG. 15–20. Dorsal view of a walnut brain *in situ*. This was a 10-month-old girl who appeared normal for the first 2 months but then failed to smile or grasp objects. She developed spasticity and microcephaly (35 cm OFC at 7 months) with attacks of sweating, tachycardia and opisthotonos which were not controlled by various drugs. The case has been described in detail (Case 1 [53]), and the photograph was provided by Dr. KM Lawrence, to whom we are greatly indebted/

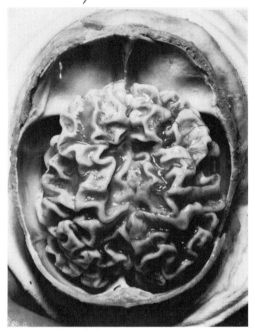

HYDRANENCEPHALY AND PORENCEPHALY

In hydranencephaly all or nearly all of the telencephalon is absent. Usually this clearly results from the destruction of previously formed brain. Within the skull there is a fluid-filled cavity surrounded by leptomeninges, usually with a gliotic molecular layer and sometimes with small islands of partly preserved cerebral cortex (Figs. 15–21 and 15–22). If any cortex persists, it is usually inferior temporal and occipital. The deep cerebral nuclei are usually partially destroyed, especially the striatum, but the diencephalon is usually somewhat better preserved and the midbrain, cerebellum, hindbrain and cranial nerves are usually normal except for the atrophy of various descending tracts.[26, 40]

Clinically the child may appear normal at birth and for several months thereafter, especially if the hypothalamus is intact. If not, the infant may die in a few days. In some cases abnormal head enlargement may become apparent after several weeks or months. The diagnosis is easily made by transillumination of the skull (Fig. 15–22c), and EEG usually shows an absence of electric activity. Optic atrophy may be present. Neurologic examination varies, but irritability, hyperreflexia and clonus are common. The Moro reflex is usually absent; response to painful stimuli is usually present, and the diagnosis can hardly be suspected on the basis of the neurologic findings themselves.

Hydranencephaly has occurred in consecutive pregnancies[40] and in twins,[42] but it usually presents as an isolated case. Environmental insults have been described in pregnancies that have resulted in a child with hydranencephaly. These include syphilis, toxoplasmosis, influenza, attempted abortion, anoxia and trauma.[24] Postnatal onset has been reported,[54, 76] but the lesion is clearly less severe than in those developing prenatally. There is no single etiologic agent, be it genetic or environmental, but the usual pattern of destruction suggests bilateral carotid artery insufficiency with preservation of the vertebrobasilar circulation. This hypothesis has some experimental evidence to support it.[24] Halsey et al.[39] relate the pathogenesis of hydranencephaly to a variety of processes that can reduce cerebral mass (e.g., vascular lesions, multiple cystic encephalomalacia, schizencephaly). A spectrum of anomalies from hydranencephaly to porencephaly has been produced in offspring of pregnant sheep vaccinated with live bluetongue virus at different stages in gestation.[64, 65] The brain destruction could be secondary to the virus acting on the vascular system. Muir[60] believes that hydranencephaly and porencephaly fall within the same spectrum of encephaloclastic disorders, and we agree that most such cases are similar, the usual porencephaly being restricted to the distribution of the middle cerebral artery.

Pathologically the nature of the membrane within the skull is critical in separating hydranencephaly from severe hydrocephaly. In the former the leptomeninges are lined internally by a layer of glial tissue (the remains of the molecular layer of the cortex) that has no ependyma, whereas in hydrocephaly there is always a greater preservation of the cerebral cortex, usually preservation also of the subcortical white matter, and ependyma may even remain in some areas.[26] Choroid plexus may be found floating within the cystic space. Other associated lesions include aqueductal stenosis (Fig. 7–7) and chorioretinitis.

Reviews of earlier studies and theories of the etiology of porencephaly are given by Globus,[35] Jaffe[48] and Patten et al.[66] In 1859, Herschl coined the term porencephalus to include those cavities within the cerebral hemispheres which communicate with either the ventricular or subarachnoid space or with both.[35] Confusion is increased if within such a broad definition are included cases with any hole within the wall of the cerebral hemisphere, whether communicating or not with the ventricular or subarachnoid space. Prenatal, natal and postnatal insults of many types can produce these holes. Trauma, vascular or infectious disorders would be especially common. Examples of porencephaly are shown in Figures 15–23 and 15–24.

As noted above, Yakovlev and Wadsworth[79] provide considerable clarification by subdividing cases of porencephaly into encephaloclastic and dysplastic types, the former occurring secondary to hemorrhage, infarction, inflammation or degenerative processes. These processes can have their onset during the fetal period, at birth or after birth; the lesions arise primarily as a

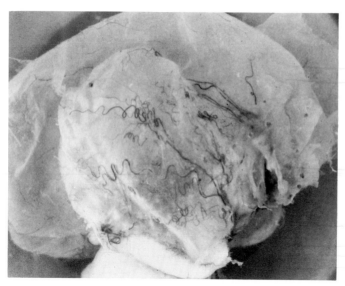

FIG. 15–21. Thin membrane surrounding a fluid-filled cavity in hydranencephaly. Note the middle cerebral artery branches. (#MCV A-206-66) Courtesy of Dr. Margaret Jones.

FIG. 15–22. **a.** Hydranencephaly in a 10-month-old girl. The membrane has been opened to reveal remnants of the brain as viewed from above. The two oval masses in the upper midline are the corpora striata. Remnants of the occipital cortex can be seen below. (#Np 2907) **b.** The membrane has been trimmed to reveal a portion of the normal cerebellum. **c.** Lateral view of the transilluminated head. The flashlight is being held on the opposite side, and light transmitted through the fluid-filled cranial cavity.

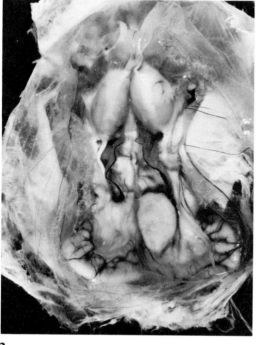

a

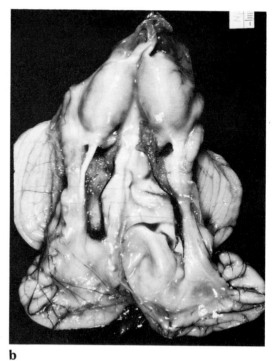

b

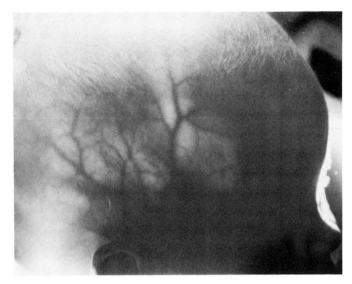

c

result of necrotic softening and destruction of brain wall. Microscopic examination reveals the proliferation of astrocytes and blood vessels around the edge of the defect. Such lesions can be unilateral but are more commonly bilateral but at least slightly asymetric in both position and degree of severity. When encephaloclastic porencephaly is associated with moderate hydrocephalus, a cone-shaped defect passes through the cortex and white matter, whereas in cases with severe hydrocephalus the lesion has a pouched-out appearance. Regardless of the age at onset, a loss of nerve cells, myelinated nerve fibers and ependyma is typical, as is ulegyria (sclerotic microgyria) at the edges of the defect, especially if the onset is prenatal. Another characteristic of encephaloclastic porencephaly is that it is not commonly associated with other CNS malformations or with malformations of other organs. Encephaloclastic porencephaly

FIG. 15–23. Lateral view of brain from a markedly retarded, spastic 4-year-old boy with bilateral large porencephalic defects. (#Np 583)

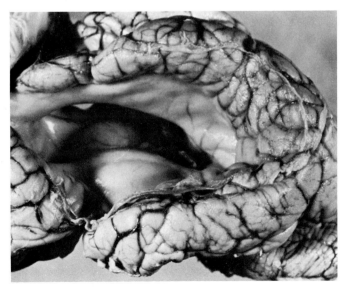

FIG. 15–24

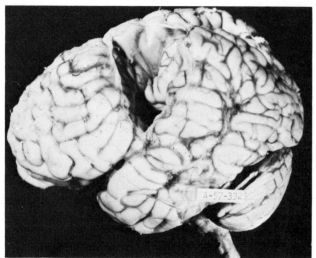

a

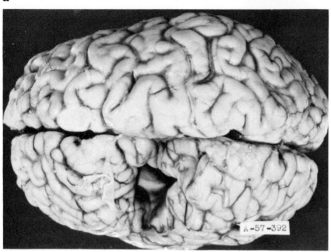

b

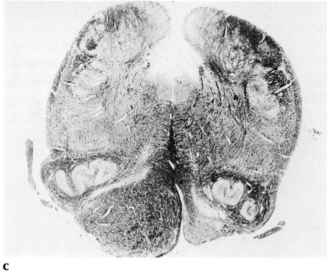

c

◄ FIG. 15–24. **a.** Lateral view of the brain of a 55-year-old hemiparetic woman with a unilateral moderate-sized porencephalic defect./(#D 550) **b.** Dorsal view of the same brain with unilateral porencephaly. **c.** Cross section of the medulla of the same brain showing marked atrophy of the left pyramidal tract (2.98 sq mm). The right pyramid is twice the normal size (20.76 sq mm, c.f., Fig. 3–7)/

has been found in association with cytomegalic inclusion disease[62] and is known to occur secondary to needle tracks passing through the cerebral mantle.[78]

MULTICYSTIC ENCEPHALOMALACIA

Aicardi *et al.*[1] have recently reviewed the subject of multicystic encephalomalacia, in which there are multiple cavities in the cerebral hemispheres/ This condition seems to occur more frequently in twins/

MULTIPLE CEREBRAL CYSTS

Cysts of various types may be found in different sites as incidental findings at autopsy (Fig. 15–25), but more commonly they are associated with epilepsy, mental retardation and hydrocephalus/[71]

INTRACRANIAL CALCIFICATIONS

A great variety of intracranial calcifications occurs, usually involving telencephalic structures, largely because of the greater mass of the telencephalon. Most such calcifications are secondary to other disease processes, as summarized in Table 15–1.[5, 29, 57, 67, 68] Rarely ossification occurs.[29] Most are not associated with entities that can be considered *developmental anomalies*. In cytomegalic inclusion disease, a subependymal periventricular calcific cast can be found in many cases several months after birth, but diagnosis has usually been suspected from other findings prior to recognition of the calcification (see Chapter 23). The calcifications of toxoplasmosis usually appear as dense, round foci scattered in the periventricular white matter, basal ganglia and elsewhere. A small midline calcification along the roof of the third ventricle is found in some cases of lissencephaly and may be of diagnostic help. Intracranial calcification is common in tuberous sclerosis, usually being found in discrete nodules along the roof of the lateral ventricle. Widespread punctate calcifications are found in idiopathic familial cerebrovascular ferrocalcinosis.[5] Choroid plexus papillomas, tera-

FIG. 15–25. Small cyst, 2.5 cm diameter, lined by glial tissue and arising from the fimbria of the fornix. This was an incidental finding at autopsy of a one-year-old boy/(#Np 1118)

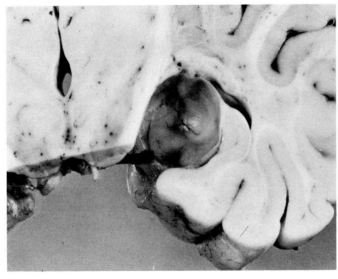

TABLE 15–1. INTRACRANIAL CALCIFICATIONS

Etiology	Site(s) and/or Characteristics of Calcification
Normal	
Pineal gland	Usually calcifies in adolescent years
Choroid plexus	Lateral ventricles; rare in third and fourth; common in adults
Falx cerebri	Found in 7% of adults; uncommon in children
Tentorium cerebelli	Outer margins in some adults
Diaphragma sellae	
Petroclinoid ligaments	
Arachnoid granulations	After middle age
Habenular commissure	C-shaped on anterior margin
Infections	
Cytomegalovirus	Periventricular, subependymal casts
Toxoplasmosis	Periventricular, dense, round foci; also basal ganglia (curvilinear)
Cryptococcosis	Surface of brain, faint and punctate; some curvilinear
Echinococcosis	Parietooccipital region, large (several centimeters) round cysts
Cysticercosis	Disseminated foci of punctate calcifications
Trichinosis	Widespread, punctate (1–2 mm) or ovoid (5–7 mm)
Paragonimiasis	Rare
Coccidioidomycosis	Rare
Tuberculosis	Rare: small nodular intracerebral foci; large (1–3 cm) deposits with irregular margins; small suprasellar plaques (basal cisterns)
Herpes simplex	Rare
Syphilis	Rare: wavy peripheral densities separated from a central nucleus (gumma)
Abscess	Rare
Malformations/Syndromes	
Tuberous sclerosis	Subcortical white, along roof of lateral ventricle; punctate or high-density lesions with irregular margins
Lissencephaly	Anterior roof of third ventricle; punctate (1–3 mm)
Idiopathic Familial Cerebrovascular Ferrocalcinosis	Disseminated; punctate
Sturge–Weber	Parietooccipital region; hairpin loops parallel to sulci
Vascular	
Aneurysms	Location depends on vessel involved; microscopic calcification occurs in 85% but is radiographically seen in only 15%
Angiomas	Rare
Arteriovenous fistulas	Variable
Subdural hematoma	Elliptic or wedge-shaped shadow with irregular outline over cerebral cortex
Intracerebral hematoma	Rare: dense mass of calcium
Arteriosclerosis	Plaques along vessels
Neoplasms	
Meningioma	Various sites and characteristics
Gliomas	Various sites and characteristics
Medulloblastoma	Rare: roof of fourth ventricle
Pinealoma (teratoma)	"Ball of thread"
Craniopharyngioma	Variable patterns of supracellar calcification
Chromophobe adenoma	Rare
Chordoma	Around clivus; large, grossly nodular densities
Lipoma	Corpus callosum most common; curvilinear streaks in shape of parenthesis
Choroid plexus papilloma	Rare
Endocrine	
Hypoparathyroidism	Basal ganglia and/or dentate nucleus of cerebellum; granular or dense, homogeneous shadows
Hyperparathyroidism	Basal ganglia; meninges and falx occasionally
Miscellaneous	
Radiation	Rare
Idiopathic basal ganglia calcification	Basal ganglia; dentate nucleus
Hypervitaminosis D	Meninges and falx
Carbon monoxide	Rare
Lead	Rare
Leptomeningeal cysts	Rare

tomas and craniopharyngiomas are examples of intracranial neoplasms that frequently calcify but would rarely enter into the differential diagnosis of the calcifications discussed above.

REFERENCES

1. Aicardi J, Goutières F, Hodebourg DeVerbois A: Multicystic encephalomalacia of infants and its relation to abnormal gestation and hydranencephaly. J Neurol Sci 15:357–373, 1972

2. Alberca-Serrano R, Fabiani F, Deneve V, Mecken J: Familial spastic diplegia due to anoxic encephalopathy (Alpers). J Neurol Sci 2:419–433, 1965

3. Alpers BJ: Diffuse progressive degeneration of the gray matter of the cerebrum. Arch Neurol Psychiatr 25:469–505, 1931

4. Alpers BJ: Progressive cerebral degeneration of infancy. J Nerv Ment Dis 130:442–448, 1960

5. Babbitt DP, Tang T, Dobbs J, Berk R: Idiopathic familial cerebrovascular ferrocalcinosis (Fahr's disease) and review of differential diagnosis of intracranial calcification in children. Am J Roentgenol Radium Ther Nucl Med 105:352–358, 1969

6. Bartelmez GW, Dekaban AS: The early development of the human brain. Contrib Embryol 37:13–32, 1962

7. Blackwood W, Buxton PH, Cumings JN, Robertson DJ, Tucker SM: Diffuse cerebral degeneration in infancy (Alpers disease). Arch Dis Child 38:193–204, 1963

8. Bolton JS, Moyes JM: The cytoarchitecture of the cerebral cortex of a human foetus of 18 weeks. Brain 35:1–25, 1912

9. Borit A, Herndon RM: The fine structure of plaques fibromyelinques in ulegyria and in status marmoratus. Acta Neuropathol 14:304–311, 1970

10. Brun A: The subpial granular layer of the foetal cerebral cortex in man: its ontogeny and significance in congenital cortical malformations. Acta Pathol Microbiol Scand [Suppl] 179:1–98, 1965

11. Christensen A, Krabbe KH: Poliodystrophia cerebri progressiva (infantilis). Arch Neurol Psychiatr 61:28–43, 1949

12. Cohn R, Neumann MA: Porencephaly. A clinicopathologic study. J Neuropathol Exp Neurol 5:257–270, 1946

13. Conel JL: The Postnatal Development of the Human Cerebral Cortex (7 vols). Cambridge, Harvard Univ Press, 1939–1963

14. Cooper ERA: Development of human red nucleus and corpus striatum. Brain 69:34–44, 1946

15. Courville CB: The pathogenesis of nodular cortical atrophy. Bull Los Angeles Neurol Soc 22:120–130, 1957

16. Courville CB: Etiology and pathogenesis of laminar cortical necrosis. Arch Neurol Psychiatr 79:17–30, 1958

17. Courville CB: Widespread softening of the cerebral gray matter in infancy. Bull Los Angeles Neurol Soc 25:72–87, 1960

18. Courville CB: Pathogenesis of nodular atrophy of the cerebral cortex. Arch Pediatr 77:101–129, 1960

19. Courville CB: Birth and Brain Damage. Pasadena, Calif, Margaret Farnsworth Courville (Publisher), 1971

20. Courville CB, Marsh C: Neonatal asphyxia. Bull Los Angeles Neurol Soc 9:121–135, 1944

21. Crome L: Microgyria. J Pathol Bacteriol 64:479–495, 1952.

22. Crome L: Pachygyria. J Pathol Bacteriol 71:335–352, 1956

23. Crome L: Brain warts. J Ment Defic Res 13:60–65, 1969

24. Crome L: Hydrencephaly. Dev Med Child Neurol 14:224–234, 1972

25. Crome L, Stern J: The Pathology of Mental Retardation. London, J & A Churchill, Ltd, 1967

26. Crome L, Sylvester PE: Hydranencephaly (hydrencephaly). Arch Dis Child 33:235–245, 1958

27. Daube JR, Chou SM: Lissencephaly: two cases. Neurology (Minneap) 16:179–191, 1966

28. Dekaban A: Large defects in cerebral hemispheres associated with cortical dysgenesis. J Neuropathol Exp Neurol 24:512–530, 1965

29. Dennis JP, Alvord EC Jr: Microcephaly with intracranial calcification and subependymal ossification: radiologic and clinico-pathologic correlation. J Neuropathol Exp Neurol 20:412–426, 1961

30. Dieker H, Edwards RH, Zu Rhein G, Chou SM, Hartman HA, Opitz JM: The lissencephaly syndrome. Birth Defects 5:53–64, 1969

31. Dreifuss FE, Netsky MG: Progressive poliodystrophy. Am J Dis Child 107:649–656, 1964

32. Druckman R, Chao D, Alvord EC Jr: A case of atonic cerebral diplegia with lissencephaly. Neurology (Minneap) 9:806–814, 1959

33. Duckett S, Pearse AGE: The cells of Cajal–Retzius in the developing human brain. J Anat 102:183–187, 1968

34. Fitz-Gerald PAMF: Defective development of the cerebral cortex involving symmetrical bilateral areas. Contrib Embryol 28:193–217, 1940

35. Globus JH: A contribution to the histopathology of porencephalus. Arch Neurol Psychiatr 6:652–668, 1921

36. Grcevic N, Robert F: Verrucose dysplasia of the cerebral cortex. J Neuropathol Exp Neurol 20:399–411, 1961

37. Greenfield JG, Wolfsohn JM: Microcephalia vera: a study of two brains illustrating the agyric form and the complex microgyric form. Arch Neurol Psychiatr 33:1296–1316, 1935

38. Haberland C, Brunngraber E: Micropolygyria: a histopathological and biochemical study. J Ment Defic Res 16:1–6, 1972

39. Halsey JH Jr, Allen N, Chamberlin HR: The morphogenesis of hydranencephaly. J Neurol Sci 12:187–217, 1971

40. Hamby WB, Krauss RF, Beswick WF: Hydranencephaly: clinical diagnosis. Presentation of seven cases. Pediatrics 6:371–383, 1950

41. Hanaway J, Lee SI, Netsky MG: Pachygyria: relation of findings to modern embryologic concepts. Neurology (Minneap) 18:791–799, 1968

42. Haque IU, Glassauer FE: Hydranencephaly in twins. NY State J Med 69:1210–1214, 1969

43. Hesdorffer MB, Scammon RE: Growth of human nervous system. I. Growth of cerebral surface. Proc Soc Exp Biol Med 33:415–418, 1935

44. Hewitt W: The development of the human caudate and amygdaloid nuclei. J Anat 92:377–382, 1958

45. Hewitt W: The development of the human internal capsule and lentiform nucleus. J Anat 95:191–199, 1961

46. Hines M: Studies in the growth and differentiation of the telencephalon in man. The fissura hippocampi. J Comp Neurol 34:73–171, 1922

47. Humphrey T: The development of the human hippocampal fissure. J Anat 101:655–676, 1967

48. Jaffe RH: Traumatic porencephaly. Arch Pathol 8:787–799, 1929

49. Josephy H: Congenital agyria and defect of corpus callosum. J Neuropathol Exp Neurol 3:63–68, 1944

50. Kershman J: Genesis of microglia in the human brain. Arch Neurol Psychiatr 41:24–50, 1939

51. Kramer W: Poliodysplasia cerebri. Acta Psychiatr Scand 28:413–427, 1953

52. Larroche JC: Development of the nervous system in early life. Part II: The development of the central nervous system during intrauterine life. In Human Development. Edited by F Falkner. Philadelphia, WB Saunders, 1966, pp. 257–276

53. Laurence KM, Cavanagh JB: Progressive degeneration of the cerebral cortex in infancy. Brain 91:261–280, 1968

54. Lindenberg R, Swanson PD: Infantile hydranencephaly—A report of five cases of infarction of both cerebral hemispheres in infancy. Brain 90:839–850, 1967

55. Liu MC, Sylvester PE: Familial diffuse progressive encephalopathy. Arch Dis Child 35:345–351, 1960

56. Malamud N: Patterns of CNS vulnerability in neonatal hypoxaemia. In Selective Vulnerability of the Brain in Hypoxaemia. Edited by J. P. Schade, WH McMenemey. Oxford, Blackwell Scientific Press, 1963, pp. 211–225

57. Mascherpa F, Valentino V: Intracranial Calcification. Springfield, CC Thomas, 1959

58. Mellus EL: The development of the cerebral cortex. Am J Anat 14:107–117, 1912

59. Miller JQ: Lissencephaly in two siblings. Neurology (Minneap) 13:841–850, 1963

60. Muir CS: Hydranencephaly and allied disorders; a study of cerebral defects in Chinese children. Arch Dis Child 34:231–246, 1959

61. Myers RF: Atrophic cortical sclerosis associated with status marmoratus in a perinatally damaged monkey. Neurology (Minneap) 19:1177–1188, 1969

62. Navin JJ, Angevine JM: Congenital cytomegalic inclusion disease with porencephaly. Neurology (Minneap) 18:470–472, 1968

63. Norman RM, Urich H, Woods GE: The relationship between prenatal porencephaly and the encephalomalacias of early life. J Ment Sci 104:758–771, 1958

64. Osburn BI, Johnson RT, Silverstein AM, Prendergast RA, Jochim MM, Levy SE: Experimental viral-induced congenital encephalopathies. II. The pathogenesis of blue tongue vaccine virus infection in fetal lambs. Lab Invest 25:206–210, 1971

65. Osburn BI, Silverstein AM, Prendergast RA, Johnson RT, Parshall CJ Jr: Experimental viral-induced congenital encephalopathies. I. Pathology of hydranencephaly and porencephaly caused by blue tongue vaccine virus. Lab Invest 25:197–205, 1971

66. Patten CA, Grant FC, Yaskin JC: Porencephaly: diagnosis and treatment. Arch Neurol Psychiatr 37:108–136, 1937

67. Paul LW, Juhl JH: The Essentials of Roentgen Interpretation, ed 3. Hagerstown, Harper & Row, 1972

68. Peterson HO, Kieffer SA: Introduction to Neuroradiology. Hagerstown, Harper & Row, 1972

69. Poliakov GI: Some results of research into the development of the neuronal structure of the cortical ends of the analyzers in man. J Comp Neurol 117:197–212, 1961

70. Rabinowicz T: The cerebral cortex of the premature infant of the 8th month. Prog Brain Res 4:39–92, 1964

71. Rand BO, Foltz EL, Alvord EC Jr: Intracranial telencephalic meningo-encephalocele containing choroid plexus. J Neuropathol Exp Neurol 23:293–305, 1964

72. Streeter GL: The cortex of the brain in the human embryo during the 4th month, with special reference to the so-called "Papillae of Retzius." Am J Anat 7:337–344, 1907

73. Streeter GL: The development of the nervous system. Handbook of Human Embryology, vol

II. Edited by F Keibel and FP Mall. Philadelphia, JB Lippincott, 1912, pp. 1–156

74. Walker AE: Lissencephaly. Arch Neurol Psychiatr 48:13–29, 1942

75. Warner FJ: The histogenic principle of microgyria and related cerebral malformations. J Nerv Ment Dis 118:1–18, 1953

76. Weiss MH, Young HF, McFarland DE: Hydranencephaly of postnatal origin. J Neurosurg 32:715–720, 1970

77. Wesenberg R, Juhl JH, Daube JR: Radiological findings in lissencephaly (congenital agyria). Radiology 87:436–444, 1966

78. Williams HJ: Skull erosion complicating traumatic porencephaly in infancy. Am J Roentgenol Radium Ther Nucl Med 106:129–132, 1969

79. Yakovlev PI, Wadsworth RC: Double symmetrical porencephalies (schizencephalies). Trans Am Neurol Assoc 67:24–29, 1941

80. Yakovlev PI, Wadsworth RC: Schizencephalies: a study of congenital clefts in the cerebral mantle. I. Clefts with fused lips. J Neuropathol Exp Neurol 5:116–130, 1946

81. Yakovlev PI, Wadsworth RC: Schizencephalies: a study of congenital clefts in the cerebral mantle. II. Clefts with hydrocephalus and lips separated. J Neuropathol Exp Neurol 5:169–206, 1946

chapter 16

FOREBRAIN WHITE MATTER

The white matter of the forebrain is composed of a wide variety of myelinated axons that connect various parts of the cerebral cortex with other parts of the cerebral cortex, deep cerebral nuclei and other more-caudal regions of the CNS. The development of the anterior commissure, hippocampal commissure, corpus callosum and internal capsule has been relatively well defined, but the development of many other forebrain tracts is not so well defined. Indeed, the human internal capsule, one of the largest and most complicated tracts of the brain, has been the subject of only one modern study.[4] Then, too, although the development of the commissures has been the subject of embryologic studies for over 100 years, significant ambiguity still exists. Perhaps this reflects the frequent involvement of midline structures in congenital malformations and the rarity of significant anomalies of the internal capsule. The major embryologic landmarks (Figs. 16–1 and 16–2) are derived from the studies of Bartelmez and Dekaban[1] and Streeter.[24–27]

NORMAL DEVELOPMENT*

INTERNAL CAPSULE

The internal capsule is the major pathway of fibers from the neocortex to the caudal portions of the neural tube and from the thalamus to the neocortex. Hewitt[4] has made the most-detailed morphogenetic study of the

* See Chapter 1 for background information on embryologic development and staging system.

human internal capsule. As the lateral dilatations of the prosencephalon develop in stage XV (7- to 9-mm CR), a ridge that protrudes from the side walls of each cerebral vesicle becomes the medial striatal elevation. At this stage there are no fibers in the internal capsule. By stage XVIII (13- to 17-mm CR), the medial and lateral striatal elevations can be identified. Deep to them in the developing mantle zone, a stratified lamina of cells partially surrounds a small bundle of fibers directed towards the diencephalon. These fibers are the earliest sign of the internal capsule. In stage XXII (23- to 28-mm CR), the number of fibers in the internal capsule increases markedly; three components are recognizable. The upper and lower components are directed to the diencephalon but do not extend to the pallium, while the intermediate set of fibers, which do reach as far as the pallium, are beginning to trace out the path of the adult internal capsule as it separates the caudate nucleus from the putamen and globus pallidus.

Further development of the internal capsule is related to the development of the lamina affixa, which is a secondary fusion between that portion of the hemispheric vesicle lying medial to the corpus striatum (and lateral to the choroid plexus) and the lateral superior surface of the burgeoning diencephalon. The lamina affixa is the result of rapid hemispheral enlargement so that the telencephalon completely surrounds the dorsal and lateral surfaces of the diencephalon. By 70-mm CR length, the fibers of the internal capsule have almost completely separated the caudate nucleus from the lentiform nucleus (putamen and globus pal-

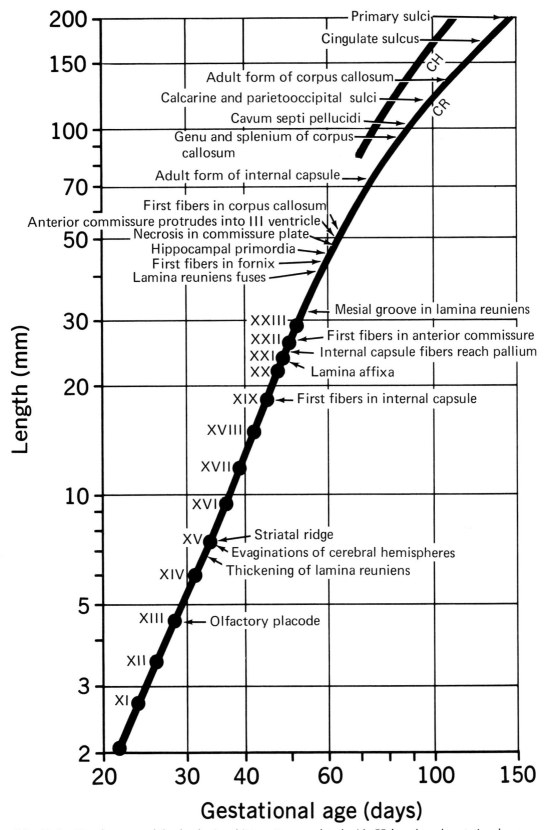

FIG. 16–1. Development of the forebrain white matter correlated with CR length and gestational age.

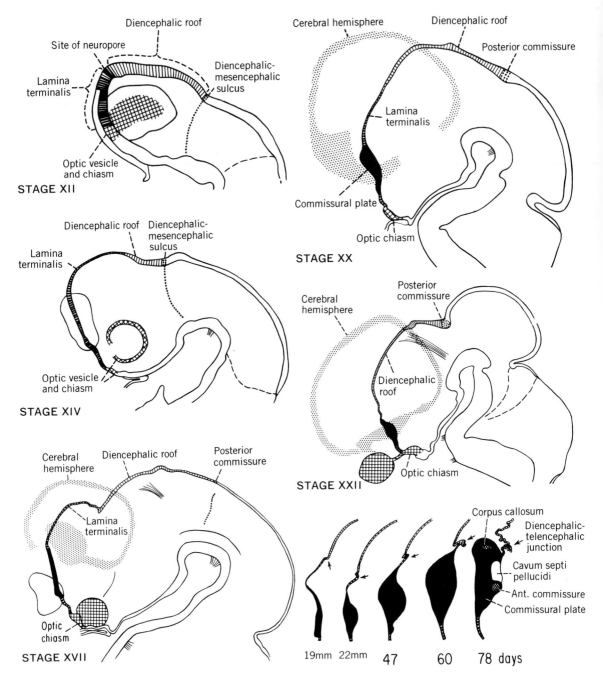

FIG. 16–2. Sagittal reconstructions of various stages in the development of the human nervous system. (Adapted from Bartelmez and Dekaban, 1962, and others) Homologous structures have been similarly shaded in all sketches: The commissural plate is solid black, the telencephalic roof is darkly striated, the diencephalic roof is lightly striated and the diencephalic–mesencephalic junction is identified by dots. The visual system is crosshatched. These drawings are not to the same scale, but each is enlarged to facilitate recognition. The arrow points to the diencephalic–telencephalic junction and emphasizes that the corpus callosum, anterior commissure and hippocampal commissure are telencephalic. (After Loeser and Alvord, 1968[12])

lidus). In general, the fibers appear to be laid down in a caudal–rostral direction. Later development of the internal capsule does not involve significant morphologic changes, and the precise development of specific fiber systems does not appear to have been studied.

COMMISSURES

Loeser and Alvord[12] have reviewed the development of the midline structures in the forebrain of the human embryo, and the study of Rakic and Yakovlev[17] provides important new data. The anterior commissure, hippocampal commissure and corpus callosum all originate from the midline of the rostral pole of the neuraxis adjacent to the site of closure of the anterior neuropore. This critical closure occurs in stage XI (2.5- to 4.5-mm CR), and morphologic errors at this time are probably expressed as anencephaly, if the embryo survives into fetal life.

After the anterior neuropore has closed, a single, spherical prosencephalic vesicle is present. By stage XV (7- to 9-mm CR), the evaginations of the cerebral hemispheres can be identified, and the telencephalon medianum can be delineated by the groove at the medial margin of the paired vesicles. At this time the region of the telencephalon lying in the midline between the optic chiasm and the paraphysis can be seen to differentiate into a ventral, inert portion (lamina terminalis or pars tenua) and a dorsal, cellularly active portion (lamina reuniens or pars crassa). The lamina terminalis remains inactive, and all of the morphologically important events occur within the more-rostral portion of the midline telencephalon, which is frequently called the *commissural plate*.

The lamina reuniens then develops a midline groove, and the two edges of this groove come together to effect a secondary fusion, within which the commissures develop. The ventral portion of the lamina reuniens is the site of the first fibers of the anterior commissure (stage XXII; 23- to 28-mm CR); it undergoes cellular differentiation to become the area praecommissuralis and eventually the septal nuclei. By 50-mm CR length, the anterior commissure has quite distinctly formed a protuberance into the telencephalic portion of the third ventricle.

A 40-mm CR length embryo contains the first fibers of the fornices, which run dorsally from the area praecommissuralis into the lamina reuniens. These are surrounded by the neuroblasts that create those paired dorsal protuberances in the lamina reuniens which are the hippocampal primordia (44-mm CR length). At approximately the same time, the two walls of the groove in the lamina reuniens begin to approach each other. They are then separated only by a single layer of meninx primativa. Proliferation of cells of the lamina reuniens obliterates the meninx, and the massa commissuralis is formed prior to the actual arrival of any of the axons that form the corpus callosum. Thus, the most-dorsal portion of the lamina reuniens, just rostral to the paraphysis, forms a bed for the fibers of the corpus callosum. The massa commissuralis is formed by 45-mm CR length, and the first callosal fibers can be seen by between 50- and 60-mm CR length. Additional fibers rapidly develop in all three commissures so that adult morphology is achieved by 140-mm CR length. However, the genu of the corpus callosum grows more rapidly in fetal life, whereas the body and splenium develop their full complement of fibers later.

The development of the cavum septi pellucidi (Fig. 16–3) is intimately related to the formation of the corpus callosum. Rakic and Yakovlev[17] believe that the cavum septi pellucidi is formed by the callosal fibers bridging over the median groove of the lamina reuniens and, therefore, that the cavum is originally open to the subarachnoid space in the region of the interhemispheral fissure. Others have thought that the cavum septi pellucidi is formed by necrosis within the massa commissuralis and never was open to the subarachnoid space. That necrosis occurs in this region is now widely accepted,[8] but Rakic and Yakovlev[17] believe the necrotic cells to be remnants of the meninx primativa that have been trapped by the developing massa commissuralis. Our observations do not support this viewpoint; we believe that necrosis occurs within the commissural plate and does not involve the meninx primativa. Histologic studies of this region reveal abundant gitter cells (foamy macrophages), and the absence of pial cells lining the cavum septi pellucidi also argues against Rakic and Yakovlev's thesis.

The two leaves of the septum pellucidum

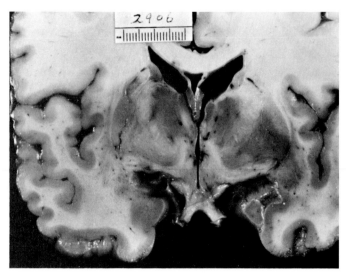

FIG. 16–3. Coronal section of the brain of a 46-year-old mentally retarded, epileptic man with a hypertrophic corpus callosum 12–15 mm thick (normal 5–7 mm), and with a cavum septi pellucidi. (#Np 2906)

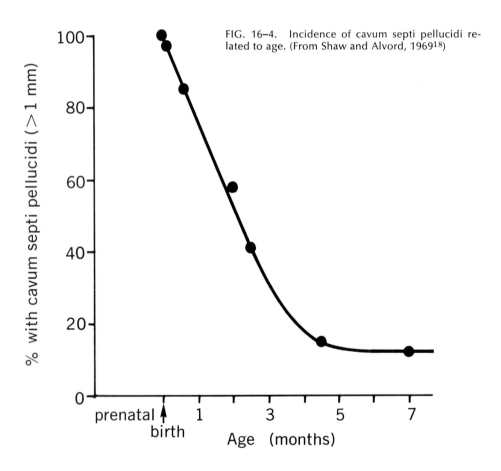

FIG. 16–4. Incidence of cavum septi pellucidi related to age. (From Shaw and Alvord, 1969[18])

are attenuated by the rapid growth of the hippocampi and corpus callosum; a cavum is present in every normal fetus up to six months gestation (250-mm CR length) and is typically about 1 cm wide, but it gradually narrows from the splenium toward the genu so that the posterior portion is normally obliterated by the time of birth[8] and the anterior by about 3 months after birth (Fig. 16–4). From this time on, it remains open to variable degrees in only 20% of children and adults.[18] If the anterior portion persists, the cavity is known as the cavum septi pellucidi. If the posterior portion persists, the cavity is called the cavum Vergae. The dividing line is arbitrarily taken as the plane of the foramen of Monro, so that the cavum Vergae lies caudal to the foramen of Monro and between the fornices, but it is embryologically equivalent to the posterior part of the cavum septi pellucidi. Grossly similar cysts that can only be differentiated microscopically are leptomeningeal cysts of the cavum veli interpositi, which normally is in continuity with the cysterna ambiens and lies between the roof of the third ventricle and the fornices.[6] In any event, these various cysts are rarely symptomatic, and their usual importance lies in the radiographic differentiation of these incidental cysts from tumors or other cysts in the midline.

The morphology of the hippocampal commissure and corpus callosum is influenced by the growth of the hippocampi and the pattern of fiber development in the corpus callosum. The first fibers of the corpus callosum lie anterior and inferior to the foramina of Monro; they appear after the earliest fibers of the hippocampal commissure are seen within the hippocampal primordia in the dorsal portion of the lamina reuniens. The rapid acquisition of fibers in the corpus callosum causes it to grow rostrally and posteriorly above the more slowly proliferating hippocampal commissure. While this process is occurring, the crescentic growth of the hippocampi carries them into the temporal lobes. The fibers of the fornices reflect this migration, and the hippocampal commissure shifts posteriorly to overlie the roof of the diencephalon subjacent to the body and splenium of the corpus callosum. The rostrum of the corpus callosum, whose development may be responsible for the formation of the cavum

septi pellucidi if Rakic and Yakovlev[17] are correct in believing that the meninx primitiva is trapped in the cavum, is formed after the initial fibers of the body of the corpus callosum.

ABNORMAL DEVELOPMENT

INTERNAL CAPSULE

The internal capsule is malformed or malpositioned in a wide variety of forebrain anomalies, but in none of these does the defect reside primarily in the capsule. In the holoprosencephalic brain, fibers interconnect the isocortex, thalamus and brain stem; these are generally markedly reduced in number and are obviously abnormally located. Isolated developmental anomalies of the internal capsule must be exceedingly rare, as we have no example in our autopsy series and cannot find any such cases in the literature beyond the rare epidermoid cyst ("pearly tumor") which must represent the displacement and lodging of epidermal cells in the junctional point between telencephalon and diencephalon as the internal capsule is forming (see Chapter 22).

COMMISSURES

Congenital anomalies of the three telencephalic commissures are quite common. The paucity of neurologic signs and symptoms that can be attributed to their total absence perhaps indicates little selective pressure against this type of anomaly. Although agenesis of the corpus callosum can be a hereditary trait in subhuman species[7] and occasionally in man,[14] most human cases seem to be sporadic. Teratogens can lead to this anomaly in experimental animals if delivered to the fetus at a critical period,[5] but so far the reported human cases can rarely be shown to have been exposed to any of these agents.

The most common type of agenesis of the corpus callosum is one in which there is complete absence of the corpus callosum and a complete separation of the two cerebral hemispheres except in the region of the anterior commissure and lamina terminalis (Figs. 16–5 through 16–7). In most such cases there is a large anterior–posterior fiber tract, Probst's bundle, which consists of

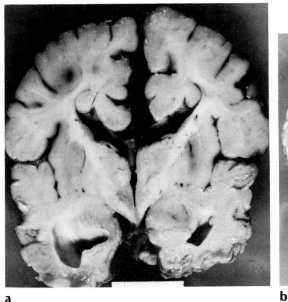
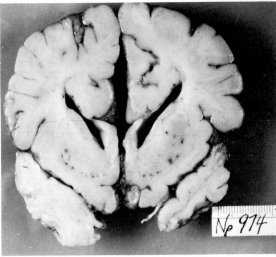

a   b

FIG. 16–5. **a.** Coronal section of the brain of a 16-month-old girl with complete agenesis of the corpus callosum. A thin T-shaped membrane spreads from the lamina terminalis to the apex of the lateral ventricles in continuity with Probst's bundles. Note the enlarged foramina of Monro. The cortex of this brain was poorly developed, and there were multiple defects in lamination. (From Loeser and Alvord, 1968[12]) (#Np 974) **b.** Agenesis of the corpus callosum with prominent parolfactory gyri and septal nuclei attenuating to form thin membranes that are probably homologous with the two leaves of the septum pellucidum. (#Np 974)

FIG. 16–6. Coronal section of the brain from another 16-month-old girl with agenesis of the corpus callosum with abnormally shaped frontal horns and prominent Probst's bundles in the apex of the lateral ventricles. Note the massive fusion of the thalami across the third ventricle. (#Np 813; see Fig. 12–11)

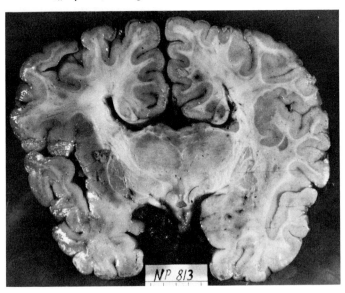

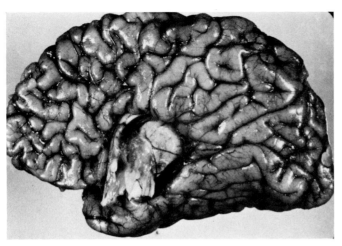

FIG. 16–7. Midsagittal section of the brain of a 17-month-old boy with complete agenesis of the corpus callosum demonstrating the radial sulcal pattern and a rudimentary hippocampal commissure immediately above the anterior commissure. (#Np 477)

axons terminating ipsilaterally. It is nowhere near the size of the normal corpus callosum, but is approximately the size of the normally decussating fibers, *i.e.*, those which connect nonisologous points of one cerebral hemisphere with the other. Only the commissural fibers are absent, *i.e.*, those which connect isologous points of the two cerebral hemispheres. It would appear as though the potentially decussating fibers arrive later, cannot find even a membranous substratum in which to cross and continue on to connect heterologous points on the same side. In general, Probst's bundle bears the same gross relationship to the fornix as does the normal corpus callosum, being interconnected by the septum pellucidum, which may be relatively short or occasionally quite attenuated (Fig. 16–8).

In this common form of agenesis of the corpus callosum, the anterior commissure is usually present, perhaps larger or smaller than normal, but at least supportive of the embryologic evidence that it develops in a separate portion of the lamina reuniens and therefore usually escapes being involved. The hippocampal commissure, normally located beneath the splenium of the corpus callosum, is of course absent, but there may be some fibers remaining near the anterior commissure, another indication that this part of the lamina reuniens escapes being involved.

It is important to recognize that the acallosal brain does not arise from a defect in the medial walls of the hemispheres but from a defect in the structures that develop from the lamina reuniens. Anterior to the foramen of Monro the major change is the absence of the genu and rostrum of the corpus callosum and the wide separation of the frontal horns of the lateral ventricles. As in the normal, the lamina terminalis separates the third ventricle from the subarachnoid space. A thick band of gray matter (septal nuclei) runs from the parolfactory cortex up to Probst's bundle; posteriorly this becomes attenuated to form the septum pellucidum (Fig 16–7).

The foramen of Monro is usually elongated and permits extensive communication between the third and lateral ventricles. As in the normal brain, the roof of the third ventricle is attached to the most-mesial portion of the telencephalic lateral vesicles. The fornix marks this transitional zone, and it is connected to Probst's bundle by the septum pellucidum. The roof of the third ventricle is greatly dilated (Fig. 16–9) and may even present at the surface of the interhemispheral fissure; however, its relationships to the telencephalon are not significantly altered.

Posterior to the foramen of Monro the mesial walls of the hemispheres consist of the fornix–hippocampal system and the Probst's bundle–cingulate gyrus complex.

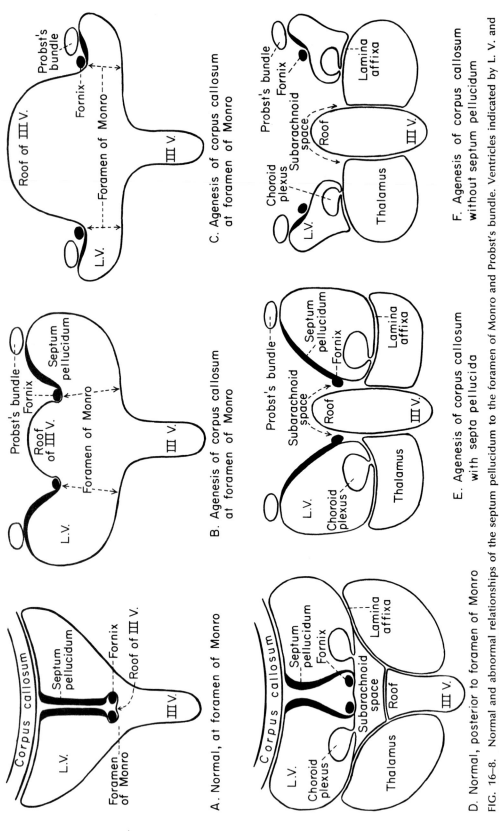

A. Normal, at foramen of Monro

B. Agenesis of corpus callosum at foramen of Monro

C. Agenesis of corpus callosum at foramen of Monro

D. Normal, posterior to foramen of Monro

E. Agenesis of corpus callosum with septa pellucida

F. Agenesis of corpus callosum without septum pellucidum

FIG. 16–8. Normal and abnormal relationships of the septum pellucidum to the foramen of Monro and Probst's bundle. Ventricles indicated by L. V. and III V. (After Loeser and Alvord, 1968[12])

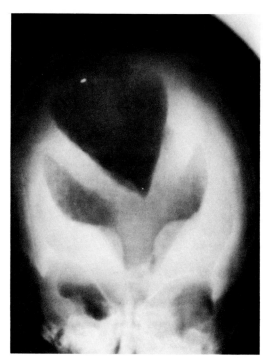

FIG. 16–9. Pneumoencephalogram of a hydrocephalic child with agenesis of the corpus callosum and a large interhemispheral cyst continuous with the third ventricle.

The absence of the splenium is responsible for the enlarged trigone of the lateral ventricle; this is not a sign of hydrocephalus. The continuity of the mesial walls of the hemisphere is not altered in the acallosal brain. The hippocampus is separated from the midline by the tela chorioidea, which is adjacent to the lamina affixa.

Whenever the corpus callosum is absent, the sulcal pattern of the mesial hemispheres is abnormal (Fig. 16–7). This has been described as a "radiating" pattern, as each sulcus runs from the surface of the interhemispheral fissure to the most inferior edge of the hemisphere adjacent to the diencephalic roof. This is not the persistence of a fetal form of sulcal patterns since such a pattern never normally exists, and since these sulci do not form until later in gestation; rather it reflects the absence of the corpus callosum and its organizing effects upon the cerebral gyri.[16, 31]

Although many patients with agenesis of the corpus callosum have neurologic or psychologic abnormalities (e.g., seizures, mental retardation, hydrocephalus), these signs and symptoms must be due to the other associated CNS anomalies.[13] Subtle testing techniques can reveal the lack of interhemispheral transfer of information, but this is rarely clinically apparent.[3]

Agenesis of the corpus callosum need not be complete. Focal absence of the corpus callosum may affect any part, most commonly the splenium and/or rostrum (Fig. 16–10). In one case we found numerous cysts (Fig. 16–11) attached to the falx at the site of focal agenesis of the corpus callosum.

Hypoplasia of the corpus callosum may be quite extreme (Fig. 16–12), with virtually no axons in the glial membrane forming the commissural bed.

If the corpus callosum is not formed, the conventional statement is that the septum pellucidum is also absent (Figs. 16–5 through 16–7). However, we have noted the unilateral absence of the septum pellucidum with unilateral arhinencephaly (Fig. 7–11), and we have also noted a septum pellucidum-like attenuation of the tissue between Probst's bundle and the fornix in some cases of agenesis of the corpus callosum (Figs. 16–5 and 16–8). Thus we see the two leaves of the septum pellucidum as relatively independent structures, interconnecting the fornix and either the usual corpus callosum or its partial equivalent (Probst's bundle).

Furthermore, the septum pellucidum may be absent, even though the corpus callosum appears normal (Fig. 16–13). The gliosis in the midline probably indicates that this was due to an acquired, encephaloclastic process occurring after the septum pellucidum had formed.

Table 16–1 summarizes many of the common findings in anomalies of the mesial telencephalon. Focal agenesis of the corpus callosum is due to a limited defect in the lamina reuniens and is less frequently seen than complete agenesis. The etiology of agenesis of the corpus callosum must be diverse. Most cases seem to be related to defects in only one anatomic structure, the lamina reuniens. Mass lesions, such as lipoma or colloid cyst of the diencephalic roof, seem able to play a role only in partial agenesis, and even here their effect remains controversial since they may be merely concomitant lesions.

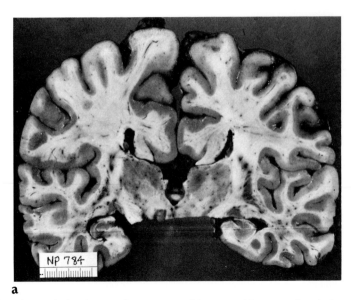

a

FIG. 16–10. **a.** Coronal section of the brain of a 49-year-old man with agenesis of the posterior portion of the corpus callosum. (#Np 784) **b.** Coronal section of the same brain showing the anterior corpus callosum to be present superiorly. The obliquely running fibers on the superior surface of the corpus callosum appear gray but should not be mistaken for cortex. **c.** Midsagittal reconstruction of the brain showing agenesis of the rostrum and splenium of the corpus callosum. A long thin membranous continuation of the lamina terminalis connects the anterior commissure vertically with the body of the corpus callosum.

TABLE 16–1. ANOMALIES OF TELENCEPHALIC COMMISSURES

Embryologic Defect	Anatomic Manifestation	Diagnosis
Failure of midline telencephalon and vesicles to develop normally	No forebrain commissures; hippocampi malpositioned; single prosencephalic ventricle	Holoprosencephaly (see Chapter 14)
Failure of lamina reuniens to develop normally	No forebrain commissures; Probst's bundle present; dorsal dilatation of third ventricle; hippocampi normal	Total agenesis of corpus callosum, anterior commissure and hippocampal commissure
Failure of dorsal portion of lamina reuniens to develop normally	Absence of corpus callosum and hippocampal commissure; Probst's bundle present; anterior commissure present; dorsal dilatation of third ventricle; hippocampi normal	Agenesis of corpus callosum
Focal defect in dorsal lamina reuniens, often associated with a lipoma of corpus callosum or colloid cyst of diencephalic roof	Focal absence of corpus callosum; Probst's bundle and dorsal dilatation of third ventricle present where corpus callosum absent	Focal agenesis of corpus callosum (usually of splenium or rostrum)
Cortical neuroblast abnormalities	Membranous corpus callosum without axons; no Probst's bundle; septum pellucidum, fornix and third ventricle normal	Hypoplasia of corpus callosum, frequently associated with agyria or mild arhinencephaly

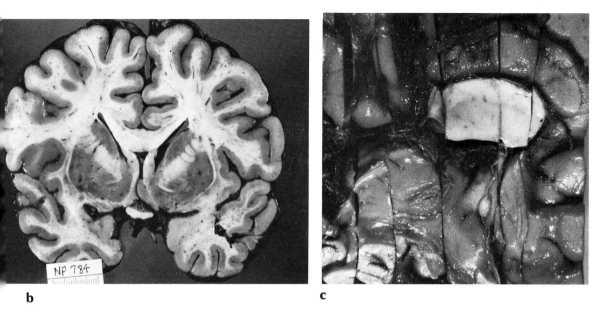

b   c

FIG. 16–11.   Anatomic dissection of the falx cerebri from a newborn with multiple arachnoid cysts attached to its inferior margin. The brain manifested focal agenesis of the corpus callosum in the region of the cysts. (From Loeser and Alvord, 1968[12] (#Np 415)

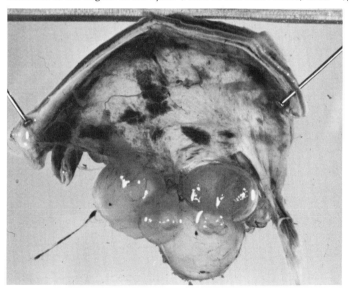

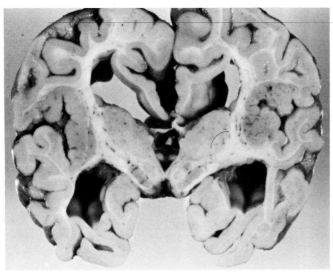

a

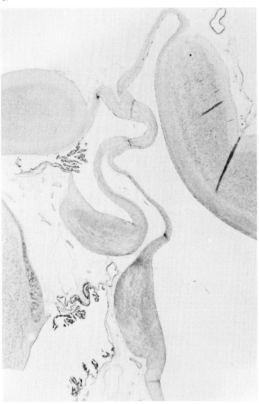

b

FIG. 16–12. **a.** Coronal section of the brain of a 10-month-old girl with arhinencephaly and hypoplasia of the corpus callosum, consisting of a glial membrane without axons. **b.** Photomicrograph of the membranous corpus callosum, septum pellucidum and fornices. (#Np 430)

FIG. 16–13. Coronal section of the brain of a 3-year-old girl who died of acute polyradiculitis with infectious mononucleosis. The brain was slightly large (1390 g after fixation), the corpus callosum hypertrophic and the septum pellucidum absent. A diffuse gliosis was present above the fornices (seen just above the rostrum of the corpus callosum) and under the middle 1 cm of the body of the corpus callosum. The olfactory bulbs and tracts were normal. (#Np 356)

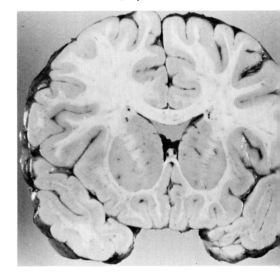

OTHER ABNORMALITIES OF THE DEVELOPING CEREBRAL WHITE MATTER

GLIAL FATTY METAMORPHOSIS AND PERIVENTRICULAR LEUCOMALACIA

Leech and Alvord,[10, 11] Sumi[28] and Sumi *et al.*[29, 30] have been investigating the accumulations of lipids in immature glial cells that occur in practically all human newborns coming to autopsy and comparing them with similar accumulations observed in certain immature monkeys. These lipid accumulations occur in two forms, focal accumulations in macrophages (usually seen in periventricular leucomalacia, or PVL; Fig. 16–14) and more diffuse accumulations (glial fatty metamorphosis, or GFM; Fig. 16–15) in glial cells too immature to be classified morphologically as committed to one or another form of differentiation. Although a certain amount of "necrobiosis" occurs normally in development, so that not all macrophages can be considered abnormal, most investigators agree that PVL is abnormal. However, considerable disagreement persists concerning the significance of GFM. Since no truly normal human infants die and come to autopsy, the question whether the diffuse type of lipid accumulation (GFM) is a stage in normal pre-myelin lipidogenesis,[15] or whether it is an abnormal reaction to metabolic stress,[10, 11] cannot be resolved until an experimental model becomes available, and this was delayed for many decades since subprimates do not show these sudanophilic lipids. Recently, however, monkeys have been found to be remarkably similar to humans in showing both necrotic lesions of PVL and subnecrotic lesions of GFM (Fig. 16–16) under abnormal situations (*e.g.*, stillbirth, death during infancy, transplacental exposure to experimentally induced maternal hypertension or hypotension). They generally do not show these changes under strictly normal situations (*e.g.*, immediate fixation by perfusion of formaldehyde or glutaraldehyde).[28, 29, 30] Although the experiments are still incomplete, the implications seem obvious: the immature glial cell is highly sensitive to metabolic stress, most likely hypoxia–acidosis. Such stress can be induced in the fetus by maternal hypertension or hypotension,

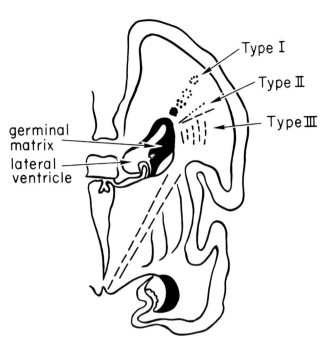

FIG. 16–14. Morphologic types of periventricular leukomalacia (PVL) include discrete foci of necrosis (Type I), linear zones of necrosis (Type II) and less well-delineated zones of necrosis (Type III). (From Leech and Alvord, 1974)

and these in turn can probably even be induced by such psychogenic factors as environmental stress. These stresses are so commonly experienced as to be considered "normal" and, as such, are generally overlooked by both patient and physician, or not recorded in the obstetrical records.

The possible importance of these lesions for the production of mental retardation and minimal brain damage (or minimal cerebral dysfunction) probably lies in the damage to the developing white matter (multifocally in PVL and either diffusely or focally, especially in the corpus callosum, in GFM). In cases of mental retardation coming to autopsy many years after birth, the difficulty in quantitating the amount of cerebral white matter is well known, and the difficulty in detecting small glial scars is almost as well known; but the degree of reversibility of GFM is as yet completely unknown. Patients with minimal brain damage simply do not die while they demonstrate the syndrome, and in fact they tend to recover from it, so that the syndrome has long since been overlooked when the patient finally dies of some

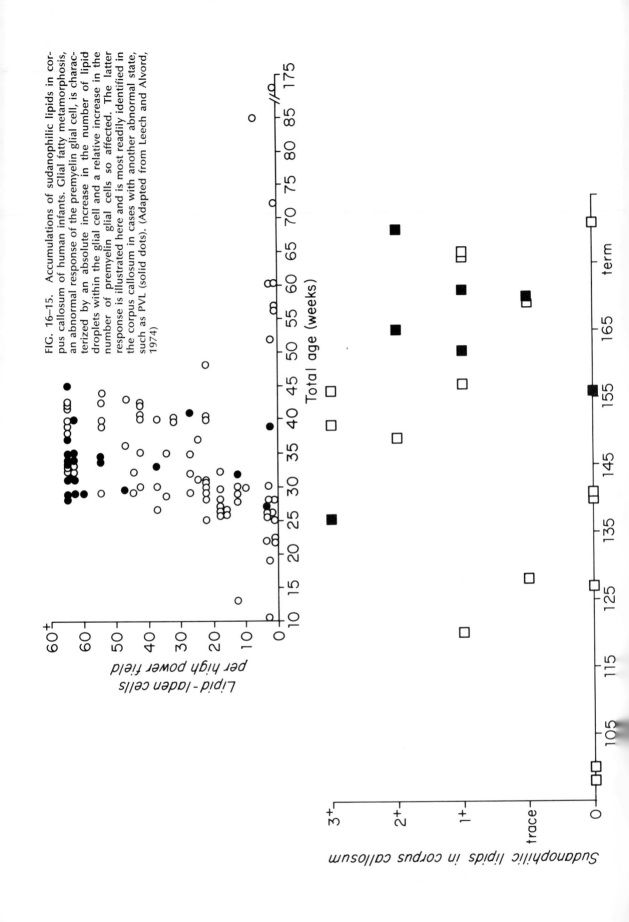

FIG. 16-15. Accumulations of sudanophilic lipids in corpus callosum of human infants. Glial fatty metamorphosis, an abnormal response of the premyelin glial cell, is characterized by an absolute increase in the number of lipid droplets within the glial cell and a relative increase in the number of premyelin glial cells so affected. The latter response is illustrated here and is most readily identified in the corpus callosum in cases with another abnormal state, such as PVL (solid dots). (Adapted from Leech and Alvord, 1974)

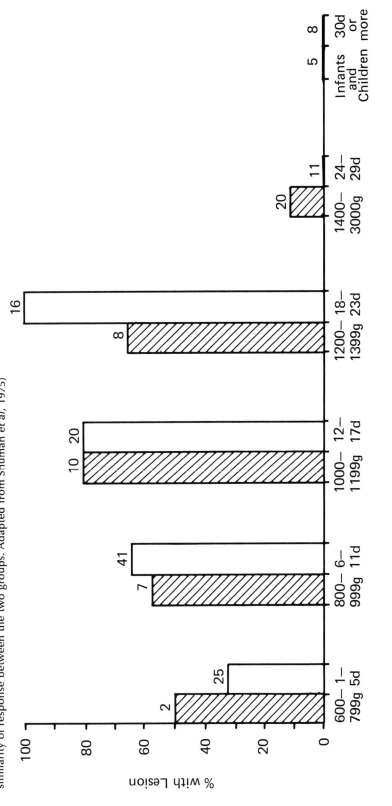

FIG. 16–17. Frequency of vacuolar encephalopathy in brain stem reticular formation in 52 human infants and 21 newborn rats following two or more baths in 3% hexachlorophene. The vertical shaded bars represent humans, the unshaded, rats. Note similarity of response between the two groups. Adapted from Shuman et al, 1975)

other disease. Thus, it seems unlikely that the pathoanatomic substrate will ever be defined in actual clinicopathologic studies. Gazzaniga[2] has recently suggested that at least some of the elements of the syndrome may relate to delayed maturation of the corpus callosum, which is exactly the site where GFM most strikingly occurs. Such a lead is most tempting to follow both experimentally and clinically.

HEXACHLOROPHENE-INDUCED VACUOLAR ENCEPHALOPATHY

Hexachlorophene (HCP) has been recently discovered to be a myelinotoxic agent that can be absorbed through normal mucosa or abnormal skin (*e.g.*, burns, desquamating dermatitis) at any age or through normal skin in small premature infants (under 1400 g birth weight). Since most myelin is formed after birth, the potential damage to the developing nervous system would seem to be relatively limited. However, since myelin is being formed *in utero*, it can be damaged if small premature infants are bathed in 3% HCP, as described by Shuman *et al.*[19, 20, 22] As few as two such whole body baths can produce a vacuolar encephalopathy of the brain stem reticular formation with fatal apnea and no other lesions detectable at autopsy. Fig. 16–17 illustrates the remarkable age–dose relationships that have been found in humans and confirmed experimentally: two-week-old baby rats are extremely sensitive, as few as two baths a day apart being sufficient to kill them.[21, 23]

In older children the lesion is much more diffuse, death resulting from massive cerebral edema due to the vacuolization of myelin sheaths throughout the CNS. Had such lesions been named "hexachlorophene encephalopathy" rather than "burn syndrome,"[9] it is likely that cases would no longer be occurring.

REFERENCES

1. Bartelmez GW, Dekaban AS: The early development of the human brain. Contrib Embryol 37:14–32, 1962
2. Gazzaniga MS: Brain theory and minimal brain dysfunction. Ann NY Acad Sci 205:89–92, 1973
3. Gazzaniga MS, Bogen JE, Sperry RW: Observations on visual perception after disconnection of the cerebral hemispheres in man. Brain 88:221–236, 1965
4. Hewitt W: The development of the human internal capsule and lentiform nucleus. J Anat 95:191–199, 1961
5. Hicks SP: Developmental malformations produced by radiation. Am J Roentgenol Radium Ther Nucl Med 69:272–293, 1953
6. Hughes RA, Kernohan JW, Craig W McK: Caves and cysts of the septum pellucidum. Arch Neurol Psychiatr 74:259–265, 1955
7. King LS: Hereditary defects of the corpus callosum in the mouse, Mus musculus. J Comp Neurol 64:337–363, 1936
8. Larroche JC, Baudey J: Cavum septi lucidi, cavum vergae, cavum veli interpositi: cavités de la ligne médiane. Biol Neonate 3:193–236, 1961
9. Larson DL: Studies show hexachlorophene causes burn syndrome. J Am Hosp Assoc 42:63, 1968
10. Leech RW, Alvord EC Jr: Glial fatty metamorphosis: an abnormal response of premyelin glia. Am J Pathol 74:603–613, 1974
11. Leech RW, Alvord EC Jr: Morphologic variations in periventricular leucomalacia. Am J Pathol 74:591–602, 1974
12. Loeser JD, Alvord EC Jr: Agenesis of the corpus callosum. Brain 91:553–570, 1968
13. Loeser JD, Alvord EC Jr: Clinicopathological correlations in agenesis of the corpus callosum. Neurology (Minneap) 18:745–756, 1968
14. Menkes JH, Philippart M, Clark DE: Hereditary partial agenesis of the corpus callosum. Arch Neurol 11:198–208, 1964
15. Mickel HS, Gilles FH: Changes in glial cells during human telencephalic myelinogenesis. Brain 93:337–346, 1970
16. Nobler MP, Shapiro JH, Fine DIM: The cerebral angiogram in agenesis of the corpus callosum. Am J Roentgenol Radium Ther Nucl Med 90:522–527, 1963
17. Rakic P, Yakovlev PI: Development of the corpus callosum and cavum septi in man. J Comp Neurol 132:45–72, 1968
18. Shaw CM, Alvord EC Jr: Cava septi pellucidi et Vergae: Their normal and pathological states. Brain 92:213–224, 1969
19. Shuman RM, Leech RW, Alvord EC Jr: Neurotoxicity of hexachlorophene in human infants (abstracted). Am J Pathol 70:19a, 1973
20. Shuman RM, Leech RW, Alvord EC Jr: Neurotoxicity of hexachlorophene in the human: I. A clinico-pathologic study of 248 children. Pediatr 54:689–695, 1974

21. Shuman RM, Leech RW, Alvord EC Jr, Sumi SM: Experimental neurotoxicity of pHisoHex (abstracted). J Neuropathol Exp Neurol 33: 195, 1973

22. Shuman RM, Leech RW, Alvord EC Jr: Neurotoxicity of hexachlorophene in humans. II. A clinico-pathologic study of 46 premature infants. Arch Neurol 32:320–325, 1975

23. Shuman RM, Leech RW, Alvord EC Jr: Neurotoxicity of topically applied hexachlorophene in the young rat. Arch Neurol 32:315–319, 1975

24. Streeter GL: Developmental horizons in human embryos. Contrib Embryol 30:211–245, 1942

25. Streeter GL: Developmental horizons in human embryos. Contrib Embryol 31:27–63, 1945

26. Streeter GL: Developmental horizons in human embryos. Contrib Embryol 32:133–203, 1948

27. Streeter GL: Developmental horizons in human embryos. Contrib Embryol 34:165–196, 1951

28. Sumi SM: Periventricular leukoencephalopathy in the monkey, a search for the "normal control" and the "early lesion." Arch Neurol 31: 38–44, 1974

29. Sumi SM, Alvord EC Jr, Parer J, Eng M, Ueland K: Accumulation of sudonophilic lipids in the cerebral white matter of premature primates: An experimental inquiry into the pathogenesis of the Virchow–Schwartz–Banker–Larroche lesion (abstracted). J Neuropathol Exp Neurol 31:183, 1972

30. Sumi SM, Leech RW, Alvord EC Jr, Eng M, Ueland K: Sudanophilic lipids in unmyelinated primate cerebral white matter after intrauterine hypoxia and acidosis. Res Publ Assoc Res Nerv Ment Dis 51:176–197, 1973

31. Zingesser L, Schecter M, Gonatos N, Levy A, Wisoff H: Agenesis of the corpus callosum associated with an inter-hemisphere arachnoid cyst. Br J Radiol 37:905–909, 1964

CNS ASSOCIATED STRUCTURES

chapter 17

MENINGES

The brain and spinal cord are enclosed within three membranes collectively known as the meninges. In common usage, these have two divisions: 1) the *pachymeninx,* or dura mater, and 2) the *leptomeninges,* or pia mater and arachnoid. Excellent discussions of their anatomic relationships are given by Millen and Woollam[17] and Barr.[3]

ANATOMY OF THE MENINGES

DURA MATER

The outermost of the three meninges, the dura mater, consists of a thick membrane composed of dense collagen lined with mesothelium. Although the dura of the spinal canal and the skull is continuous, their relationships to associated structures are quite different. Within the spinal canal, the dura is not adherent to the vertebrae or intervertebral discs, so that there are both epidural and subdural spaces. The epidural space is filled with fat and a network of veins, whereas the subdural space is obliterated by the adherence of the two moist membranes, arachnoid and dura. Beginning at the level of the foramen magnum, the dura adheres to the periosteum of the skull (another connective tissue of collagen frequently referred to as the outer layer of the dura), which lines the cranial bones. Thus, there is no natural epidural space within the skull, but a subdural space exists in the same manner as the spinal canal.

Dural Venous Sinuses

Dural venous sinuses develop in the midline superiorly and around the sides of the skull posteriorly. They are lined internally by endothelium. In association with these venous channels, two layers of dura become fused in what are termed *dural reflections,* the tentorium cerebelli, falx cerebelli and falx cerebri.

TENTORIUM CEREBELLI. The tentorium cerebelli is an obliquely placed dural septum that separates the middle and posterior cranial fossas. Immediately above it lie the occipital lobes and below it, the cerebellum. It is attached superiorly to the posterior portion of the falx cerebri and is higher in the midline than laterally at the skull insertions.

Three major dural venous sinuses are associated with the tentorium: the straight sinus and the two transverse sinuses. Their posterior point of juncture is termed the torcular Herophili. The incisura tentorii (tentorial notch) allows the midbrain to connect the forebrain (supratentorial) with the hindbrain (infratentorial).

FALX CEREBELLI. The falx cerebelli is a small midline vertical dura septum in the posterior fossa. It separates the two cerebellar hemispheres and contains the occipital sinus.

FALX CEREBRI. The falx cerebri is a dorsal midline, vertically placed dural septum that extends from the straight sinus and torcular posteriorly to the crista galli (ethmoid bone) anteriorly. It separates the cerebral hemispheres along the length of the longitudinal fissure, encloses the superior and inferior sagittal sinuses and forms the superior wall of the straight sinus posteriorly.

PIA MATER

The pia mater is a thin transparent membrane that provides the innermost covering of the brain and spinal cord. As with the dura mater, the pia mater within the spinal canal and that within the skull differ from one another.[16,17] The pia mater associated with the spinal cord consists of two components: 1) the *intima pia,* a continuous layer of reticular collagenous connective tissue that immediately surrounds the cord and is incorporated ventrally in the anterior longitudinal sulcus, and 2) the *epipial tissue,* consisting of an irregular network of delicate collagenous fibers that extends from the intima pia to the arachnoid as *arachnoid trabeculae* and a thick, regular set of from 18 to 23 denticulate ligaments laterally (which attach to the arachnoid and inner surface of the dura mater).

The epipial tissue is also found within the anterior longitudinal sulcus. In addition to the denticulate ligament, the epipial tissue is thickened over the anterior spinal artery and termed the *linea splendens.* The blood vessels supplying the spinal cord are found within the epipial tissue.

Beginning at the level of the foramen magnum, there is a gradual reduction in the amount of epipial tissue such that the medulla has less than the cord, the pons less than the medulla, the midbrain less than the pons and the cerebrum least of all. The cranial pia mater is thinner than the spinal pia, and blood vessels lie directly on the intima pia, being connected to it by fine trabeculae.

There are several places (called the *tela chorioidea*) where the intima pia is in direct apposition to the ependyma. The tela chorioidea are found in the roofs of the third and fourth ventricles and in the choroidal fissure of the cerebral hemispheres.

ARACHNOID

The leptomeninx lying between the dura mater and pia mater is called the arachnoid.

This transparent avascular membrane is composed of both collagen and modified fibroblasts (arachnoid cells); it is surrounded by two spaces: 1) the subarachnoid space (which contains trabeculae connecting the arachnoid to the pia and CSF) and 2) the potential subdural space between the arachnoid and dura.

As with the two other meninges, the arachnoid has different relationships within the skull and the vertebral column. The spinal arachnoid surrounds a fairly uniform subarachnoid space along its length; the cranial arachnoid is irregular and forms the external boundaries of various-sized cisterns. The only normal enlargement of the subarachnoid space found over the spinal cord is the lumbar cistern, which is the site of the common diagnostic "lumbar puncture." Within the skull, there are numerous cisterns, *i.e.,* places where the arachnoid does not follow the convexities of the brain. The cisterna magna is located dorsal to the medulla and just caudal to the cerebellum. CSF passing from the fourth ventricle through the foramen of Magendie enters the cisterna magna, from which the CSF then circulates rostrally or caudally. Rostral to the cerebellum, at the level of the tentorial notch dorsal and lateral to the colliculi, lies the cisterna ambiens. On the ventral side of the brain stem, the pontine cistern (at the pontomedullary junction) and interpeduncular cistern (ventral to the midbrain) are collectively referred to as the basal cisterns. Other subarachnoid cisterns are located in the Sylvian fissure and the cerebellopontine angle.

At innumerable places in the dural venous sinuses, the arachnoid penetrates the dura mater in the form of arachnoid villi (or "Pacchionian granulations" as they hypertrophy with age). Through this route the most significant amount of CSF is reabsorbed into the vascular system. The largest number of villi are in the superior sagittal sinus, and decreasing numbers in the transverse, cavernous and superior petrosal sinuses.

About the optic nerves are extensions of all three meninges through the optic foramen. Since the central vein of the retina (in the distal portion of the optic nerve) crosses an extension of the subarachnoid space to join the ophthalmic vein,[3] it may be compressed with increased intracranial pressure. This impedes the venous flow, leading to the engorgement of retinal veins and contributing to the production of papilledema.

NORMAL DEVELOPMENT*

Sensenig[20] credits Tiedemann in 1816 as the first to describe the embryology of the meninges, but numerous hypotheses persist that the meninges develop: 1) from the peripheral layers of the neural tube, 2) from both the neural tube and the skeleton-forming layer, 3) from a cranial mass of embryonal tissue comparable to Warton's jelly and from spinal primitive vertebrae, 4) as derivatives of somites, 5) as derivatives of mesoderm (according to the hypothesis of three germ layers for all embryonic parts), and 6) from both neural crest and mesoderm (pia) and from mesoderm (arachnoid and dura). Sensenig[20] has provided the most-reasonable analysis and accurate observations in a series of 75 human embryos and fetuses at the Carnegie Institute of Embryology. Most of the following information of normal development of the meninges is derived from his study. The temporal relationships are presented in Figure 17–1.

MENINX PRIMITIVA

The meninx primitiva is not an actual meninx, but rather a loose, sparsely cellular area lying between the neural tube, somites and notochord. It provides the matrix for the migration and condensation of cells that will contribute to the formation of both the meninges and vertebrae, and it also contributes precursor cells directly involved in the development of the meninges. It is of mesodermal origin and is first seen as a distinct zone lateral to the neural tube in stage XV (7- to 9-mm CR). By stage XVI (8- to 11-mm CR), the meninx primitiva extends around the entire neural tube; during stage XVIII (13- to 17-mm CR), it becomes stratified between the neural tube and the vertebral centra. In stage XIX (16- to 18-mm CR), the meninx primitiva begins to cavitate, with its cells having a reticular arrangement. This temporal sequence is true for the

* See Chapter 1 for background information on embryologic development and staging system.

upper thoracic region; more-caudal areas show this pattern somewhat later.

In stage XII (3- to 5-mm CR), before the meninx primitiva develops, vascularization begins in tissue around the neural tube, and condensations of neural crest cells begin to form the spinal ganglia that begin a ventral migration in stage XIII (4- to 6-mm CR). In stage XV the neural tube is completely surrounded by developing vessels, and condensations of primordial vertebral cells are found, appearing denser than the meninx primitiva. In stages XVI–XVII vascular channels surround the spinal ganglia and penetrate the neural tube, carrying cells of the meninx primitiva as their adventitia. In stage XVIII the spinal canal becomes distinguishable due to beginning chondrification of the vertebrae.

DURA MATER

The dura mater develops from mesodermal cells of sclerotomic (and/or meninx primitiva) origin. The first indication of cervical and thoracic dura is seen in stages XIX–XX (16- to 22-mm CR), mainly ventral to the cord, but with some lateral extension to the spinal ganglia. The dura is continuous with cells of the vertebral centra and the intervertebral discs. By stage XXII (23- to 28-mm CR) the dura (now found through the lumbar level) surrounds the spinal ganglia, which are migrating to the intervertebral foramina. Not until stage XXIII (17- to 31-mm CR) is the dura mater complete around the neural tube and clearly distinguishable from the perichondrium. In a few places ventrolaterally it is already separating from the latter, thus producing the first indication of an epidural space. This separation is not complete until early fetal life (50-mm CR length). By 80-mm CR length, the dura mater has most of the characteristics seen in the newborn except for its relationship with the arachnoid[20] and the fact that it is thicker ventrally (8–10 cells) than laterally or dorsally (2–3 cells).[11]

Sensenig[20] provides an explanation for the difference in relationships between cranial and spinal dura. Separation of the spinal dura from the perichondrium to form an epidural space is necessary to allow movement within the functional articulations be-

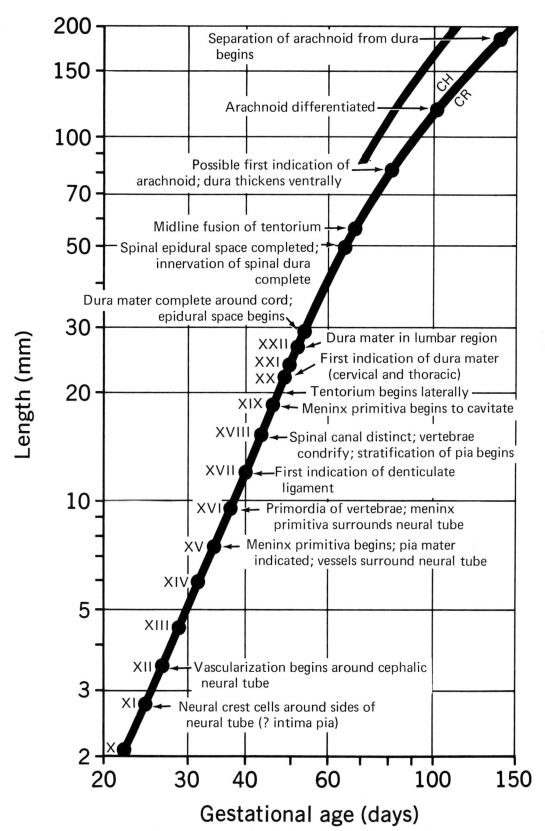

FIG. 17–1. Development of the meninges correlated with CR length and gestational age.

tween the vertebrae. Within the skull, there are no sites of functional articulation, and the dura can remain adherent to the endocranium.

Although apparently not important in the consideration of malformations of the meninges, the innervation of the dura mater is an interesting developmental relationship that should be mentioned. In a study of 22 specimens between 20- and 106-mm CR length, Kimmel[11] found that innervation of the spinal dura is derived from the meningeal rami of spinal nerves that are seen first in the thoracic region at stage XX (20-mm CR). By 47-mm CR length, all segmental levels are innervated with from two to four rami per segment, each having ascending and descending branches providing a maximum of two segments overlap in the lumbar dura. Although CR length relationships are not mentioned, the dura mater on the floor of the posterior fossa is innervated by rami of spinal nerves C1 to C3 and the sympathetic trunk. These enter through the foramen magnum, hypoglossal canal and jugular foramen. The lateral and dorsal dura mater of the posterior fossa receives rami from C1 and C2 and the superior cervical ganglion (via the hypoglossal canal and jugular foramen). The dura of the anterior and middle fossae is innervated by branches of the trigeminal nerves.

PIA MATER

At present there seems to be ample evidence that the pia mater is mainly derived from the meninx primitiva and is thus mostly of mesodermal origin, although Sensenig[20] believes that some cells of neural crest origin also participate in the formation of the intima pia.

In stage XI (2.5- to 4.5-mm CR), a single layer of cells, continuous with the neural crest, is first seen along the lateral aspect of the neural tube. They differ morphologically from the surrounding mesodermal cells and may be migrating from the neural crest. The uncertainty persists largely because it is not until four stages later, i.e., stage XV, that the first indication of pia mater (which can then be sequentially followed) is found on the ventrolateral aspect of the neural tube as an intermittent single cell layer. By stage XVII (11- to 14-mm CR), the primordia of the denticulate ligaments can be identified by a condensation of meninx primitiva and pia. In stage XVIII (13- to 17-mm CR) some pia is found in the anterior longitudinal sulcus in the cervical region. This is the first indication that the pia mater will later have two components, the intima pia and epipial tissue. Except for this area the pia mater is only one cell layer thick around the cord at the end of the embryonic period. By 50-mm CR length, the epipial tissue has a discrete plexus of small vessels from which some (with pial sleeves) are found to penetrate the cord.

ARACHNOID

Whereas it is possible to provide a few definitive statements about the development of dura mater and pia mater, the sequence of arachnoid development is much less certain. From the limited information available on humans it can be said that: 1) it is of mesodermal origin, 2) it develops from the inner aspect of the dura mater with nothing to suggest interaction with the pia mater except for the development of the trabeculae derived from the meninx primitiva, and 3) it is the last of the meninges to differentiate.

Because of the cavitation of the meninx primitiva in stage XIX (16- to 18-mm CR), the subarachnoid space actually starts to form before any arachnoid is identifiable. Since this is also the first time that the dura can be distinguished, it is obvious, but potentially confusing, that the embryonic subdural space develops first and only later becomes the fetal and adult subarachnoid space. Sensenig[20] first found identifiable arachnoid in "restricted" areas of an 80-mm CR length fetus, and he cites a previous study indicating that it was completely differentiated in some specimens by 120-mm CR length. Therefore, during the period from 80- to 120-mm CR length the embryonic subdural space becomes the adult subarachnoid space. For the true subdural space to develop, the arachnoid must separate from the dura mater, but the timing of this event has not yet been worked out. Whereas no separation was found in one 230-mm CR length fetus cited, Sensenig[20] observed isolated areas of arachnoid–dura separation in other specimens of 180- and 245-mm CR length. Our limited observations (Table 17–1) generally agree with his findings and

TABLE 17–1. AGES OF FETUSES SHOWING SEPARATION OF ARACHNOID FROM DURA MATER

CR Length (mm)	Level of the Spinal Cord		
	Cervical	Thoracic	Lumbar
180	Not separated	Not separated	. . .
200	Separating in several places	Separating in several places	Complete separation
225	Separating in several places	Attached at one point	Separating in several places
280	Complete separation	Complete separation	Complete separation
290	Complete separation	Separating in several places	Separating in several places
330	Complete separation	Complete separation	Complete separation

suggest that the separation begins approximately at 180-mm CR length.

CRANIAL MENINGES

Hochstetter[10] shows that, as the dural reflections develop, the posterior point of attachment between the tentorium cerebelli and the falx cerebri gradually moves to a more caudal position in the skull, thus producing a continual reduction in the size of the posterior cranial fossa relative to the supratentorial fossae. This migration is practically completed between 35- and 90-mm CR length. Klintworth[12] found that the tentorium was first seen microscopically as a bilateral, three-layered structure in a stage XX (20-mm CR) embryo. The two tentorial precursors were visible grossly by stage XXIII (30-mm CR), and they fused at 55-mm CR length to create the straight sinus.[21] It is important that any considerations of malformations involving enlargement of the posterior fossa take into account the possible lack of fusion of the tentorium and the position of the torcular.

Robertson[19] notes that ventral to the brain stem the arachnoid is not closely approximated to the pia mater. Dorsally and laterally, however, the arachnoid is closely applied to the pia on the inferior surface of the cerebellum. Although we do not know when the cranial arachnoid separates from the dura mater, the studies of Brocklehurst[4] and our own unpublished observations suggest that a subarachnoid space (cisterna magna) occurs before the end of the embryonic stages when the foramen of Magendie is

formed. By this time, the ventral, but not the dorsal, pia mater is closely approximated to the arachnoid. In the later consideration of dorsal midline cysts in the posterior fossa, the histologic development of the meninges assumes importance. If the cyst arises from an early dilatation of the fourth ventricle, the pia mater (or tela chorioidea) should be in direct apposition to the arachnoid, whereas these layers should be separated in leptomeningeal ("subarachnoid" or "arachnoid") cysts of the cisterna magna. Grossly, a second membrane should be seen separating the latter cyst from the fourth ventricle. This relationship, as well as the incomplete fusion of the bilateral tentorial anlage and the position of the torcula, may be helpful in determining the relative timing of certain malformations.

ABNORMAL DEVELOPMENT

The meninges appear to be involved in most congenital abnormalities secondarily, although it is often difficult to make the distinction between primary and secondary abnormalities. Additional difficulties occur based upon apparent inconsistencies between postnatal histologic appearances and the presumed sequence of normal development. This may be due to the degeneration of membranes late in fetal life, modification of cells lining cysts, errors in the developmental studies, differences in development in certain regions of the neuroaxis or misinterpretations of histologic appearances. There are many situations in which two or three meninges are involved in the anomaly, thus creating difficulty in resolving the primary role.

MENINGOCELE (SPINAL AND CRANIAL)

This well known but relatively uncommon (as compared with meningomyelocele) entity is characterized by a prolapse of the arachnoid and dura mater through a bony defect in the spine or skull (*e.g.*, "sacral meningocele," "occipital meningocele"). It therefore usually represents an enlarged subarachnoid space on the dorsal aspect of the neural tube, although it can occur ventrally.

MYELOCYSTOCELE AND MYELOCYSTOMENINGOCELE

Myelocystoceles are skin-covered cystic lesions arising from an abnormal dilatation of the central canal, usually found in association with cloacal exstrophy or exomphalos. Ballantyne[2] states that the wall of the sac "consists of thin spinal membranes (without any trace of the dura mater)." A meningocele may coexist with such a lesion, in which case it is termed myelocystomeningocele.

INTRACRANIAL MENINGEAL CYSTS

Meningeal cysts within the skull are one of the most perplexing anomalies to discuss as a group. Haymaker and Foster[9] described a 34-year-old patient who had what they considered to be an intradural cyst arising in the posterior fossa and displacing the tentorium. They considered it to be of embryonic origin, *i.e.*, that the dura mater had not fused with the periosteum (or outer layer of dura). Since there is a question as to whether the periosteum should be considered as part of the dura mater, one could question whether such a cyst should be described as intradural or epidural.

The dura mater is most commonly involved by a cystic protrusion of other structures from the posterior fossa through an enlarged tentorial notch.[6,13] The dural defect in these cases involves incomplete development of the tentorium anteriorly, but whether it is primary or secondary is questionable. Robertson[19] presents several pneumoencephalographs in which air in the cisterna magna is shown to rise above the level of the inion, thus inferring a defect in the posterior aspect of the tentorium. A post mortem examination in one patient revealed that the torcular was far above the level of the inion, but the lateral attachments (*i.e.*, the origin) of the tentorium were in the normal position. There were also anomalies of the dural venous sinuses, and the anterior portion of the falx cerebri was missing.

Arachnoidal cysts have been reported at the spinal, cerebral (Figs. 17–2 and 17–3) and cerebellar levels.[15] There seems to be a

FIG. 17–2. Inferior–lateral view of the indentation associated with an arachnoid cyst (*arrow*) in a 78-year-old man. Note the shortened temporal pole. This was an incidental observation at autopsy. (#VA N-298-56)

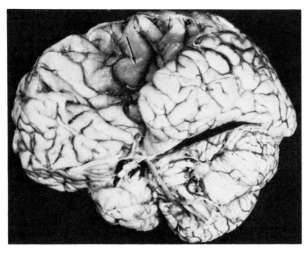

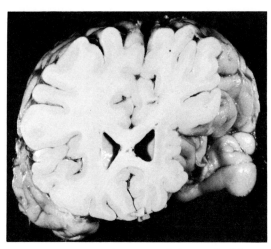

FIG. 17–3. Coronal section of the cerebral hemispheres showing the asymmetry and displacement associated with an arachnoid cyst incidentally discovered at autopsy of a 52-year-old woman. (#Np 466)

predilection for the posterior fossa, mainly the dorsal midline[6] and the cerebellopontine angle.[7] In one series of 20 infratentorial arachnoid cysts mainly in adults, 6 were in the cerebellopontine angle, 6 in the inferior midline, 1 in the superior midline, 4 over the cerebellar hemispheres, 1 associated with the clivus and 2 within the tentorial notch.[14] In only one case was the etiology thought to have a congenital basis. The recognition of these cysts is increasing, although many are still confused with the Dandy–Walker syndrome. The diagnosis is usually made because of an abnormally enlarging head (hydrocephalus), but it is also discovered incidentally at autopsy.

Histologically, the arachnoidal cyst wall varies.[6] In some areas it may be collagenous and contain capillaries; in other areas ependyma on an astroglial membrane can be found, and in still others there is "a gradual transition from low cuboidal epithelium to an arachnoid-like membrane." The combination of islands of ependyma with leptomeninges has lead to the hypothesis that many of these cysts in the posterior fossa may be caused by a persistence of Blake's pouch.[6] Histologic examination of the cyst wall is essential to separate those of developmental origin from cysts occurring secondary to infection, hemorrhage and/or trauma.[8] Neuhauser *et al.*[18] report "juxta-sellar"

arachnoid cysts in four autopsied cases of Hurler and one of Scheie syndrome.

HETEROTOPIAS

Heterotopic CNS tissue found in the spinal or cranial meninges rarely is clinically significant *per se*, but it usually indicates a more severe malformation. Freeman[5] describes a 55-year-old patient in whom an incidental finding at autopsy was a small, soft, pearly, pink mass, lying in the meninges and connected to the pons by a strand of pia mater. Histologically some of it looked like hippocampal gyrus; in other regions there were well-defined molecular layer, glia and myelin bodies. Willis[23] reviews eight other reports (1907–1955), some of which had cortex, astrocytic nests, spongioblasts, neuroblasts and neuroglial nodules in the leptomeninges. He also presents a case of a 12-year-old boy who died from meningitis and who had a strip of neural tissue embedded in the leptomeninges and extending from the cervical to lumbar region. Histologically the heterotopic neural tissue was composed of neuroglia, medullated nerve fibers and small islands of gray matter without any architectural pattern. Heterotopic tissue from other organs can be found in the meninges, but the mechanism by which they arise is unclear.[22]

MISCELLANEOUS ANOMALIES

In the typical thoracolumbar meningomyelocele there is an abnormally large ventral subarachnoid space lying under the dysplastic cord. In diastematomyelia there are variations in meningeal morphology; in some cases each cord is invested with a separate dural sheath, whereas in others a single dural sheath surrounds both. The intracranial angiomas of the Sturge–Weber syndrome involve the leptomeningeal vessels. Although there is less-direct evidence for hamartomatous origin, "melanosis"[22] and "lipomatosis" of the meninges are other examples of unusual conditions that involve the meninges. In the latter situation, Baker and Adams[1] report a one-year-old girl with hydrocephalus and several meningeal lipomas over the spinal cord and in the cerebellopontine angle. She also had bilateral aniridia, which is a primary malformation of the CNS. Finally, there may be marked hypoplasia of portions of the falx cerebri in holoprosencephaly or Arnold–Chiari malformation.

REFERENCES

1. Baker AB, Adams JM: Lipomatosis of the central nervous system. Am J Cancer 34:214–219, 1938

2. Ballantyne JW: Manual of Antenatal Pathology and Hygiene. The Embryo, vol II. New York, William Wood, 1905, pp. 406–420

3. Barr ML: The Human Nervous System. New York, Harper & Row, 1972

4. Brocklehurst G: The development of the human cerebrospinal fluid pathway with particular reference to the roof of the fourth ventricle. J Anat 105:467–475, 1969

5. Freeman W: Cortical heterotopia in the pontile meninges. Arch Pathol Lab Med 2:352–354, 1926

6. Gilles FH, Rockett FX: Infantile hydrocephalus: retrocerebellar "arachnoidal" cyst. J Pediatr 79:436–443, 1971

7. Gomez MR, Yanagihara T, MacCarty CS: Arachnoid cyst of the cerebello-pontine angle and infantile spastic hemiplegia. J Neurosurg 29:87–90, 1968

8. Gruber FH: Post-traumatic leptomeningeal cysts. Am J Roentgenol Radium Ther Nucl Med 105:305–307, 1969

9. Haymaker W, Foster ME Jr: Intracranial dural cyst. J Neurosurg 1:211–218, 1944

10. Hochstetter F: Über die Entwicklung und Differenzierung der Hüllen des meschlichen Gehirnes. Morphol Jahrb 83:359–394, 1939

11. Kimmel DL: Innervation of spinal dura mater and dura mater of the posterior cranial fossa. Neurology (Minneap) 11:800–809, 1961

12. Klintworth GK: The ontogeny and growth of the human tentorium cerebelli. Anat Rec 158:433–442, 1967

13. Lewis AJ: Infantile hydrocephalus caused by arachnoid cyst. J Neurosurg 19:431–434, 1962

14. Little JR, Gomez MR, MacCarty CS: Infratentorial arachnoid cysts. J Neurosurg 39:380–386, 1973

15. McDonald JV, Colgan J: Arachnoidal cysts of the posterior fossa. Neurology (Minneap) 14:643–646, 1964

16. Millen JW, Woollam DHM: Observations on the nature of pia mater. Brain 84:514–520, 1961

17. Millen JW, Woollam DHM: The Anatomy of the Cerebrospinal Fluid. New York, Oxford Univ Press, 1962

18. Neuhauser EBH, Griscom NT, Gilles FH, Crocker AC: Arachnoid cysts in the Hurler–Hunter syndrome. Ann Radiol (Paris) 11:453–469, 1968

19. Robertson EG: Developmental defects of the cisterna magna. J Neurol Neurosurg Psychiatry 12:39–51, 1949

20. Sensenig EC: The early development of the meninges of the spinal cord in human embryos. Contrib Embryol 34:145–157, 1951

21. Streeter GL: The development of the venous sinuses of the dura mater in the human embryo. Am J Anat 18:145–178, 1915

22. Wiener MF, Dallgaard SA: Intracranial adrenal gland (abstracted). J Neuropathol Exp Neurol 18:330–332, 1959

23. Willis RA: The Borderland of Embryology and Pathology. Washington DC, Butterworth, 1962

chapter 18

SKULL

The skull is divided into the *neurocranium,* which is the portion that surrounds the brain, and the *viscerocranium,* the part in which the facial bones develop. The neurocranium itself is subdivided into: 1) the bones of the base (chondrocranium) which undergo endochondral ossification (*i.e.,* they pass through a cartilaginous stage) and 2) those membranous or flat bones which ossify directly and are never cartilage. The more commonly identified clinical developmental anomalies pertain to the membranous bones. Although numerous anomalies are found in the cartilaginous bones, they are less often clinically diagnosed; they are, however, important in the pathogenesis of certain defects, especially those of sutures or those associated with more-severe defects in the membranous portions.

NORMAL DEVELOPMENT*

DEVELOPMENTAL LANDMARKS

Developmental landmarks (Fig. 18–1) begin with stage XI (2.5- to 4.5-mm CR), when the otic plate is visible externally and marks the position of the future temporal bone. During stage XII (3- to 5-mm CR) this plate transforms into a vesicle. Also at this time, the notochord separates from the neural tube in the cranial and cervical areas with the rostral portion of the notochord marking the boundary between the future sphenoid and occipital bones. Mesodermal condensa-

tions around it, referred to as prechordal and parachordal, are destined to differentiate into nearly all of the major bones of the base of the skull.

Other important changes commence during stages XII and XIII (4- to 6-mm CR). The first vascularization around the cephalic neural tube, which will give rise to both the chondrocranium and the membranous neurocranium, occurs in the mesoderm. The four occipital segments (the most-rostral four somites) become identifiable as such and a "sclerotomic fissure" is found in the most-caudal occipital somite.[41] All sclerotomes caudal to this eventually develop similar fissures that divide them into rostral and caudal portions. The rostral portion of one sclerotome then combines with the caudal portion of the next sclerotome to form a vertebral segment. In the caudal occipital somite, this process contributes to the formation of the atlas.

Further landmarks in the development of the skull occur during stage XIV (5- to 7-mm CR), when the meninx primitiva is first seen, and during stage XV (7- to 9-mm CR), when the first cervical segmental artery demarcates the skull from the vertebral column.[41] By stage XVI (8- to 11-mm CR), there is a membranous roof to the cranial cavity.

The first chondrification begins during stage XVII (11- to 14-mm CR) in both the basiocciput and the body of the sphenoid. This process of chondrification continues rapidly, and by stage XX (18- to 22-mm CR), the hypoglossal nerve passes through a chondrified foramen. This is when the first indication of dura mater is seen within the skull, the pia mater having been formed con-

---

* See Chapter 1 for background information on embryologic development and staging system.

289

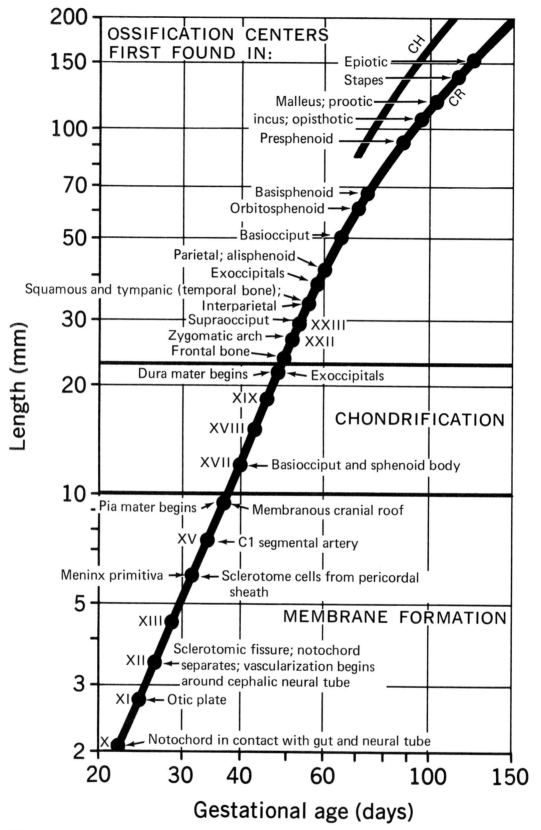

FIG. 18–1. Development of the skull correlated with CR length and gestational age. The period of membrane formation is featured between 2- and 10-mm CR length, the period of chondrification between 10- and 22-mm CR length and the onset of ossification thereafter.

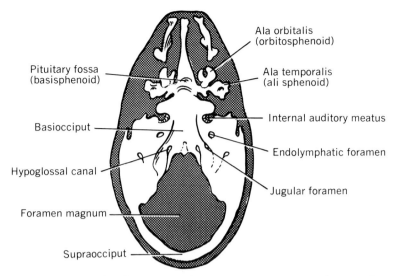

FIG. 18–2.   The chondrocranium of stage XX (20-mm CR) embryo. (Adapted from Kernan, 1916)

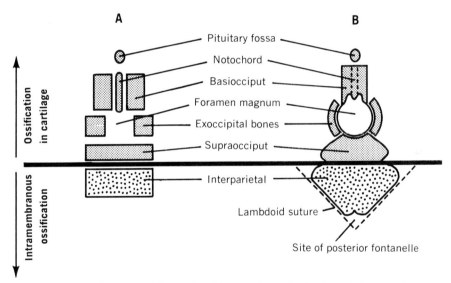

FIG. 18–3.   Development of the occipital bone. Above the horizontal line are those parts that undergo endochondral ossification; the interparietal portion, below the line, undergoes intramembranous ossification. A, the various components while they are still isolated entities; B, after the basioccipitals have fused in the midline, incorporating the notochord, and after the supraocciput has fused with the interparietal. (Adapted from Bardeen, 1910)

siderably earlier, during stages XV–XVI. Figure 18–2 reconstructs the chondrocranium at this stage of development.[22]

After stage XVI the changes in the bones of the skull are too numerous to list in a sequential manner. Therefore, a description of several bones will be presented individu-

ally. Most of the information has been derived from the studies of Mall,[29] Bardeen,[5] deBeer,[10] Noback[36] and Patten[37] and from aliziran red "S"-stained specimens in the collection of The Central Laboratory for Human Embryology at the University of Washington.

OCCIPITAL BONE

The occipital bone is derived from both chondrocranium and membranous bone. The previously mentioned parachordal mesodermal cells, which begin to proliferate bilaterally, migate toward the midline during stage XIII (4- to 6-mm CR) and gradually fuse around the notochord to form that portion of the base of the skull from the pituitary fossa to the foramen magnum at the level of the future jugular foramen. This tissue undergoes chondrification, then ossification at 50-mm CR length, and is known as the basiocciput. Immediately lateral to it are the otic vesicles; in its caudal aspect are the bilateral exoccipitals, which are also formed from parachordal mesoderm (ossifying at 37-mm CR length) and which eventually become the lateral boundaries of the foramen magnum. The hypoglossal canals form within the exoccipitals.

The two portions of the occipital bone that remain are the supraoccipital, which forms the caudal boundary of the foramen magnum (ossifying at 30-mm CR length), and the interparietal, which is immediately above it and begins ossification at 32-mm CR length. The interparietal portion is the only part of the occipital bone that undergoes membranous ossification. Some fusion is found between the supraoccipital and interparietal at 34-mm CR length, but the others do not fuse until much later (the supraoccipital and exoccipitals fuse two years postnatally, and the exoccipitals fuse with the basiocciput four years postnatally). The primary development of the occipital bone is shown schematically in Figure 18–3, and the ossification patterns of the skull in general are shown in Figure 18–4. The occipital bone begins to develop earlier than the other bones and is frequently involved in congenital anomalies.

SPHENOID BONE

The sphenoid bone has four major components. Fawcett,[13] Bardeen[5] and deBeer[10] give detailed discussions of their individual developments. The basisphenoid (whose pharyngeal canal closes during stage XX) arises in prechordal mesoderm immediately rostral to the basiocciput, to which it eventually begins to fuse 18 months after birth,[10] and completes the fusion at 18 years.[20]

Median pairs of centers of ossification are found at 65-mm CR length, and lateral centers at 90-mm CR length, on each side of the pituitary fossa. Ossification of the anterior clinoid process occurs directly from the lateral centers, whereas the dorsum sellae arises later, the timing still being unclear. Just lateral to the basisphenoid is the alisphenoid (greater wing), with which it fuses at birth. The temporal ossification center of the alisphenoid is seen at 37-mm CR length and the lateral pterygoid center at 54-mm CR length. Both the foramen rotundum and the foramen ovale are formed in this portion of the sphenoid. It is uncertain whether the lateral pterygoid process undergoes intramembranous ossification or not, but the median process does.

Just rostral and somewhat inferior to the basisphenoid is the presphenoid, in which the sphenoid sinuses eventually form, and which contributes the floor of the optic foramen. The presphenoid has five centers of ossification: two lateral (ossifying at 90-mm CR length), two median (117-mm CR length) and a median unpaired (168-mm CR length). The presphenoid has fused with both the basisphenoid and orbitosphenoid by 165-mm CR length, although the median and lateral paired centers do not fuse with the unpaired median center until 180-mm CR length.

The orbitosphenoid (lesser wing) develops both laterally and rostrally to the anterior clinoid processes of the basisphenoid. It forms the roof of the optic foramen. Through a large unfused fissure between the orbitosphenoid and the alisphenoid (the orbital fissure) pass cranial nerves III, IV, and VI. Paired ossification centers are found at 60-mm CR length.

FRONTAL BONE

Not much has been written about the development of the frontal bone before the onset of intramembranous ossification. Inman and Saunders[19] describe this ossification as beginning at from 32- to 36-mm CR length, but it has been seen as early as 23-mm CR (stage XXI) in at least one embryo.[37] The right and left halves of the developing frontal bone are separated by the metopic suture. The primary ossification centers are located in the region of the future superciliary arches; ossification then spreads dorsally

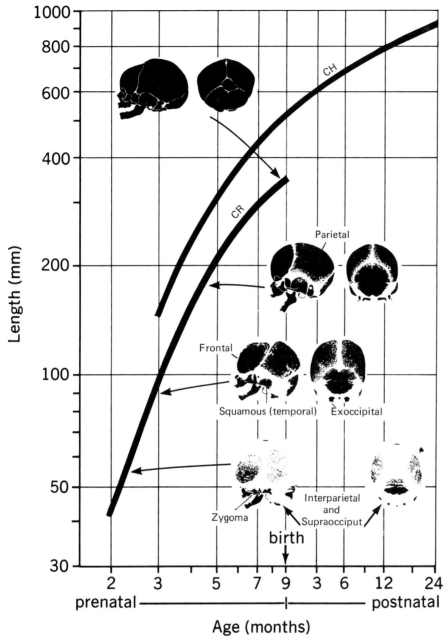

FIG. 18–4.   Lateral and corresponding posterior views of ossifying fetal skulls from 56-mm CR length to birth. (Adapted from Noback, 1944)

over the pars frontalis and into the pars orbitalis at 42-mm CR length. The latter then continues to ossify more rapidly at the lateral margins, and by 49-mm CR length the portion between it and the zygomatic process is ossified.

There has been a controversy as to whether or not more than two primary ossification centers exist,[5] but the more recent study of Inman and Saunders[19] does not demonstrate any others. However, accessory ossicles have been found in the metopic fontanelle. The middle portion of the metopic suture ossifies during the second year after birth and is closed over its entire length by the eighth year. The frontal sinuses appear during the first postnatal year and continue to enlarge throughout adolescence.

TABLE 18–1. ONSET OF OSSIFICATION IN PORTIONS OF THE TEMPORAL *cambial –*
BONE THAT UNDERGO ENDOCHONDRAL OSSIFICATION

Name of Bone	Position	First Ossification*
Styloid Portion		
Tympanohyal	Medial to tympanic	Birth
Stylohyal	Styloid process	Postnatal (third year)
Petrosal Portion (arising from otic capsule)		
Opisthotic	Cochlear–canalicular and cochlear center	110 130
Prootic	Anterior canalicular center	117
	Posterior canalicular center	130
	Intermediate canalicular center	134
Epiotic	Mastoid center	161
Ossicles		
Incus	Middle ear	110
Malleus	Middle ear	125
Stapes	Middle ear	139

* First ossification measured in mm CR length.

PARIETAL BONE

The paired parietal bones each contain two centers of ossification (intramembranous) that are first seen at 37-mm CR length. These eventually merge, and subsequent ossification radiates from this single locus.

TEMPORAL BONE

The bones in the auditory region are so numerous and complex that a detailed discussion of their development is beyond the scope of this chapter. The squamous portion, to which the zygomatic arch connects, begins membranous ossification at 36-mm CR length; the arch itself starts earlier, during stage XXII (25-mm CR). The tympanic portion lying immediately inferior begins ossification at 32-mm CR length and is the only other part of the temporal area bones that undergoes membranous ossification. The various times at which ossification is found in those that pass through a cartilaginous stage are listed in Table 18–1.

SUTURES AND FONTANELLES

The nonossified connective tissues between the edges of the developing cranial bones are termed sutures. At many points these sutures are widened and form fontanelles. With the exception of the metopic and parietal fontanelles, this widening occurs at the junction of three or more bones. The size and contour of the sutures and fontanelles are clinically important and are discussed later.

Pritchard *et al.*[38] have shown that the sutures of the face (viscerocranium) originate as five separate layers between the bone edges; there are two cambial layers, two fibrous layers and a "loose" middle cellular layer (Fig. 18–5). The cambial layers are the

FIG. 18–5. Sutures of the face and neurocranium: *A*, layers involved in the development of the sutures of the face; *B*, layers involved in the development of the membranous neurocranium. (Adapted from Pritchard et al., 1956)

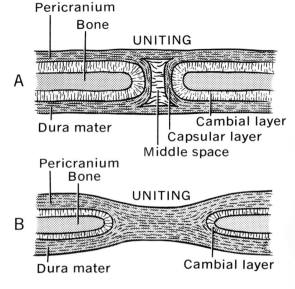

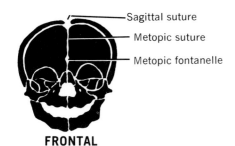

FRONTAL

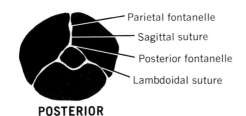

POSTERIOR

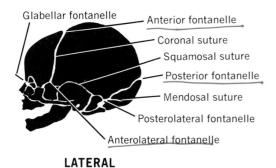

LATERAL

FIG. 18-6. Major fontanelles and sutures in the newborn skull.

perpendicular to the bone is not known, nor is the mechanism for the development of the middle layer known.

Most clinicians are familiar with two fontanelles, the "anterior" (junction point of the two parietal and two frontal bones) and the "posterior" (junction point of the two parietal bones with the interparietal portion of the occipital bone). While the former has more significance with respect to aiding in the assessment of changes in intracranial pressure, it should be mentioned that many other fontanelles exist at the time of birth. Most can be palpated or demonstrated on radiographs and are named as follows: glabellar, metopic, anterior lateral (sphenoid), parietal (sagittal), posterior lateral and cerebellar. These and the major sutures are shown in Figure 18-6.

The resolution, or gradual closure, of the anterior fontanelle has been studied after birth in several large series of children. Aisenson[2] found that 90% closed between 7 and 19 months of age, and Acheson and Jefferson[1] determined the mean age of closure to be 16.3 months clinically and 17.9 months radiologically in males, and 18.8 and 19.7 months in females. Delayed closures of sutures and fontanelles are found in several malformations of the skull.

sites of quite active osteogenesis where pro-osteoblasts and osteoblasts are found in abundance. In addition, collagen is found oriented in a radial manner around the bone edge.

The fibrous capsules are composed of collagen and fibroblasts that run at right angles to the advancing bone edges. In contrast, the sutures of the membranous neurocranium originally do not have the fibrous layers oriented perpendicularly between the bone edges. Instead, the dura mater and pericranium are fused at this point with fibers oriented parallel to the bone edges (Fig. 18-5). However, as the bone edges gain close approximation, bringing the cambial layers closer together, the layers between them transform into two capsular and a middle layer as seen in the facial sutures. The manner in which the connective tissues within the capsular layers become oriented

MEASUREMENTS

The cephalometric studies of Ford[14] and Scammon and Calkins[40] provide the following information on the growth of the skull during the fetal period. When the fetus is 60-mm CR length, the occipitofrontal circumference (OFC) is approximately 60 mm. From then until the time of birth it increases between five- and six-fold. Initially the frontal region is more prominent and the skull is higher as compared with the length and width. As development proceeds, the skull becomes more square, but the width is always less than the length. Within the cranial base (chondrocranium) the prechordal portion grows more than the parachordal during gestation with a six- to seven-fold increase of the former as compared to a four- or five-fold increase for the latter.

Three external measurements have clinical importance as related to both prenatal and postnatal growth of the skull. These are the OFC, the width (biparietal diameter) and the length (occipitofrontal diameter). Figure 18–7 provides these dimensions during the fetal period as based on the studies of Scammon and Calkins.[40]

At the time of birth, the mean OFC is 34 cm for girls and 34.6 cm for boys. The subsequent development is influenced by many factors; most studies have been done on selected ethnic or socioeconomic classes. Nellhaus[35] compiles many recent studies into composite international and interracial graphs for boys and girls. Utilizing these graphs, one can follow the progression of head growth into adolescence in any individual.

The cephalic index (CI), utilizing the width and lengths of the skull, becomes clinically useful, especially in a certain type of abnormal development (craniosynostosis), if followed over several weeks. The CI is calculated as follows:

$$CI = \frac{W}{L} \times 100$$

The CI tells whether the head is growing too rapidly in one or the other dimension and can be used to confirm clinical suspicions. Normal values for the CI over the first few months vary from 75% to 85%; Table 18–2 gives approximations of subsequent values. From the clinical standpoint, it cannot be emphasized enough that a single measurement of any dimension of the head has only limited value. Serial measurements must be taken and plotted to determine that abnormal growth is occurring. Another important measurement that can be meaningful in assessing certain malformations relates to those taken from radiographs. Standards for normal growth are available in many radiologic texts.

ABNORMAL DEVELOPMENT

Moss[34] points out five developmental stages at which malformations could potentially arise in the sphenoid bone, but these stages probably apply to the other bones of the

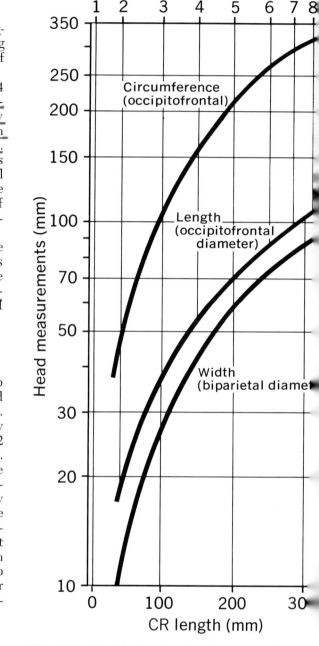

FIG. 18–7. Occipitofrontal circumference, occipitofrontal diameter and biparietal diameter correlated with CR length and gestational age.

TABLE 18–2. CEPHALIC INDEX VALUES THROUGH CHILDHOOD

Age	CI
Birth	84%
6 months	83%
1 year	82%
5 years	78%
15 years	80%

skull as well 1) during mesenchymal condensation, 2) during chondrification, 3) during the fusion of separate chondral centers, 4) during ossification and 5) during the fusion of ossification centers.

In many cases, malformations of the skull are either associated with maldevelopment of the brain or are part of a more generalized mesodermal syndrome. There are, however, some cases in which the cranial bone anomaly is an isolated feature in an otherwise normal individual. The following discussion will not separate these as it is much more useful clinically to approach a classification from a different viewpoint.

ABNORMALITIES OF THE CRANIAL VAULT

The following list* presents malformations of the membranous neurocranium (cranial vault) as they relate to: 1) pattern of ossification (decreased or increased), 2) size of head (decreased or increased) and 3) fusion of sutures (premature or delayed). Some diagnoses that are not true malformations are included because they are clinically important and fall within the differential diagnosis. Other diagnoses could be listed under more than one category.

I. Abnormal patterns of ossification
    Deficiencies in ossification
        Anencephaly (acrania)
        Encephalocele
    Decreased ossification
        Osteogenesis imperfecta
        Hypophosphatasia
        Lacunar skull (Lückenshädel)
        Hydranencephaly
        Aminopterin embryopathy
        Parietal foramina
        Eosinophilic granuloma
        Metopic fontanelle
    Increased ossification
        Osteopetrosis
        Albers–Schönberg disease
        Pyknodysosteogenesis
        Idiopathic hypercalcemia
        Myotonic dystrophy
II. Abnormal size of the head
    Increased size (macrocrania)
        Hydrocephalus
        X-linked aqueductal stenosis
        Intracranial cysts
        Encephalocele
        Subdural hematoma
        Familial idiopathic macrocephaly
        Achondroplasia
        Hurler syndrome
        Neoplasms
    Decreased size (microcephaly)
        Gene associated
            Seckel's bird-headed dwarfs
            Inborn errors of metabolism
                 (e.g., phenylketonuria)
        Chromosome anomalies
            Trisomies (Down syndrome)
            Deletions (cat cry syndrome)
            Translocations
        Environmental causes
            Intrauterine infections (e.g., rubella)
            Irradiation in utero
            Birth asphyxia
            Kernicterus
            Hydranencephaly
            Neonatal meningitis
            Subdural hematoma
        Dysmorphic syndromes of unknown etiology
            de Lange syndrome
III. Abnormalities of fusion of sutures
    Premature fusion (craniosynostosis)
        Idiopathic
        Apert syndrome, Carpenter syndrome, Crouzon syndrome
        Hyperthyroidism
        Hypophosphatasia
    Delayed fusion or separation
        Hydrocephalus
        Hypothyroidism
        Rickets
        Cleidocranial dysostosis
        Deprivational dwarfism (treated)
        Pyknodysosteogenesis

Anencephaly

Anencephaly (acrania) is discussed in Chapter 4 as a defect of neurulation. From the standpoint of the skull alone, there are defects in development of both the membranous neurocranium and chondrocranium. These have been studied in detail by Marin-Padilla.[30, 31] Depending on the severity of the defect, the occipital bone presents in two different ways. If the cranial defect extends

* Modified from Lemire and Shurtleff.[25]

FIG. 18–8.   Radiograph of skull with a small mid-line hole through which a very small encephalocele protruded.

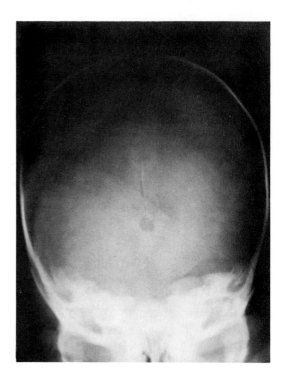

through the foramen magnum, the supra-occipital portion may be represented by only two small fragments articulating with the exoccipitals on each side. If the cranial defect is incomplete and placed more rostrally (as in meroacrania), the supraoccipital, basioccipital and exoccipitals are present but irregular. The basiocciput has been noted to be increased in thickness. Both the parietal and frontal bones are rudimentary, being mainly recognizable where they articulate with other bones. In some cases, the frontal bone is only represented by the superior portion of the orbits, whereas in others it is rotated posteriorly and lies on the sphenoid. The temporal bones have an abnormal orientation, being oblique and internally rotated. Marin-Padilla states that the sphenoid is the most severely malformed bone, showing complete distortion of all portions and being anomalous in position and greatly reduced in the transverse diameter.

Encephalocele

Between 60% and 75% of encephaloceles occur in the occipital region; the remainder occur in the frontal, nasofrontal, parietal, temporoorbital and nasopharyngeal regions (Figs. 18–8 to 18–12). They can originate anywhere along suture lines within the skull, even in the middle ear. A simple hole existing in the skull with no prolapse of meninges or cortex is referred to as cranium bifidum occultum. If only meninges are found within an external skin-covered sac, it is termed a meningocele (e.g., occipital meningocele). The term encephalocele (or meningoenceph-alocele) is reserved for those cases in which brain substance is within the sac. When a ventricle is also included, hydranencephalo-cele or encephalocystocele is applied.

The pathogenesis of encephaloceles as a group is not known. The earliest onset could be stage XII (3- to 5-mm CR), after the cephalic neural tube has closed, but they can develop at any later time depending on the size and degree of involvement. They have been produced experimentally[21] with tera-togenic agents given to various rodents and

primates, the effective timing being early, shortly after closure of the neuroectoderm in the cases of the larger lesions.

Encephaloceles occur from 5 to 10 times less commonly than meningomyeloceles, i.e., about 1/10,000 live births in the United States and as high as 1/2,500 live births in England.[23] The prognosis depends on the degree of involvement. Large hydranen-cephaloceles permit very few long-term survivals; occipital encephaloceles (i.e., with cortex but no ventricle in the sac) allow a 50% survival, whereas occipital meningo-celes carry a very good prognosis (nearly 100% survival). In some cases, the occipital encephalocele is part of a more severe syndrome (see Chapter 10), in which case the prognosis is poor.[18] Figures 18–13 and 18–14 illustrate typical occipital encephaloceles.

Other Clinical Syndromes

Varying degrees of decreased ossification are found in many situations in which there is no necessary involvement of the CNS (e.g., osteogenesis imperfecta, cleidocranial dysostosis, hypophosphatasia, syphilis and rickets) and in other situations with some neural involvement (e.g., hydranencephaly

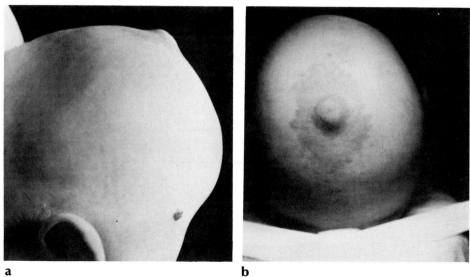

a   **b**

FIG. 18–9. **a.** Lateral view of a small interparietal encephalocele. **b.** Dorsal view of the encephalocele shown in Figure 18–9a. Note capillary hemangioma around the lesion.

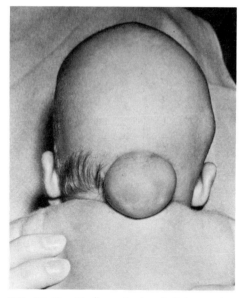

FIG. 18–10. Medium-sized occipital encephalocele.

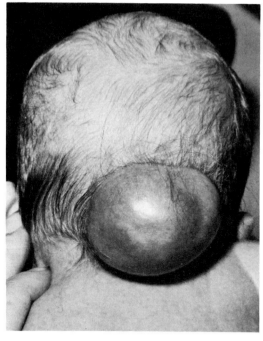

FIG. 18–11. Moderate-sized occipital encephalocele which is under some tension. Note the shine of the skin as compared with that illustrated in Fig. 18–10. (From Lemire and Shurtleff, 1971[25])

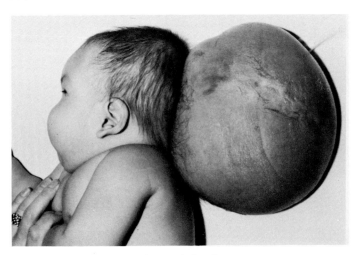

FIG. 18–12.   Large occipital encephalocele.

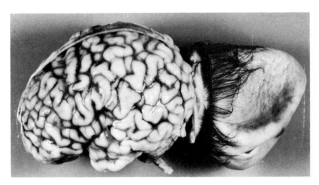

FIG. 18–13.   The brain and occipital encephalocele of a newborn boy. The sac originated from the roof of the third ventricle. (#Np 2072)

and aminopterin-induced embryopathy). Focal deficiencies, appearing as punched-out lesions, are seen in eosinophilic granuloma, Hand–Schuller–Christian and Letterer–Siwe diseases. In addition, markedly decreased ossification of the frontal bones around the metopic suture can present as a large irregular metopic fontanelle that persists into early adulthood.

Other deficiencies in ossification are seen in the form of parietal foramina that are only delays in physiologic ossification (up to 25% of neonates have these). In contrast, the lucunar skull (Lückenshädel) has multiple areas of thinning of the inner table and is frequently associated with the Arnold–Chiari malformation. A recent article by Epstein and Epstein[12] discusses many of these situations in more detail.

Macrocephaly vs. Macrocrania

A large head (macrocrania) may or may not be associated with a large brain (macrocephaly, as in idiopathic familial cases, achondroplasia, Hurler syndrome or certain leukodystrophies[46, 50]), other intracranial lesions (e.g., hydrocephalus, subdural hematoma, intracranial cyst or neoplasm) or a thickened skull (pyknodysostosis).

Microcephaly

The classification of microcephaly proposed by Böök et al.[6] divides all conditions in which the skull is abnormally small into two basic categories: 1) those due to specific nongenetic disease of the brain and 2) those due to the effects of specific genes. Warkany

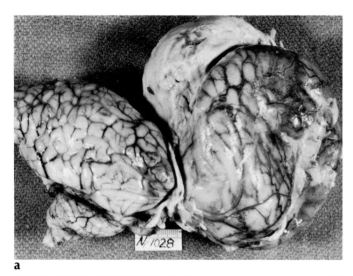

a

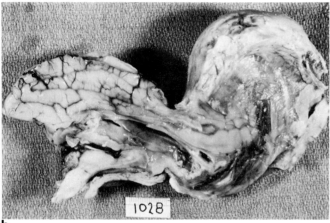

b

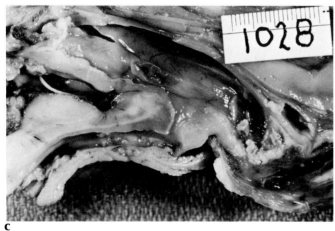

c

FIG. 18–14. **a.** Large occipital encephalocele (right) which contains a large amount of cerebral cortex and other elements derived from the diencephalon, mesencephalon and cerebellum. The infant lived 19 days. (#Np 1028) **b.** Midsagittal section through the specimen illustrated in Fig. 18–14**a. c.** Closer view of the same specimen.

and Dignan[47] provide a more complete separation of etiologies as follows: 1) gene mutations, 2) chromosomal changes and 3) environmental damages. While it is usually easy to categorize most cases appropriately, the definition of microcephaly itself is more difficult. There is little disagreement in calling a given case microcephaly when the OFC is three or more standard deviations below the mean for age, but some studies have included cases that are only two standard deviations below the mean. The problem is further compounded by patients whose height is also reduced; in such situations the OFC, though small, would not be strictly three standard deviations for that particular height.

GENE MUTATIONS. "Genetic micrencephaly" is associated with underlying cerebral hypoplasia. Unlike the other types of microcephaly where the skull can be of nearly normal shape but small, these patients may have a sloping forehead and flat occiput. Most of these heterogeneous conditions have autosomal recessive inheritance and include such diagnostic categories as Seckel's bird-headed dwarfs as well as many of the inborn errors of metabolism. Warkany and Dignan[47] provide a complete listing of these conditions. The specific patterns of cranial bone malformation vary, but in general there is hypoplasia of the entire membranous neurocranium. It is important to correctly differentiate these entities (which are associated with a high risk of severe mental retardation) from oxycephaly (see "Craniosynostosis" below), with which they can be confused.

Some patients with chromosomal anomalies have microcephaly. This is especially true of the trisomy 13 syndrome, which is associated with many primary malformations of the CNS. Many patients with Down syndrome have small brachycephalic skulls. Microcephaly is found associated with several types of chromosome deletions (e.g., cat cry syndrome, 4p−, 18q−) and is also found in some patients with ring chromosomes or translocations.[46]

ENVIRONMENTAL AGENTS. Environmental agents which may damage the brain include intrauterine infections, of which the congenital rubella syndrome and cytomegalic inclusion disease are the best known (see Chapter 23). In both situations a generalized viremia affecting multiple organ systems is transmitted from mother to fetus. In the rubella syndrome, there is generalized growth retardation (including the brain) when the infection occurs within the first two months in utero; this retardation is especially severe when infection occurs between the third and fifth gestational weeks. The small skull is usually associated with a small brain that shows cortical atrophy, degenerative lesions, focal ischemic necrosis and cerebral vascular damage. There is frequently degeneration of one or more layers of the vessel wall and replacement by acellular material that is sometimes metachromatic and sometimes PAS-positive.[39]

Toxoplasmosis and Type 2 herpesvirus[44] are also associated with microcephaly. In herpesvirus disease it is suspected that the infection occurs early in pregnancy, whereas in toxoplasmosis and cytomegalic inclusion disease the infection may occur as late as the fourth or fifth gestational month. Undoubtedly many other viruses will ultimately be implicated in cases of microcephaly in which the small skull size is only one aspect of a more generalized problem, including cortical atrophy.

The association of early ionizing irradiation in utero with microcephaly is well known. Factors during extrauterine life that may be associated with subsequent lack of normal head growth are birth asphyxia, kernicterus, neonatal meningitis and subdural hematoma, the last of which is more frequently associated with an enlargement of the skull.

As with most systems of classification, a fourth group might be added, that of cases of microcephaly in which the etiology is presently unknown. The de Lange syndrome is an example of anomalies in this category.[43]

Craniosynostosis

The premature fusion of one or more sutures is a condition of interest to the basic scientist as well as to the clinician. Experimental and descriptive studies[34] have helped clarify the probable basis of craniosynostosis as a primary defect in the cranial base (chondrocranium) at the sites of initial attachment of the dura mater. Thus, premature sutural synostosis is considered a secondary phenomenon, not a cause. With respect to the sagittal suture, it is postulated that an anomalous spatial relationship between the midline anterior attachment of the falx with the crista galli may cause abnormal tensile stresses to occur sagittally within the tissues and be directly transmitted to the sagittal suture. Moss[34] cites other studies showing that tension itself is capable of initiating osteogenic processes within the sutural tissue. Such osteogenesis subsequently bridges the area between the approximating parietal bones. In the case of the coronal suture the initial spatial abnormality involves the dural attachment to the developing lesser wings of the sphenoid, the subsequent tension being transmitted transversely vertically to the coronal suture. The abnormality in attachment of the dura mater is considered secondary to anomalous development of the chondrocranium.

Anatomically it is easiest to classify craniosynostosis by a system that combines descriptive names with the suture(s) involved (Table 18–3). Cohen[9] provides a different classification that is useful for an overall genetic counseling approach, particularly for syndromes with multiple defects of which the craniosynostosis is only a part.

As a general rule, normal bone growth is inhibited in a plane perpendicular to the fused suture, and therefore, the skull increases in a plane parallel to the fused suture. Thus, the OFC is frequently not abnormal initially, but one should make serial recordings of the CI when an infant is suspected of having a craniosynostosis. A

decreasing numerical value of the CI indicates elongation in an anteroposterior plane (scaphocephaly), whereas an increasing value of the CI indicates increasing width (brachycephaly). McLauren and Matson[33] point out the advantage of using the CI, but radiographic studies are most helpful in establishing the diagnosis of synostosis. Absence of a suture and a ridge of dense bone at the normal suture site are diagnostic. Recent articles dealing with all types of craniosynostosis are provided by Anderson and Geiger,[3] Anderson and Gomes,[4] Shilloto and Matson[42] and Cohen.[9]

SCAPHOCEPHALY. Scaphocephaly (dolichocephaly) accounts for from 50% to 60% of all craniosynostoses. This name usually applies to fusion of the sagittal suture alone, which results in a skull that elongates in an anteroposterior plane (Figs. 18–15 to 18–17), with the occiput growing downward and backward and deforming the posterior fossa. Some cases have been found to be familial, and a male preponderance has been noted, suggesting a genetic factor. However, unlike other varieties of craniosynostosis, this form is not usually associated with other clinical syndromes. Many articles in recent years have emphasized the importance of surgery within the first three or four months. Shillito and Matson[42] recommend operation at from four to six weeks, with the supposition that

FIG. 18–15. Lateral view of an infant with scaphocephaly, secondary to premature fusion of the sagittal suture.

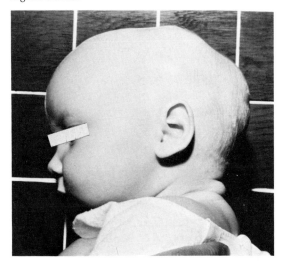

TABLE 18–3. CLASSIFICATION OF CRANIOSYNOSTOSIS

Popular Name	Suture(s) Affected
Scaphocephaly and dolichocephaly	Sagittal
Brachycephaly	Coronal (bilateral)
Plagiocephaly	Coronal (unilateral) or lamboid (unilateral) or both; with or without accompanying sagittal suture involvement
Trigonocephaly	Metopic
Oxycephaly	All sutures
Acrocephaly and turricephaly or turribrachycephaly	Any combination that gives a pointed or "tower"-shaped head

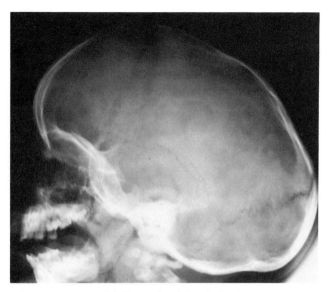

FIG. 18–16.   Lateral radiograph of the skull of another patient with scaphocephaly. Note the anteroposterior elongation of the skull.

FIG. 18–17.   Anteroposterior radiograph of the skull of a patient with premature fusion of the sagittal suture.

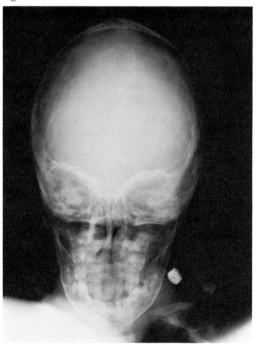

both cosmetic results and intellectual achievement can be favorably influenced.

BRACHYCEPHALY AND PLAGIOCEPHALY. Brachycephaly (bilateral fusion of the coronal sutures) and plagiocephaly (unilateral fusion of the coronal or lambdoid sutures) are less common than scaphocephaly (each accounts for approximately 10% of craniosynostoses in the United States), but they are much more commonly associated with other syndromes. The skull is increased in width and height. Moss[34] found that the clivus is hypoplastic.

Because of the other associated disorders, cases that involve the coronal suture pose questions as to whether or not operative intervention is indicated. As reviewed by Cohen,[9] many of these cases represent syndromes with an underlying genetic basis: for example, Apert syndrome (autosomal dominant) and Carpenter syndrome (autosomal recessive). Since the optimal time for operation is too early to firmly establish the intellectual potential of the individual, there are grounds for controversy as to whether the subsequent mental retardation is ameliorated by surgical procedure. Fortunately in Crouzon syndrome (inherited as an autosomal dominant) mental retardation is not frequent. The diagnosis is frequently made shortly after birth because of associated dysmorphic features or a history of previous family involvement. In many cases, the skull deformity itself is obvious at birth, but radiographic confirmation is indicated.

TRIGONOCEPHALY. Trigonocephaly, premature fusion of the metopic suture producing a V-shaped frontal abnormality of the skull, accounts for 10% of the craniosynostoses.

OXYCEPHALY. The term *oxycephaly* is a term sometimes used for cases with premature closure of the coronal suture plus any other suture, but it is better used when "all sutures" are fused. This occurs in less than 10% of all cases of craniosynostosis in the United States, but in other countries, such as Egypt, it may be the most common form.[11]

Oxycephaly represents the most severe clinical problem in this type of malformation. Aside from the necessity to consider early surgery to relieve increased intracranial pressure, it presents an important diagnostic consideration because of its frequent association with genetic micrencephaly, which is invariably associated with severe mental retardation. In such cases, surgery cannot be recommended as the surgery necessary to correct the maldevelopment of the skull is too extensive. Unfortunately it is sometimes difficult to make the distinction between oxycephalies that are associated with genetic micrencephaly and those that are not, and this difficulty has resulted in errors in both directions.[4]

Craniosynostosis is also found in Hallerman–Strieff syndrome, Kleeblattschädel anomaly, hypophosphatasia, hypercalcemia and hyperthyroidism.

Delayed Fusion of Sutures

This is not a malformation, but an abnormality of skull growth in which sutures fail to fuse properly, usually not as an isolated entity but as part of another process. Suture separation (such as is found in hydrocephalus with increased intracranial pressure) is different from delay (such as in hypothyroidism, cleidocranial dysostosis and rickets). Delayed closure of the anterior fontanelle is associated with a variety of conditions: Down syndrome, hypophosphatasia, aminopterin embryopathy, cerebrohepato-

renal syndrome, Hallerman–Strieff syndrome and trisomy 13 and 18 syndromes.[43]

ABNORMALITIES OF THE CRANIAL BASE

Numerous malformations involving the cranial base are of both clinical importance and scientific interest. Most are secondary to abnormalities of other structures (*e.g.*, atresia of the external auditory canal, hypoplastic optic foramina and hypoplasia of the pituitary fossa). At least four conditions are recognized with increased ossification in the skull, mainly in the chondrocranium: 1) pyknodysosteogenesis, 2) Albers–Schönberg disease, 3) idiopathic hypercalcemia and 4) myotonic dystrophy. Although none involves a primary malformation of the nervous system, secondary compression of the cranial nerves can occur when excess bone builds up around the foramina of the skull. In the case of the optic nerve, this can lead to blindness.

Platybasia and Basilar Impression

Because these conditions frequently occur in the same patient and are sometimes erroneously regarded as being synonymous, they will be presented together. They are separate entities.

Platybasia is probably the easiest to understand since it merely implies a flattening of the base of the skull and can be defined by an increase in an angle measurable on a lateral radiograph. If one line is drawn from the nasion to the middle of the pituitary fossa and a second line from the latter to the anterior margin of the foramen magnum (basion), the "basal angle" created should be between 125° and 143°.[45] If this angle is greater than 143°, the skull is considered to have platybasia. There is some ethnic variation in the normal limits of the basal angle,[32] so that the extreme range of normals may be from 115° to 150°.

Basilar impression, unlike platybasia, only involves the basal bones surrounding the foramen magnum. In basilar impression an invagination of these bones upward into the posterior fossa creates a smaller volume to accommodate the cerebellum and brain stem and often results in compromise of the cervicomedullary junction because of impingement by the odontoid process. This condition is frequently compounded by fusion of the atlas with the occiput and by rostral projection of the odontoid process (axis). Methods of diagnosing basilar impression utilize various points on both lateral and anteroposterior radiographs. The extension of the odontoid process above Chamberlain's line,[8] a line drawn from the posterior margin of the hard palate to the posterior margin of the foramen magnum, is perhaps the best-known method of diagnosing basilar impression. However, it has fallen into some disrepute due to difficulty in establishing the posterior point. Although each type of measurement has some drawback,[7] they are all directed at establishing the relationship of the odontoid process to the foramen magnum. The study of Hinck et al.[16] provides normal values from the third postnatal year to adulthood.

It is difficult to establish the time of onset of either platybasia or basilar impression from a pathogenetic viewpoint. Although numerous cases occur in which these are the only anomalies and were undoubtedly present at birth, neurologic symptoms resulting from compression may not occur until adolescence. In the case of platybasia appearing alone, no symptoms may result. In many other situations these conditions are part of a more generalized syndrome (e.g., osteogenesis imperfecta, cretinism, cleidocranial dysostosis) or are secondary to diseases associated with softening of bones (e.g., osteomalacia, rickets, Paget's disease and hyperparathyroidism).

Iniencephaly

Newborns with iniencephaly seldom live more than a few hours, and less than 200 cases have been reported. However, it remains one of the most interesting of all anomalies even though the skull defect is relatively slight. The typical iniencephalic has: 1) a defect in the occipital bone around the foramen magnum, 2) spina bifida of a considerable degree and 3) retroflexion of the head on the spine (Fig. 18–18). It has been produced experimentally in the offspring of rats given streptonigrin[48] and has features to associate it with the Klippel–Feil syndrome[15] and with anencephaly with spinal retroflexion.[17, 24] The associations with the Klippel–Feil syndrome and anencephaly

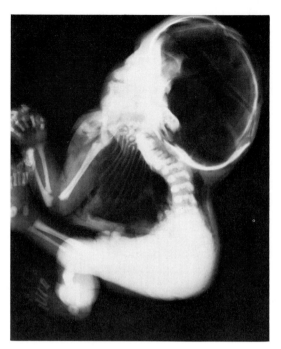

FIG. 18–18. Lateral radiograph of a case of iniencephaly clausus.

with spinal retroflexion are based on a number of features (Table 18–4) that are uncommon to other conditions. While it does not seem likely that these entities comprise a real spectrum, the association of so many features is curious at least.

To infer that the skull defect is the major component of this condition is misleading. In fact, there are numerous malformations of the spine and viscera.[24] However, because of the occipital defect and the retroflexion of the head on the spine, an unusual cavity (the cephalorhachidian space) that houses the brain stem is formed. Its boundaries consist of cervical vertebrae–basiocciput ventrorostrally, supraocciput dorsocaudally, cervical–thoracic vertebral laminae laterally and the malformed bodies of cervical–thoracic vertebrae ventrally. Lewis[26] divides these cases into those that have encephalocele (apertus) and those that do not (clausus). In cases of iniencephalus apertus, the defect of the supraocciput is significant and the encephalocele itself forms the caudal boundary of the space.

The major alterations are in the development of the vertebrae. Iniencephaly is a

TABLE 18–4. CHARACTERISTICS OF INIENCEPHALY, ANENCEPHALY (WITH SPINAL RETROFLEXION) AND KLIPPEL–FEIL SYNDROME

Characteristic	Iniencephaly (Clausus/Apertus)	Anencephaly (with spinal retroflexion)	Klippel–Feil Syndrome
NEURAL			
Myeloschisis	+	+	(±)
SKELETAL			
Retroflexion	+	+	(±)
Absent or short neck	+	+	+
Enlarged foramen magnum	+	(±)	(±)
Posterior cervical spina bifida	+	+	+
Anomalies of occipital bone	+	(+)	+
Hypoplasia of cervical vertebrae	+	+	+
Cephalorachidian space	+	0	(±)
Anterior spina bifida	+	(+)	0
Hemivertebrae	+	+	+
Rib anomalies	+	+	+
Enlarged upper extremities	+	+	(?)
Fusion of cervical vertebrae	+	+	+
VISCERAL			
Adrenal hypoplasia	(±)	+	(±)
Diaphragmatic hernia	+	+	0
Hypoplastic lungs	+	+	0
GENERAL			
Female sex preponderance	+	+	+
Hydramnios	+	+	(±)
Common experimental tertogen	+	(+)	0

Note: ( ) = Not commonly found, but reported

good example of the interaction between the chondrocranial portion of the occipital bone with the cervical vertebrae. That the defect arises during embryogenesis is evidenced by its presence in 8-mm CR length[28] and 20-mm CR length[49] specimens. Since the cranial lesions are skin covered, it has to occur after stage XI, most likely during stages XII or XIII. The evidence supporting this hypothesis is based on the fact that many specimens have a caudal myeloschisis, which probably does not arise later than stage XII (see Chapter 4).

The CNS is variably abnormal, depending on whether an encephalocele or a myelocele is present. Hydrocephalus has been reported but is not frequent, and the nature of the other malformations of the brain has not been thoroughly studied even though individual case reports are available.

Clinically, several facts are of interest. There is a marked female preponderance (about 8 to 1) and a high incidence of maternal hydramnios (approximately 20%). Although the average birth weight is from four to six pounds, dystocia is common, probably due to the nonmobile head. The arms are disproportionately elongated relative to the legs[24] (a condition frequently found in anencephalics).

Klippel–Feil Syndrome

As previously noted, certain factors relate the development of the cervical vertebrae to the development of the base of the skull. The Klippel–Feil syndrome is one of these conditions, but in most cases there is no actual malformation of the skull. In the discussion of iniencephaly, we alluded to certain characteristics suggesting that the Klippel–Feil syndrome might be a variant of that condition (Table 18–4). Both platybasia and basilar impression have been described in this syndrome. However, in the usual situation it consists of varying degrees of fusion of cervical vertebrae alone, including fusion of the atlas with the occiput. The many variations of the Klippel–Feil syndrome (and of other syndromes[27]) provide morphologic evidence that there is a large overlap between the developing base of the skull, vertebral column and nervous system.

REFERENCES

1. Acheson RM, Jefferson E: Some observations on the closure of the anterior fontanelle. Arch Dis Child 29:196–198, 1954

2. Aisenson MR: Closing of the anterior fontanelle. Pediatrics 6:223–226, 1950

3. Anderson FM, Geiger L: Craniosynostosis: A

survey of 204 cases. J Neurosurg 22:229–240, 1965

4. Anderson H, Gomes SP: Craniosynostosis, review of the literature and indications for surgery. Acta Paediatr Scand 57:47–54, 1968

5. Bardeen CR: Development of the skeleton and of the connective tissues, E. The skull, hyoid bone and larynx. Manual of Human Embryology, vol I. Edited by F Keibel and FP Mall. Philadelphia, JB Lippincott, 1910, pp. 398–453

6. Böök JA, Schut JW, Reed SC: A clinical and genetical study of microcephaly. Am J Ment Defic 57:637–660, 1953

7. Bull JWD, Nixon WLB, Pratt RTC: The radiological criteria and familial occurrence of primary basilar impression. Brain 78:229–247, 1955

8. Chamberlain WE: Basilar impression (platybasia). Yale J Biol Med 11:487–496, 1939

9. Cohen MM Jr: An etiologic and nosologic overview of craniosynostosis syndromes. Birth Defects, 1975 (in press)

10. deBeer GR: The Development of the Vertebrate Skull. Oxford, Clarendon Press, 1937

11. El-Sheriff H, Khalifa AS, Abou-Senna AM, Ghaly AF: Craniosynostosis in Egypt. J Neurosurg 33:29–34, 1970

12. Epstein JA, Epstein BS: Deformities of the skull surfaces in infancy and childhood. J Pediatr 70:636–647, 1967

13. Fawcett E: Notes on the development of the human sphenoid. J Anat Physiol 44:207–222, 1910

14. Ford EHR: The growth of the foetal skull. J Anat 90:63–72, 1956

15. Gilmour JR: The essential identity of Klippel–Feil syndrome and iniencephaly. J Pathol Bacteriol 53:117–131, 1941

16. Hinck VC, Hopkins CE, Savara BS: Diagnostic criteria of basilar impression. Radiology 76:572–585, 1961

17. Howkins J, Lawrie RS: Iniencephalus. J Obstet Gynaecol Br Commonw 46:25–31, 1939

18. Hsia YE, Bratu M, Herbordt A: Genetics of the Meckel syndrome (dysencephalia splanchnocystica). Pediatrics 48: 237–247, 1971

19. Inman VT, Saunders JB de CM: The ossification of the human frontal bone. J Anat 71:383–394, 1937

20. Irwin GL: Roentgen determination of the time of closure of the spheno-occipital synchondrosis. Radiology 75: 450–453, 1960

21. Kalter H: Teratology of the Central Nervous System. Chicago, Univ Chicago Press, 1968

22. Kernan JD: The chondrocranium of a 20 mm human embryo. J Morphol 27:605–646, 1916

23. Leck I, Record RG, McKeown T, Edward JH: The incidence of malformations in Birmingham, England, 1950–1959. Teratology 1:263–280, 1968

24. Lemire RJ, Beckwith JB, Shepard TH: Inien-

cephaly and anencephaly with spinal retroflexion: A comparative study of eight human specimens. Teratology 6:27–36, 1972

25. Lemire RJ, Shurtleff DB: Malformations of the skull (ch 28). Brennemann–Kelley Practice of Pediatrics, vol IV. Edited by V Kelley. Hagerstown, Harper & Row, 1971

26. Lewis HF: Iniencephalus. Am J Obstet 35:11–53, 1897

27. List CF: Neurologic syndromes accompanying developmental anomalies of occipital bone, atlas and axis. Arch Neurol Psychiatr 45:577–616, 1941

28. Lockwood CB: Retroflexion of an early human embryo associated with absence of the spinal medulla and imperfection of the vertebral column. Trans Obstet Soc London 29:234–243, 1887

29. Mall FP: On ossification centers in human embryos less than one hundred days old. Am J Anat 5:433–458, 1906

30. Marin-Padilla M: Study of the sphenoid bone in human cranioschisis and craniorachischisis. Virchows Arch pathol Anat 339:245–253, 1965

31. Marin-Padilla M: Study of the skull in human cranioschisis. Acta Anat (Basel) 62:1–20, 1965

32. McGregor M: The significance of certain measurements of the skull in the diagnosis of basilar impression. Br J Radiol 21:171–181, 1948

33. McLaurin RL, Matson DD: Importance of early surgical treatment of craniosynostosis: review of 36 cases treated during first six months of life. Pediatrics 10:637–652, 1952

34. Moss ML: The pathogenesis of premature cranial synostosis in man. Acta Anat (Basel) 37:351–370, 1959

35. Nellhaus G: Head circumference from birth to eighteen years. Pediatrics 41:106–114, 1968

36. Noback CR: The developmental anatomy of the human osseous skeleton during the embryonic, fetal and circumnatal periods. Anat Rec 88:91–125, 1944

37. Patten BM: Human Embryology, ed 2. New York, Blakiston, 1953

38. Pritchard JJ, Scott JH, Girgis FG: The structure and development of cranial and facial sutures. J Anat 90:73–86, 1956

39. Rorke LB, Spiro AJ: Cerebral lesions in congenital rubella syndrome. J Pediatr 70:243–255, 1967

40. Scammon RE, Calkins LA: The Development and Growth of the External Dimensions of the Human Body in the Fetal Period. Minneapolis, Univ Minnesota Press, 1929, pp. 105–117

41. Sensenig EC: The development of the occipital and cervical segments and their associated structures in human embryos. Contrib Embryol 36:141–152, 1957

42. Shillito J, Matson DD: Craniosynostosis: a review of 519 surgical cases. Pediatrics 41:829–853, 1968

43. Smith DW: Recognizable Patterns of Human Malformation. Philadelphia, WB Saunders, 1970

44. South MA, Tomkins WAF, Morris CR, Rawls WE: Congenital malformations of the central nervous system associated with genital type (type 2) herpesvirus. J Pediatr 75:13–18, 1969

45. Taveras JM, Wood EH: Diagnostic Neuroradiology. Baltimore, Williams & Wilkins, 1964

46. Vogel FS, Hallerworden J: Leukodystrophy with diffuse Rosenthal fiber formation. Acta Neuropathol 2:126–143, 1962

47. Warkany J, Dignan P St J: Congenital malformations and mental retardation: microcephaly. Ment Retard Rev 5:113–135, 1973

48. Warkany J, Takacs E: Congenital malformations in rat from streptonigrin. Arch Pathol 79:65–79, 1965

49. Willis RA: The Borderland of Embryology and Pathology, ed 2. Washington DC, Butterworths, 1962

50. Wohlwill FJ, Bernstein J, Yakolev PI: Dysmyelinogenic leukodystrophy. J Neuropathol Exp Neurol 18:359–383, 1959

chapter 19

VERTEBRAE

NORMAL DEVELOPMENT*

Sensenig[38] provides a detailed analysis of the early development of the human vertebrae. Normal development is such that the differentiation at each vertebral level varies at any given point in time. Details about specific levels will be presented following a description of the general patterns of development (Fig. 19–1).

PERIOD OF MEMBRANE FORMATION
Vertebrae Stage I

During embryonic stages X and early in stage XI (3-mm CR), the notochord is in contact with the neural tube dorsally and the gut roof ventrally. The somites lie lateral to the neural tube, and within each somite a cavity termed the myocele separates the somite into medial and lateral halves. The rostral and caudal boundaries of each somite are delimited by intersegmental fissures. From the medial half of the somite, sclerotomic cells begin to migrate toward the notochord. The first such cells to do so eventually orient themselves around the notochord and contribute to the bodies of the vertebrae and the intervertebral discs. To accomplish this the notochord loses contact first with the gut and then with the neural tube. Both of these events occur during stage XI in the cervical segments, thus creating subchordal and epichordal zones, respectively. The sequence of separation then progresses in a rostral to caudal direction.

In stage XII (3- to 5-mm CR), sclerotomic

* See Chapter 1 for background information on embryologic development and staging system.

cells migrate into both the subchordal and epichordal zones. Those closest to the notochord orient themselves around it to form a perichordal tube. Two other important changes commence during this stage: 1) the first indication of sclerotomic cells migrating dorsally (to eventually form the neural arch) occurs and 2) sclerotomic fissures are found in cervical and in some thoracic segments.

The significance of sclerotomic fissures should be explained before proceeding to the next stage. As the embryo is viewed from above, the segmentation is in the form of somites, which, as mentioned above, have their rostral and caudal limits somewhat marked by intersegmental fissures. These somites, when viewed in cross section, have a medial portion (sclerotome) and a lateral portion (myotome). The sclerotome provides the cells that will eventually form the vertebral column, whereas the myotome, in general, develops into the supporting musculature. The final segmentation of the vertebral column does not conform to the segmentation of the somites. Instead, the caudal half of one somite unites with the cranial half of the next somite to form a vertebral segment. For this to occur, each sclerotome must be divided into rostral and caudal portions, which process defines the sclerotomic fissure.

Vertebrae Stage II

During embryonic stage XIII (4- to 6-mm CR) sclerotomic cells migrate ventrolaterally and become the primordia of the ribs. Those cells moving dorsally have a smaller area because of the progressive enlargement of

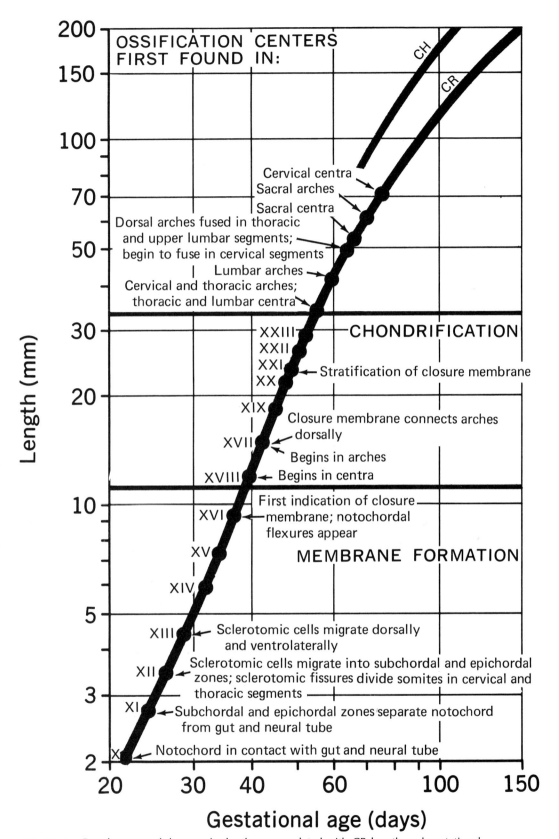

FIG. 19–1. Development of the vertebral column correlated with CR length and gestational age. The period of membrane formation (lower portion) is followed by the periods of chondrification (middle portion) and ossification (upper portion).

the neural crest (sensory ganglia). By stage XIV (5- to 7-mm CR), the space between the sensory ganglion and the myotome begins to increase, thus allowing the migration of more cells that will form the neural arches of the vertebrae. Most of the sclerotomic cells involved in this dorsal migration originate from the caudal half of the sclerotome, while the sensory ganglion lies medial to the cranial half. Viewed in cross section, the cells that are forming the neural arches are seen to connect directly with those around the notochord, whereas the laterally placed cells are involved in the formation of ribs and zygapophyseal processes.

Vertebrae Stage III

In embryonic stages XV and XVI (7- to 11-mm CR) most of the aforementioned areas show an increased number of migrating cells, thus better defining structure. Some less well-defined cells migrate over the neural tube and provide the first indication of a "closure membrane," which will be discussed below. Another indistinct but definite change is found ventrally. The notochord, which up to this time has been of uniform thickness, shows a change in diameter that provides more contrast between the vertebral bodies (centra) and the intervertebral discs. This occurs in the form of notochordal flexures, the furrows of which are associated with the bodies and the crests with the discs. By the end of stage XVI, the segmentation of the vertebrae is still incomplete, i.e., both sclerotomic and intersegmental fissures still exist. The final segmentation is completed later, during the period of cartilage formation.

PERIOD OF CARTILAGE FORMATION

Chondrification begins first in the vertebral centra during embryonic stage XVII (11- to 14-mm CR) and occurs in portions of the arches during stage XVIII (13- to 17-mm CR). The neural arches are completed dorsal to the spinal cord in the following manner. As noted above, in vertebrae stage III some cells are found dorsal to the neural tube. By embryonic stage XVIII these cells have increased and stratified into two layers, the inner of which is termed the membrana reuniens dorsalis, or "closure membrane."

This closure membrane is continuous laterally with the neural arches, which at this time are well defined opposite the midportion of spinal cord. The dorsal portion of the spinal canal is slowly formed by the proliferation of cells at the tips of these arches. By stage XXII (23- to 28-mm CR), the tips (which remain membranous) extend above the level of the sensory roots but show no medial deflection. The closure membrane now stratifies into two layers, the outer of which is continuous with the lateral tips, and the inner of which will later form dura mater. During stage XXIII and shortly thereafter (30- to 35-mm CR) the tips of the neural arches begin a medial deflection, and by 50-mm CR length they are almost united across the dorsal surface of the spinal cord in the upper cervical region, in contact in the lower cervical region and completely fused in the thoracic and upper lumbar regions.[38]

PERIOD OF BONE FORMATION

The onset of ossification overlaps the period of chondrification. Mall[27] found ossification of the vertebral arches to follow a rostro-caudal pattern, beginning in the cervical and thoracic regions at from 33- to 34-mm CR length, in the lumbar at 41-mm CR length and in the sacral at from 50- to 70-mm CR length. In contrast, ossification of the vertebral bodies begins in the thoracolumbar region at 34-mm CR length and spreads rostrally and caudally to involve the sacral bodies at about 55-mm CR length and the cervical at 70-mm CR length. The period of bone formation extends well beyond birth.

SEGMENTAL DIFFERENCES

The preceding description of the general processes involved in the formation of the vertebrae has been generally applicable to the thoracic segments except where otherwise indicated. Two regions, the cervical and sacrococcygeal, deserve further consideration because of the nature and frequency of malformations in these regions.

Cervical Vertebrae

Sensenig[39] studied the development of the occiput (see Chapter 18), atlas, axis and other cervical vertebrae.

By stage XII (3- to 5-mm CR), the notochord has separated from both the neural tube and gut in all cervical segments, some sclerotomic cells are found in the epi- and subchordal zones, and intersegmental vessels lie in the intersegmental fissures. During stages XIII and XIV (4- to 7-mm CR), rudimentary neural processes are present. Concentrations of sclerotomic cells now mark the perichordal discs and primary centra. Although still within the period of membrane formation, some delineation of the occipitocervical junction occurs.

The first four somites contribute to the development of the occipital bone. An intersegmental fissure separates the fourth from the fifth somite and contains the first cervical intersegmental artery. The fifth somite is then subdivided into rostral and caudal halves by a sclerotomic fissure. The rostral half of this somite becomes the primordium of the proatlas, while the caudal half will eventually unite with the rostral half of the sixth somite to form the atlas. This union is not effected at this stage because of the presence of the second intersegmental artery lying in its respective fissure, but this artery disappears by stage XVII and the atlas fuses. The intricacy of the relationships of the fourth and sixth somites, their intersegmental vessels and fissures and their sclerotomic fissures at this stage provide an adequate basis for understanding how early maldevelopment of any one of these formations can cause an anomaly of the occipitocervical junction.

In stages XVII and XVIII (11- to 17-mm CR), chondrification is found in the bodies of the cervical vertebrae, and the membrana reuniens dorsalis (closure membrane) connects the arches dorsally. Some cartilage formation is present in the pedicles of the atlas, and the primordium of the odontoid process develops. During stages XIX and XX (16- to 22-mm CR), all parts of the cervical vertebrae show cartilage formation. The first indications of the atlantooccipital and atlantoaxial articulations also appear during this period.

Sacrococcygeal Vertebrae

The manner in which the caudal neural tube develops many segments that undergo retrogressive differentiation has already been discussed (see Chapter 5). The development of the sacrococcygeal vertebrae similarly includes retrogressive differentiation to decrease the number of segments to the small number present postnatally. The studies of Bardeen[4] and Kunitomo[22] give good descriptions of the developmental relationships of the caudal vertebral column.

By stage XVII (11- to 14-mm CR), maximum segmentation has been achieved, and thereafter the regressive changes occur. The usual maximum number of somites found is 38, of which from 7 to 8 are located in the embryonic tail. In addition, there is a more-caudal portion of the tail that does not contain somites and is referred to as the nonvertebrated tail. However, this portion does contain neural tube, which in fact extends to its tip. Opposite the 25th and 26th primitive vertebrae (sacral 1 and 2), the iliac blastema is found in near approximation, but not yet in contact. The primordium of the sacrum is further marked at this stage by the fusion of the lateral costal processes of vertebral segments 25 through 29 into a continuous, solid mass. Usually the next 6 or 7 segments are regarded as the membranous coccyx at this time, leaving 2 or 3 segments undesignated if one rigidly adheres to a count. The fate of these extra somites is unknown, but they have disappeared by the end of the following stage. Kunitomo[22] believes they fuse into the last existing vertebra.

During stage XVIII (13- to 17-mm CR), the developing iliac blastema makes contact with S1 and S2. The sacral bodies now have some chondrification, as do the neural processes of S1 and S2 (which are still separated from the bodies). The total number of vertebrae present at the end of this stage is usually 35, the 30th through the 35th comprising the coccygeal segments. Some early fusion of coccygeal 3 and 4 begins at this time. By stage XIX (16- to 18-mm CR), there are usually 34 vertebral segments, and some early cartilage formation is found in the arches of the coccygeal segments. All sacral arches show chondrification.

The coccygeal curve found in adults is first noted in stage XXII (23- to 28-mm CR) embryos as an angle between the 30th and 31st vertebral segments. This angle develops such that by 37-mm CR length it is nearly 90°.

ABNORMAL DEVELOPMENT

Malformations of the spine are found in many syndromes, such as achondroplasia and Hurler, and are sometimes helpful in their early diagnosis. Smith[40] compiles these entities. The following discussion generally considers various types of vertebral malformations from the point of view of when and how the faulty development occurs and generally does not emphasize the differential diagnostic features of the associated clinical syndromes.

OCCIPITOCERVICAL REGION

Platybasia, basilar impression and iniencephaly have been discussed in Chapter 18. These anomalies mainly involve defects in the occipital bone. Sometimes they are associated with anomalies of the upper cervical vertebrae, as in iniencephaly, where an integral part of the diagnosis includes spina bifida of many vertebrae.

Occipitalization of the Atlas

If the atlantooccipital joint is rendered non-functional by any degree of fusion of the atlas with the occiput, the term *occipitalization,* or *assimilation,* is used. In most cases, a bony continuity is found between the anterior portion of the atlas and the basiocciput. Sometimes this appears in the form of bony spicules; in other cases there can be cortical or cortical and medullary consolidation. Varying degrees of fusion of the transverse processes with the exoccipitals are also found, and sometimes the posterior arch is absent (spina bifida posterior). Platybasia and basilar impression are found in some cases, and fusion of the second to the third cervical vertebrae is frequent.[16, 30]

Klippel–Feil Syndrome

The spectrum of congenital "fusions" of the cervical vertebrae can best be covered under the Klippel–Feil syndrome. From the previous discussion of the embryology of the vertebral column, it is apparent that the term "fusion" is frequently inappropriate since the primary anomaly can involve a lack of proper segmentation. However, fusion is so often used clinically in the descriptive sense

that we will use it here. Most cases of fused cervical vertebrae are acquired secondary to osteoarthritis, which is found in 4.6% of cadavers ranging from 17 to 102 years, with the incidence of those considered congenital being from 0.6% to 0.7% of all cases of fusion.[9] In both types of disease the most common level is C2–C3, and the second most common is C5–C6. The separation of acquired fusions from congenital fusions can usually be made rather easily since the acquired forms involve only the bodies, whereas the congenital forms involve the laminae, pedicles and spines.

Gunderson *et al.*[18] utilize Feil's classification to subdivide the original syndromes described by Klippel and Feil into three types: Type I encompasses patients with "block vertebrae," that is, there is a massive fusion of multiple cervical and higher thoracic vertebrae into solid blocks of bone. In Type II there are fusions at only one or two cervical levels, whereas in Type III the cervical fusion is accompanied by lower thoracic or lumbar fusions. The classic clinical triad of short neck, low hairline and limitation of neck movement is nearly always associated with Type I lesions. Type II lesions include those cases that have atlantooccipital fusion in addition to having fusion of two cervical vertebrae and autosomal dominant (if C2–C3 fusion) or possibly recessive (if C5–C6 fusion) inheritance. Type II lesions are by far the most common form of Klipple–Feil syndrome.

There is a marked variety of associated clinical findings and malformations. Patients with Type II lesions are generally unaffected by their relatively minor vertebral fusion, but they can develop neurologic symptoms, such as radiculitis or vertebral artery compression in older age with the onset of superimposed osteoarthritis. Unfortunately, most studies have not separated Types I and II in the discussion of the associated clinical problems. Sprengel deformity is a common accompaniment, as are facial asymmetry and torticollis. Synkinesis occurs frequently and paresthesias, ataxias and muscle atrophies are found. Anomalies of most organ systems have been reported in some cases of Klippel–Feil syndrome.[32] Those related to the vertebral column and nervous system include lordosis, scoliosis, hemivertebrae, meningomyelocele and hydrocephalus.

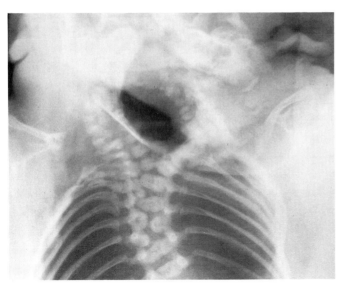

FIG. 19–2. Anteroposterior radiograph showing anterior cervical rachischisis in a case of iniencephaly clausus.

Although many patients with this syndrome have died, very few autopsy reports have described dissections of the vertebrae, so that most of our information is derived from radiographic studies. Mitchell,[31] in two Type I cases, found all intervertebral foramina to be present in spite of the fact that the fusion was so extensive that the individual vertebrae could not be distinguished from one another. In addition, the arches in the cervical region were directed caudally and all fused in an irregular mass at approximately the C6–C7 level, creating a large triangular space with a rostral base and a caudal apex. Radiographically, such a trianglular space is rare, being present in only 1 of 13 Type I cases in one series;[15] but as suggested by Gilmour,[14] it is an important consideration, being reminiscent of the cephalorachidian space found in iniencephaly.

Anterior Cervical Rachischisis

Clefts in the bodies of the cervical vertebrae permit communication of the spinal canal with such structures as the esophagus. This condition is very rare as an isolated lesion,[43] but it is not infrequent in cases of iniencephaly (Fig. 19–2) or in anencephaly with spinal retroflexion.[25]

Absence of Cervical Pedicles

An uncommon but intriguing malformation is unilateral congenital absence of a pedicle in the cervical spine so that the nerve roots of two consecutive segments share a common dural pouch. Radiographically the diagnosis should be considered when a large intervertebral foramina is found, but neoplasms and tortuosity of the vertebral artery more commonly cause destruction of a pedicle and must receive primary consideration in such cases. Only eight cases of congenital absence of a pedicle had been reported by 1966.[44]

Miscellaneous Cervical Anomalies

Bilateral absence of the arch of the atlas has been reported,[36] as well as absence of the odontoid process of the axis.[13]

THORACOLUMBAR REGION

Segmentation Variations

Stevenson[41] reports that 75% of patients with tracheoesophageal fistula and/or esophageal atresia have extra thoracic or lumbar vertebrae. Hypersegmentation has also been reported in one case of a related syndrome with imperforate anus and digital and other vertebral anomalies.[37]

As mentioned previously, fusion of thoracic and lumbar vertebrae can occur in Type III Klippel–Feil syndrome, leading to apparent numerical reduction. Hemivertebrae can also be considered a type of unilateral numerical reduction caused by faulty segmentation, or possibly by an alteration in the blood supply to one side after segmentation has occurred.[11] Congenital scoliosis can be associated with the presence of hemivertebrae and rib anomalies, usualy fusion. In extreme forms with multiple thoracic hemivertebrae and absent ribs, intrathoracic meningomyelocele can occur.[17] Intrathoracic meningoceles are more commonly associated with neurofibromatosis than not.[24] Hemivertebrae can be transmitted as an autosomal dominant or recessive trait,[29] but its occurrence in only one of identical twins indicates a nongenetic mode of etiology as well.[35]

True hyposegmentation anomalies occur with a complete absence of one or more segments. In one such case in our files, the patient had agenesis of the third and fourth lumbar vertebrae associated with a severe gibbus deformity.[26] Complete absence of the lumbar spine can occur in association with sacral agenesis (see Sacral Agenesis, below). Severe hypoplasia of the vertebral bodies can also cause kyphosis.[6, 42]

Rachischisis

Absence or nonfusion of the spinous process, with or without accompanying laminal defects, can occur anywhere along the vertebral axis. Involvement of the entire spine is found in cases of complete neural tube dysraphism, and a gradation of less-severe involvement occurs with isolated myeloschisis. Rachischisis of multiple vertebrae is a common finding in both anencephaly[28] and meningomyelocele[5] in the absence of a neural tube lesion at the involved vertebral segments. There is an increased incidence of spinal dysraphism (spina bifida occulta) in siblings of patients with anencephaly and meningomyelocele.[23]

Spina bifida occulta is considered synonymous with spinal dysraphism[2, 19] and is so

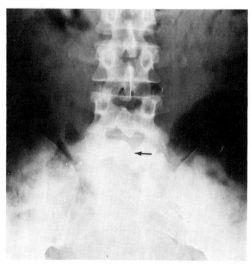

FIG. 19–3. Anteroposterior radiograph showing spina bifida occulta of the fourth and fifth lumbar vertebrae (*arrow* on fifth).

commonly present (from 10% to 20% of the population) in the fifth lumbar and first sacral vertebrae that it is considered a normal finding in the absence of any associated signs or symptoms (Fig. 19–3). When there is an overlying skin-covered subcutaneous mass, be it cystic or fatty, other diagnostic considerations (*e.g.*, meningocele,

FIG. 19–4. Anteroposterior radiograph of a patient with sacral agenesis.

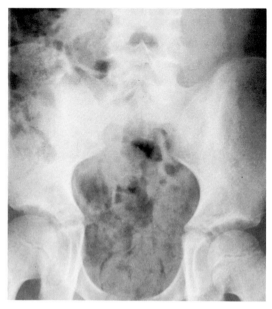

lipoma) must be entertained (see Chapter 5).

SACROCOCCYGEAL REGION

Many lesions of clinical importance that involve the lower lumbar, sacral and coccygeal segments have been discussed in relation to the development of the neural tube in Chapter 5.

Anterior Sacral Meningocele

The symptoms produced by anterior sacral meningocele vary from constipation to radicular pain. Nearly all cases occur in females (85%), and many of these become clinically apparent during pregnancy. Radiographically there is a defect in the anterior sacrum that frequently resembles a crescent or scimitar. The rectal gas shadow is displaced anteriorly in cases with a large meningeal prolapse through the bony defect.[1, 10, 20]

Sacral Agenesis

A wide spectrum of sacrococcygeal anomalies is covered under the diagnosis of sacral agenesis (Figs. 19–4 and 19–5), especially if one accepts "partial" as well as "incomplete" cases. The diagnosis may even include cases with agenesis of higher segments, such as the entire lumbar spine.[12, 34] Sacral agenesis has recently received attention among pediatricians as part of the "caudal regression syndrome" found in some infants born to diabetic mothers.[33] The question of a relationship between sacral agenesis and maternal exposure to fat solvents has been raised.[21]

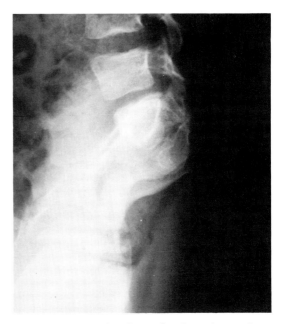

FIG. 19–5. Lateral radiograph of another patient with sacral agenesis.

Partial sacral agenesis includes those conditions in which portions of the sacrococcygeal vertebrae are missing. The missing portions may be caudal segments or lateral hemisegments. These conditions may be clinically inapparent, or they may be associated with severe entities such as myelocystocele.

Agenesis is regarded as incomplete if the fifth lumbar vertebrae is sacralized, thus forming a bridge for the iliac bones. In its true ("complete") form the iliac bones fuse with each other directly. Numerous associated malformations of nearly every organ system have been reported.[3, 7, 8, 43]

REFERENCES

1. Amacher AL, Drake CG, McLachlin AD: Anterior sacral meningocele. Surg Gynecol Obstet 126:986–994, 1968
2. Anderson FM: Occult spinal dysraphism. J Pediatr 73: 163–177, 1968
3. Banta JV, Nichols O: Sacral agenesis. J Bone Joint Surg (Am) 51A:693–703, 1969
4. Bardeen CR: Studies on the development of the human skeleton. Am J Anat 4:265–302, 1905
5. Barson AJ: Spina bifida: the significance of the level and extent of the defect to the morphogenesis. Dev Med Child Neurol 12:129–144, 1970
6. Beals RK: Familial vertebral hypoplasia and kyphosis. J Bone Joint Surg (Am) 51A:190–196, 1969
7. Blumel J, Butler MC, Evans EB, Eggers GWN: Congenital anomaly of the sacrococcygeal spine. Arch Surg 85:982–993, 1962
8. Blumel J, Evans EB, Eggers GWN: Partial and complete agenesis or malformation of the sacrum with associated anomalies. J Bone Joint Surg (Am) 41A:497–518, 1959

9. Brown MW, Templeton AW, Hodges FW III: The incidence of acquired and congenital fusions in the cervical spine. Am J Roentgenol Radium Ther Nucl Med 92:1255–1259, 1964

10. Cohn J, Bay-Neilsen E: Hereditary defect of the sacrum and coccyx with anterior sacral meningocele. Acta Paediatr Scand 58:268–274, 1969

11. Ehrenhaft JL: Development of vertebral column as related to certain congenital and pathological changes. Surg Gynecol Obstet 76:282–292, 1943

12. Frantz CH, Aitken GT: Complete absence of lumbar spine and sacrum. J Bone Joint Surg (Am) 49A:1531–1540, 1967

13. Gillman EL: Congenital absence of the odontoid process of the axis. J Bone Joint Surg (Am) 41A:345–348, 1959

14. Gilmour JR: The essential identity of the Klippel–Feil syndrome and iniencephaly. J Pathol Bacteriol 53:117–131, 1941

15. Gjørup PA, Gjørup L: Klippel–Feil's syndrome. Dan Med Bull 11:50–53, 1964

16. Gladstone RJ, Wakeley CPG: Variations of occipito-atlantal joint in relation to metameric structure of cranio-vertebral region. J Anat 59: 195–216, 1924–25

17. Goldman IR: Congenital malformation of the vertebrae (hemivertebrae) with aplasia of corresponding ribs, associated with lateral meningomyelocele. Arch Pathol 47:153–159, 1949

18. Gunderson CH, Greenspan RH, Glaser GH, Lubs HA: The Klippel–Feil syndrome: Genetic and clinical reevaluation of cervical fusion. Medicine (Baltimore) 46:491–512, 1967

19. James CCM, Lassman LP: Spinal Dysraphism: Spina Bifida Occulta. New York, Appleton-Century-Crofts, 1972

20. Kaufmann HJ: Anterior sacral meningocele. Ann Radiol (Paris) 10:121–128, 1967

21. Kučera J: Exposure to fat solvents, a possible cause of vertebral agenesis in man. J Pediatr 72:857–859, 1968

22. Kunitomo K: The development and reduction of the tail and of the caudal end of the spinal cord. Contrib Embryol 8:161–198, 1918

23. Laurence KM: Vertebral abnormalities in first degree relatives of cases of spina bifida and of anencephaly. Arch Dis Child 45:274, 1970

24. LaVielle CJ, Campbell DA: Neurofibromatosis and intrathoracic meningocele. Radiology 70: 63–66, 1958

25. Lemire RJ, Beckwith JB, Shepard TH: Iniencephaly and anencephaly with spinal retroflexion. A comparative study of eight human specimens. Teratology 6:27–36, 1972

26. Lemire RJ, Graham CB, Beckwith JB: Skin-covered sacrococcygeal masses in infants and children. J Pediatr 79:948–954, 1971

27. Mall FP: On ossification centers in human embryos less than one hundred days old. Am J Anat 5:433–458, 1906

28. Marin-Padilla M: Study of the vertebral column in human craniorachischisis. Acta Anat (Basel) 63:32–48, 1966

29. McKusick VA: Mendelian Inheritance in Man, ed 3. Baltimore, Johns Hopkins Press, 1971

30. McRae DL, Barnum AS: Occipitalization of the atlas. Am J Roentgenol Radium Ther Nucl Med 70:23–46, 1953

31. Mitchell HS: The Klippel–Feil syndrome (congenital webbed neck). Arch Dis Child 9:213–218, 1934

32. Morrison SG, Perry LW, Scott LP III: Congenital brevicollis (Klippel–Feil syndrome). Am J Dis Child 115:614–620, 1968

33. Passarge E, Lenz W: Syndrome of caudal regression in infants of diabetic mothers: observation of further cases. Pediatrics 37:672–675, 1966

34. Pearlman CK, Bors E: Congenital absence of the lumbosacral spine. J Urol 101:374–378, 1969

35. Peterson HA, Peterson LFA: Hemivertebrae in identical twins with dissimilar spinal columns. J Bone Joint Surg (Am) 49A:938–942, 1967

36. Roulleau J, Toulemond H, Costagliola M: Congenital aplasia of the posterior arch of the atlas. Rev Med Toulouse 4:733–736, 1968

37. Say B, Balci S, Pirnar T, Tuncbilek E: A new syndrome of dysmorphogenesis: imperforate anus associated with poly-oligo-dactyly and skeletal (mainly vertebral) anomalies. Acta Paediatr Scand 60:197–202, 1971

38. Sensenig EC: The early development of the human vertebral column. Contrib Embryol 33: 23–41, 1949

39. Sensenig EC: The development of the occipital and cervical segments and their associated structures in human embryos. Contrib Embryol 36:141–152, 1957

40. Smith DW: Recognizable Patterns of Human Malformation. Philadelphia, WB Saunders, 1970

41. Stevenson RE: Extra vertebrae associated with esophageal atresias and tracheo-esophageal fistulas. J Pediatr 81:1123–1129, 1972

42 Turunen A, Unnérus C-E: Spinal changes in patients with congenital aplasia of the vagina. Acta Obstet Gynecol Scand 46:99–106, 1967

43. Warkany J: Congenital Malformations. Chicago, Year Book Med Publ, 1971

44. Wilson CB, Norrell HA Jr: Congenital absence of a pedicle in the cervical spine. Am J Roentgenol Radium Ther Nucl Med 97:639–647, 1966

chapter 20

CEREBRAL VASCULATURE

NORMAL DEVELOPMENT*

GENERAL CONSIDERATIONS

Streeter[57] divides the development of the cerebral vasculature into five periods. In the first period are primordial endothelium-lined channels, which are neither arteries nor veins, but are the sources from which the arteries, veins and capillaries will eventually be derived. These endothelium-lined channels eventually become plexiform in nature and constitute the primary head plexus, but there is no circulation in these vessels at this time. This probably takes place in stage IX (1.5- to 2.5-mm CR).

The second period involves the differentiation of the above primordial system into arteries, veins and capillaries. Direct connections with the primitive aortic system feed the arteries (stage X and early stage XI), and the drainage from the brain is accomplished by the "primitive head vein," which is found in stages XII and XIII (approximately 4-mm CR). The first circulation of the head is established at this time.

The third period shows a cleavage of the blood vessels into separate systems. With the early differentiation of the supporting structures that form from mesoderm (*e.g.,* dura mater), the vascular system is subdivided into superficial and deep components. The subsequent development of a membranous skull further separates the dural system from an external network of vessels that supply the integument and soft tissues. Therefore, there are three strata of blood vessels: 1) the

---

external, 2) the dural and 3) the cerebral. Streeter states that the separation of the external vessels takes place between 12- and 20-mm CR length (corresponding to stages XVII through XIX).

The fourth period pertains to the adjustment of the blood channels to the growth and change in the form of the brain. This period has its onset in stage XIX (18-mm CR) and extends into the fetal period. During this time the arterial (at 40-mm CR length) and venous (at 80-mm CR length) systems of the head are established along lines that correspond to those found in the adult.[46]

The fifth period involves the late histologic changes in the walls of the vessels that convert them into the final adult form, a period that extends well beyond birth.

ARTERIAL SYSTEM (FIGS. 20–1 AND 20–2)

Congdon[9] divides the development of the aortic arches into a branchial phase and a postbranchial phase. The former extends from stage X to stage XVII and lasts from about 18–20 days; the latter resembles the adult arterial pattern and continues thereafter. The cerebral arteries are intimately related with the development of the aortic arch system and undergo numerous changes before the final adult pattern is realized.[9, 43]

Stages X and XI (2- to 4.5-mm CR)

The first aortic arch is formed in stage X (2-mm CR), and the second aortic arch is just beginning to develop during stage XI (3-mm CR). During these two stages the primitive internal carotid and trigeminal arteries are

---

* See Chapter 1 for background information on embryologic development and staging system.

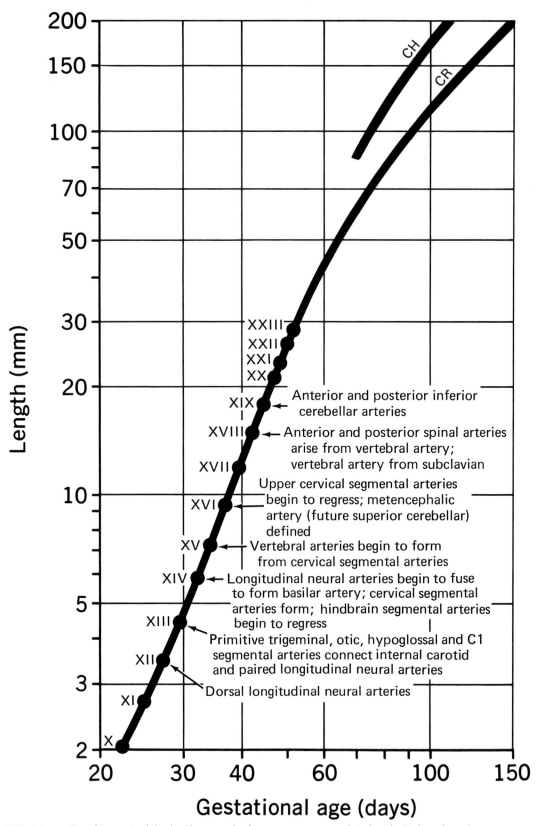

FIG. 20–1. Development of the basilar–vertebral artery system correlated with CR length and gestational age.

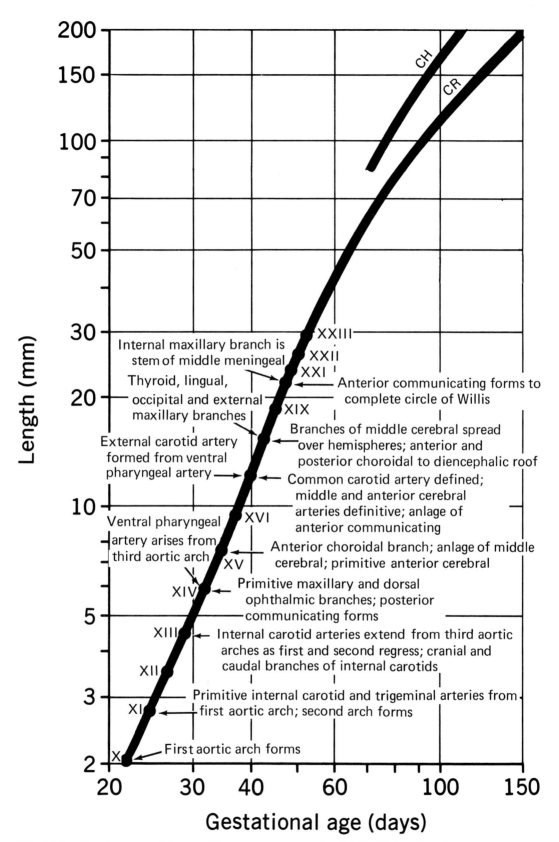

FIG. 20–2. Development of the carotid artery system correlated with CR length and gestational age. The development of the external carotid is to the left of the line, the internal carotid to the right.

found as branches of the first aortic arch. There is a large plexus of undifferentiated endothelium-lined channels dorsal to them.

Stage XII (3- to 5-mm CR)

The plexus of endothelial channels that lie dorsal to the internal carotid arteries differentiates into a pair of longitudinal neural arteries, the forerunner of the basilar artery.

Stage XIII (4- to 6-mm CR)

The first two aortic arches begin to involute and the primitive internal carotid arteries appear as extensions of the third aortic arch. Each internal carotid artery divides into a cranial branch (which can be termed the primitive olfactory artery) and a caudal branch (the future posterior communicating artery, which will join the longitudinal neural artery lying dorsally along the hindbrain wall). The longitudinal neural arteries are supplied cranially by segmental connections with the internal carotid arteries (mainly through the primitive trigeminal arteries of the anterior hindbrain segment but also through the otic and hypoglossal arteries of the middle and posterior hindbrain segments, respectively) and caudally by the first cervical segmental arteries that arise from the paired dorsal aortae.

Stage XIV (5- to 7-mm CR)

The internal carotid artery is now a well-defined extension of the third aortic arch and has primitive maxillary and dorsal ophthalmic branches. Another extension of the third aortic arch (medial to the internal carotid) is the ventral pharyngeal artery, which later will contribute to the external carotid artery. During this stage the previously bilateral longitudinal neural arteries begin to coalesce in the midline to form the primitive basilar artery. The primitive segmental hindbrain arteries show regressive changes at their origins from the internal carotid artery. The main connection of the basilar system is now via the definitive posterior communicating artery, which arises as a result of a connection between the caudal branch of the internal carotid artery with the longitudinal neural artery in stage XIII. The caudal end of the basilar artery is still bilaterally repre-

sented and fed by the first cervical segmental arteries, but additional cervical segmental arteries are also defined; the second through the sixth arise from the paired dorsal aortae, and the seventh arises from the subclavian artery.

Stages XV and XVI (7- to 11-mm CR)

Three separate systems can now be appreciated: 1) the internal carotid system containing the primitive maxillary artery coursing ventrally at the level of Rathke's pouch, the primitive dorsal ophthalmic artery supplying a capillary plexus around the optic cup, the anterior choroidal artery supplying the diencephalon, a few twigs representing the primitive middle cerebral artery and the future anterior cerebral artery arising from the stem of the primitive olfactory artery; 2) the ventral pharyngeal artery, which will be later identified with the external carotid artery system; and 3) the basilar–vertebral system with the stem of the posterior cerebral artery now defined rostrally and the first stage of the formation of the vertebral artery caudally. The latter vessel is formed by rostrocaudal anastomoses of each of the cervical segmental arteries, while the aortic connections of the first six cervical segmental arteries begin to disappear. In the final stage, the seventh cervical segmental artery retains its connection with the subclavian artery as the source of blood supply for the basilar–vertebral system. At the rostral end of the basilar artery, the metencephalic artery (future superior cerebellar artery) is now clearly defined.

Stage XVII (11- to 14-mm CR)

The common carotid artery now exists as the stem of the internal and external carotid (formerly ventral pharyngeal) arteries. The internal carotid artery has continued its differentiation (the anterior choroidal artery being its first branch, and the middle cerebral artery its second). A well-defined stem of the anterior cerebral artery is also present with the primitive olfactory artery arising from this stem and joining with its counterpart by plexiform anastomoses across the midline, the first indication of the future anterior communicating artery. The vertebral artery is still irregular, but it shows increasing differentiation in a rostrocaudal gradient.

Stages XVIII and XIX (13- to 18-mm CR)

The common carotid artery becomes elongated, and the origin of the vertebral artery (from the subclavian) shifts cranially to near its adult position. Both anterior and posterior spinal arteries arise from it. The external carotid artery, the stem of which was the former ventral pharyngeal artery, may be identified primarily by branches named the thyroid, lingual, occipital and external maxillary arteries. A proximal part of this system will show the primordium of the internal maxillary artery from which the middle meningeal artery will arise two stages later.

The middle cerebral artery is now quite prominent with many branches spreading over the cerebral hemisphere. The anterior and posterior choroidal arteries now terminate in the diencephalic roof. Changes in the basilar system include definition of the stems of the anterior and posterior inferior cerebellar arteries with some twigs extending to the developing choroid plexus of the fourth ventricle.

Stages XX and XXI (22- to 24-mm CR)

The circle of Willis is completed with the formation of the anterior communicating artery. The internal maxillary branch of the external carotid artery becomes recognizable as the stem of the middle meningeal artery.

In concluding this discussion of the development of the cerebral arterial system, it is worth commenting on one morphologic feature that is helpful in staging embryos. It was previously mentioned that the differentiation of mesodermal structures separates the vasculature into superficial (subcutaneous), dural and cerebral systems, the latter two of which we have described in part. Streeter[58] used the developing subcutaneous system as an external landmark in the later embryonic stages. In stage XXI (22- to 24-mm CR), the subcutaneous plexus extends one-half the distance to the vertex of the head, in stage XXII (23- to 28-mm CR) it extends three-fourths the distance, and in stage XXIII (27- to 31-mm CR) it extends nearly to the vertex of the head. This plexus

is derived from the external carotid artery and external jugular vein system.[16, 39]

The above patterns of development of Padget[43] and Congdon[9] are supplemented by those of Mall,[34] Streeter[57] and Lie,[32] who discuss general aspects of the development of the cerebral arteries. Evans[13] describes, and elegantly illustrates, both the cranial and spinal vasculature. Padget[45] also describes the development of the venous system and various relationships between it and the arteries. The study of Moffat[38] mainly involved rat embryos, but it also contained human fetuses whose arteries were injected with neoprene latex. Bast[3] describes the vascular supply to the otic capsule of a 150-mm CR length human fetus in detail, and Seydel[51] measured the diameter of the internal carotid artery in human fetuses ranging from 155- to 372-mm CR length. Other studies relating mainly to anatomy but containing developmental considerations have been provided by Padget,[44] Kaplan et al.,[29] Gillilan[22] and Bergström et al.[5]

VENOUS SYSTEM (FIG. 20–3)

The complex development of the cranial venous system has been most extensively studied and elegantly illustrated by Padget,[45, 46] but excellent supplements are provided by Gibbs and Gibbs,[21] Kaplan[28] and Streeter.[56, 57]

Stages XII and XIII (3- to 6-mm CR)

The first indication of the venous system is a transient midline vessel in the region of the hindbrain, the "primordial hindbrain channel."

Stage XIV (5- to 7-mm CR)

Late in stage XIII but probably more commonly in stage XIV, bilateral venous channels, the "primary head veins," are formed. These constitute the first true drainage channels from the capillary plexus. Streeter[56] divides this plexus into three parts, the anterior, middle and posterior dural plexuses. The anterior dural plexus drains both the forebrain and midbrain regions; the middle dural plexus drains the metencephalic region (future cerebellum); the posterior dural plexus drains the myelencephalic region. The

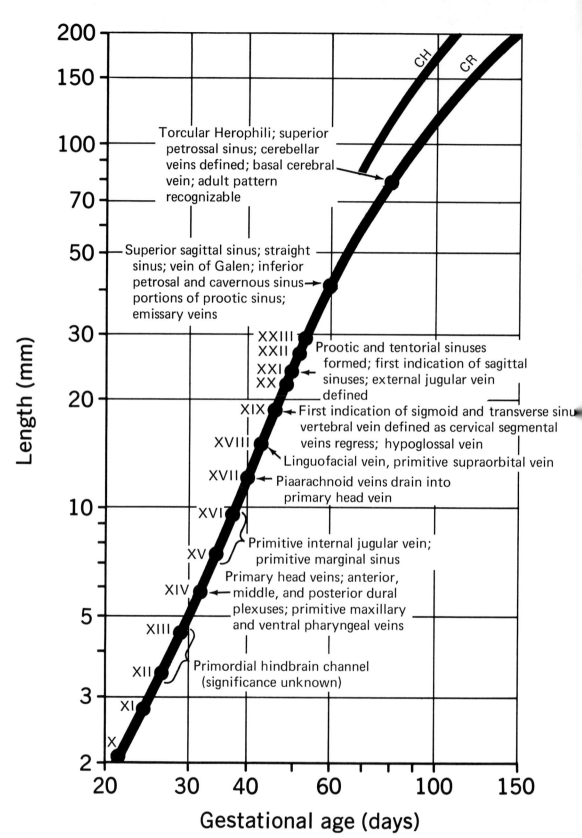

FIG. 20–3. Development of the cerebral venous system correlated with CR length and gestational age.

primary head vein draining the above plexuses (each by way of a separate stem) is directly continuous with the anterior cardinal vein that will later become the internal jugular vein. Other veins forming at this time include the primitive maxillary vein (which drains the ventral aspect of the optic vesicle into the primary head vein) and the ventral pharyngeal vein (which drains into the common cardinal vein and will later contribute to the linguofacial and external jugular veins). Intersegmental veins arising from the anterior and posterior cardinal veins are found in the future cervical region.

Stages XV and XVI (7- to 11-mm CR)

Extending over the developing telencephalic vesicle, the anterior dural plexus now has a primitive marginal sinus, which will later contribute to the formation of the superior sagittal and transverse sinuses. Below the vesicle is the telencephalic vein (later to become the superficial middle cerebral vein). Although the stems of the anterior and middle dural plexuses are separate, there are anastomoses between their peripheral portions. The stem of the posterior dural plexus joins the primary head vein at the level where the latter drains into the primitive internal jugular (anterior cardinal) vein. The stem of the posterior dural plexus will become part of the caudal end of the sigmoid sinus. In the same region, the ventral myelencephalic vein that will later give origin to the inferior petrosal sinus proliferates from the primary head vein within the leptomeninges. The primitive subclavian vein can also be identified.

Stages XVII and XVIII (11- to 17-mm CR)

The differentiation of the meninges during these stages is such that a definite series (telencephalic, diencephalic, mesencephalic, metencephalic and myelencephalic) of leptomeningeal veins can be identified draining into the primary head vein. In addition, the primordium of the central vein of the retina is present, and a primitive supraorbital vein (above the optic vesicle) is found to arise near the primitive maxillary vein (below the optic vesicle). In the adult, the primitive supraorbital vein will constitute a major portion of the superior ophthalmic vein. Also arising from the anterior dural plexus at this stage is the mesencephalic vein. The internal jugular vein has migrated to the lateral side of the hypoglossal trunk, and one of its major tributaries, the linguofacial vein (later named the common facial vein), is prominent. The linguofacial vein arises, in part, from the ventral pharyngeal vein (stage XIV).

Stage XIX (16- to 18-mm CR)

Up to this time, the main drainage channel for the anterior, middle and posterior dural plexuses has been the primary head vein. During stage XIX, a secondary anastomosis occurs between the middle and posterior dural plexuses, and there is a change in the venous drainage to this new dorsally located channel, the first indication of the sigmoid and transverse sinuses. The transverse sinus is represented by the most-cranial position of the anastomosis and is derived partly from the middle dural plexus and partly from the primitive marginal sinus. The sigmoid sinus is represented by the caudal portion of the new dorsal channel combined with the stem of the posterior dural plexus. The posterior dural plexus itself will become the marginal sinus of the foramen magnum with an additional contribution to the occipital sinus. The stem of the middle dural plexus itself will contribute to the prooptic sinus in the next stage.

The orbital veins show further differentiation. Above the developing eye the primitive supraorbital vein is now quite prominent, and below the eye the primitive maxillary (infraorbital) vein has divided. One of these divisions is the future anterior facial vein.

The cervical intersegmental areas are supplied by veins that run with the arteries and nerves. The proximal ends of these veins drop out during this stage, and the main drainage channel is composed of a secondary longitudinal anastomosis, the vertebral vein. The vertebral vein empties into the internal jugular vein, but on its cranial end there may be anastomoses with several emissary veins. One of these is the primitive hypoglossal emissary vein, a tributary of the primitive myelencephalic vein, which will later contribute to the inferior petrosal sinus. The hypoglossal emissary vein, in conjunction with the primitive mastoid emissary vein, will provide a source of collateral circulation between the sigmoid sinus and external jugular system of the adult.

Stages XX and XXI (18- to 24-mm CR)

During this period several important changes in the cranial sinuses occur. As mentioned above, part of the primary head vein has regressed as a result of the beginning formation of the sigmoid and transverse sinuses. The stem of the middle dural plexus has now undergone marked changes and may be regarded as the definitive prootic sinus, the lateral end of which is in the position of and later constitutes the adult superior petrosal sinus. The prootic sinus will also give rise to the middle meningeal sinuses (the dural veins), some of which may be differentiated during this stage.

Another addition is the tentorial sinus, which develops from the anterior dural plexus. The tentorial sinus receives the superficial and deep telencephalic (middle cerebral) veins as well as the ventral diencephalic vein. The transverse sinus is now definitive (but small), and there is the first indication of the formation of the sagittal sinuses (superior and inferior).

The first definition of the external jugular system takes place with the appearance of the anterior, posterior and common facial veins. Prior to this time, the common facial vein was known as the linguofacial, which drained into the internal jugular system.

Further Venous Development

The development of the cranial venous system lags significantly behind that of the arterial system. Padget[46] states that at the end of embryonic development only one definitive sinus has formed, the sigmoid. Although we have mentioned other sinuses above, they are poorly defined and very primitive. At approximately 40-mm CR length, the superior sagittal sinus begins to develop. As the cerebral hemispheres enlarge, the bilateral marginal sinuses are displaced caudally. They are connected in the midline by a plexus of vessels that will constitute the superior sagittal sinus. At the same time, the primitive straight sinus and the primitive great cerebral veins of Galen begin to develop. With the veins they drain, they consti-

tute the Galenic system, which provides most of the intracerebral drainage. Further definition of the inferior petrossal and cavernous sinuses also takes place. Both of these sinuses are medial derivatives of the prootic sinus, whereas the cavernous sinus is a lateral derivative. The cavernous sinus surrounds the lateral aspect of the internal carotid artery at the level of the hypophysis (40-mm CR length). The prootic sinus also has another tributary, the middle meningeal sinus, which is found in the outer part of the dural layer.

Padget[46] discusses the development of the orbital veins in considerable detail. At 40-mm CR length, the superior ophthalmic vein is the major component, joining the cavernous sinus via a common orbital vein (derived from the stem of the primitive maxillary vein). Also draining into the common orbital is the inferior ophthalmic vein.

The emissary venous system begins as the hypoglossal vein in stage XIX, which drains the veins of the upper spinal cord into the ventral myelencephalic vein, and the primitive condylar emissary vein, which drains the upper spinal cord into the sigmoid sinus. In stages XX and XXI, the primitive mastoid emissary vein drains the occipital region into the sigmoid sinus. At 40-mm CR length, these veins have developed into an extensive emissary system, the sphenoid emissary and the primitive temporal emissary veins having become very prominent. The drainage now occurs mainly laterally into the facial vein and from there into the external jugular vein, whereas previously the drainage had been medially into the internal jugular vein.

Between 40- and 80-mm CR length, the differentiation and shifting of the sinuses and veins have progressed to the point where an adult pattern is recognizable even though further growth of the brain and skull will continue to provide relative changes in their gross relationships, just as happens with most of the structures surrounding (or supporting) the CNS. By 80-mm CR length, the transverse sinus is in its definitive position, and the tentorial plexus (the junction of the transverse sinus with the superior sagittal and straight sinuses) may now be termed the definitive torcular Herophili. The drainage from the eye is into the well-defined cavernous sinus and from there into the inferior petrossal sinus. As previously mentioned, these are both derivatives of the pro-otic sinus, which still receives a remnant of the primary head sinus, now termed the superficial petrossal vein. The prootic sinus also receives a tributary of the previous ventral metencephalic vein, now called the superior petrossal sinus. This sinus is the last of the major sinuses to be defined. Another sinus created during this period is the petro-squamosal sinus, the caudal end of the pro-otic sinus leading temporarily into the sigmoid sinus and eventually incorporated into the diploic system.

The basal cerebral veins (which join with the internal cerebral veins to form the great cerebral vein of Galen) become identifiable during this same period, and the cerebellar veins differentiate into the great anterior cerebellar veins, anterior cerebellar veins and posterior cerebellar veins.

ABNORMAL DEVELOPMENT

ANOMALIES OF THE ARTERIAL SYSTEM

Lie[32] discusses anomalies of the carotid artery system. The common carotid artery has several variations in its origin. The "normal" pattern is for the right common carotid to arise from the innominate artery and for the left common carotid to arise from the aortic arch itself (65% to 70% of cases). The next most common variations are for the left common carotid to arise abnormally close to the base of the innominate artery (16%) or for both common carotid arteries to arise from the innominate (8%). More unusual is for the stem of both carotid arteries to arise independently but directly from the aorta, or independently from the subclavian arteries. In the latter situation, both common carotids can originate from the left subclavian artery. Absence of the common carotid artery is rare; the term is applied on the right side when the internal and external carotids arise separately from the innominate artery, or on the left side if the internal and external carotids arise independently from the aortic arch.

Numerous anomalies of the internal carotid artery have been described.[32] The course of the vessel may be manifested in from 12% to 15% of cases by unusual S- or C-shaped curves, called *tortuosity of the inter-*

nal carotid artery. Kinking and looping of the internal carotid artery are parts of this spectrum that have recently been associated with neurologic deficits, mental retardation and cerebral atrophy in children.[50] Unilateral and bilateral hypoplasia and even aplasia of the internal carotid arteries have been reported. In aplasia a fibrous strand and a foramen at the base of the skull are usually present, whereas in agenesis there is complete absence of the vessel and the foramen. Both internal carotid arteries may be absent, or there may be absence of the internal and external carotid arteries on one side. In other instances there may be partial absence of one segment of the internal carotid artery, either an intracranial or extracranial portion. The blood supply to the brain is not affected in these cases as long as the anterior and posterior communicating arteries are present and functional. Turnbull[61] reports absence of the left internal carotid artery in an 81-year-old male. The left middle cerebral artery arose from the basilar via the left posterior communicating artery. Hills and Sament[26] describe a case of bilateral absence of the internal carotid arteries in a child with congenital heart defects, the posterior communicating arteries giving origin to the ophthalmic, middle cerebral and anterior cerebral arteries. The entire blood supply to the brain came, therefore, from the vertebral–basilar system, which itself had a hypoplastic right vertebral artery and com-

FIG. 20–4. Lateral view of a cerebral arteriogram showing a persistent trigeminal artery (*arrow*).

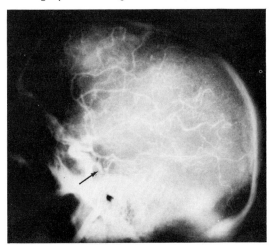

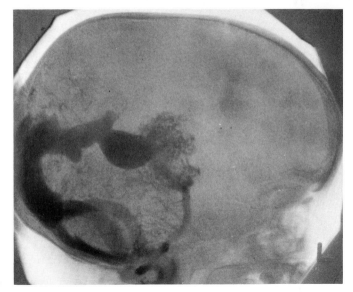

FIG. 20–5

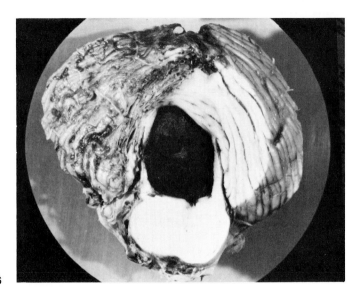

FIG. 20–6

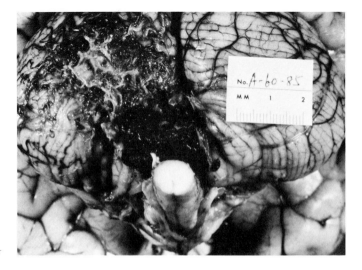

FIG. 20–7

◄ FIG. 20–5. Lateral view of the venous phase of an arteriogram showing an aneurysm of the vein of Galen and adjacent angioma.

◄ FIG. 20–6. Angioma of the right cerebellar hemisphere. The fourth ventricle is distended and filled by blood clot. This mother died unexpectedly while waiting with her baby in the well baby clinic. (#ML-56-150)

◄ FIG. 20–7. Inferior view of an angioma of the left cerebellar hemisphere from a 21-year-old woman who had episodes of subarachnoid hemorrhage 11 years apart. (#Np 139)

pensatory dilatation of the left vertebral artery.

While there is no disagreement that agenesis of the internal carotid artery (no fibrous strand and no foramen in the skull) has an embryologic origin, the evidence in aplasia is not so clear since secondary regression can occur later in life. The onset of symptoms in later life is not of critical importance in deciding whether hypoplasia of the internal carotid arteries occurred early or late since the actual changes in blood flow can rarely be defined.[2] Further support for the hypothesis of a secondary factor is found in "Moyamoya" disease, which was first recognized in young Japanese females, but which is obviously more widespread.[25] In this disease there is a progressive occlusion of the internal carotid artery at its intracranial fork[59] with the development of a radiographically fuzzy maze of additional small vessels in the base of the brain.

The cerebral arteries can give origin to vessels not ordinarily derived from them. Usually this is done by the enlargement of primitive anastomatic channels. Newton and Young[41] found three patients in whom the occipital artery arose directly from the internal carotid, whereas it normally is derived from the external carotid artery. Morris and Moffat[39] found the basilar artery to arise from the left internal carotid artery.

More commonly one finds persistence of anastomoses between the developing carotid and vertebral–basilar systems, such as the segmental hindbrain arteries. As noted above, the trigeminal artery appears in stage X (2-mm CR), joining the internal carotid artery with the bilateral longitudinal neural arteries. These eventually differentiate into the basilar system and begin to disappear during stage XIV (5- to 7-mm CR). If this regression fails to occur, a permanent carotid–basilar anastomosis results (Fig. 20–4). The incidence of this anomaly is probably from 1% to 2%,[32] and in most cases is merely an incidental angiographic or postmortem finding. However, it is statistically correlated with a propensity to develop aneurysms and arteriovenous malformations. Fields[15] found 9 persistent trigeminal arteries in 1600 patients (0.6%), and in each case the posterior communicating artery on the side of the persistent trigeminal artery was either hypoplastic or absent. The primitive hypoglossal artery, another temporary carotid–basilar anastomosis that normally regresses during stages XV and XVI (8-mm CR),[6] may persist. Usually discovered as an incidental finding on arteriograms, it too is found frequently associated with aneurysms.

Another carotid–basilar anastomosis can persist at the level of the primitive otic artery, and carotid–vertebral anastomoses can occur if the cervical intersegmental arteries do not regress. In the latter case the first cervical intersegmental artery seems to persist most commonly.[32] The carotid and basilar arterial systems also have normal anastomoses through the posterior communicating arteries as part of the circle of Willis, formed in stage XIV (5- to 7-mm CR), but many variations occur, with unilateral and bilateral hypoplasia of the posterior communicating arteries or of the stem of the posterior cerebral arteries. One of the frequent patterns is for the posterior cerebral artery to arise directly from the internal carotid artery, with absence of the connection to the basilar via the usual stem of the posterior cerebral artery. When this occurs on one side, there is frequently a contralateral "diagonally symmetric" anomaly such that the stem of the anterior cerebral artery is small or absent. The resultant pattern gives a grossly asymmetric supply of four cerebral arteries by one carotid and of two cerebral arteries by the vertebral–basilar.[4]

Aneurysms of the major intracranial arteries are commonly spoken of as congenital,[7, 12, 17] but the available evidence strongly suggests that most of them are acquired secondary to atherosclerosis and hypertension,[10] and it would be wise to call them saccular (a descriptive term without etiologic connotations). Most such aneurysms occur at the distal angle or crotch of bifurcations, where congenital defects in the media[17, 23, 53] commonly occur in perhaps as many as half of all major bifurcations.[52] However, it is the internal elastic membrane which contributes most of the strength of the vessel wall and which rarely shows a congenital defect.[52, 54] Since the elastica can be damaged by atherosclerosis, hypertension or other diseases,[10] and since aneurysms are most common in adults, affecting at least 1% of this population, it seems likely that the requirement for a superimposition of two or more lesions, which individually are much more common, may account for the relative rarity of aneurysms.[10]

Among the other diseases of the elastica should be mentioned musculoelastic pads. These may be seen even in premature infants,[52] most commonly on the front or back of a bifurcation, next on the sides and least in the crotch. Thus they tend not to overlap with the congenital medial defect. The simple statistically random overlapping of these two congenital abnormalities may still not be sufficient to produce an aneurysm without further degenerative change, e.g., with further splitting of the elastica with age or increasing blood pressure. Certain congenital variations in the diameter of the arteries making up the circle of Willis[49] further predispose to the development of aneurysms, as described above, and suggest the importance of local increased blood flow in further potentiating all of these congenital and acquired factors in the production of saccular aneurysms.[10, 14] Purely congenital aneurysms are extremely rare.[7, 10] They should contain all 3 elements of a normal artery and could represent the failure of absorption of the primitive arterial net.[12]

Anomalies of the external carotid arteries have also been found. Failure of the stem of the external carotid artery to develop can result in its complete absence, and the blood supply to the area it normally supplies is then derived from either the opposite external carotid artery or the ipsilateral internal carotid artery. Clinically this does not present any problem. Branches of the external carotid artery can arise from other vessels (e.g., the superior thyroid artery may arise

directly from the common carotid). In other cases, the external carotid artery may give rise to vessels normally considered part of the internal carotid or vertebral–basilar systems, e.g., the ophthalmic artery arising from the middle meningeal artery,[20] or the vertebral artery arising from the right external carotid.[24] Lie[32] describes a condition in which the external carotid arteries do not undergo their usual migration and are positioned dorsolateral to the internal carotid artery.

ANOMALIES OF THE VENOUS SYSTEM

True malformations of the cranial venous system usually have an arterial component that categorizes them under arteriovenous anomalies. Even in cases of aneurysm of the great vein of Galen (Fig. 20–5), the aneurysm is fed by anomalous branches of the carotid and/or basilar circulation.[33] Calabro and Palmieri[8] report a patient with anomalous duplication of the posterior part of the internal cerebral vein and the great vein of Galen. The etiology of this condition was not delineated, and the diagnosis was by angiography, not autopsy. "Venous angiomas," commonly found in the posterior fossa, may represent true venous malformations. McCormick et al.[36] studied 164 posterior fossa angiomas (Figs. 20–6 and 20–7) and found 70 arteriovenous malformations, 38 telangiectasias, 21 cavernous angiomas, 4 varices and 31 venous angiomas. Of the venous angiomas, 20 involved the cerebellum, 7 the pons and 3 the midbrain, while 1 was found to be extensive over the brain stem.

It is surprising that more isolated venous malformations of the CNS have not been reported since the venous system undergoes many more modifications during development and one would expect many more abnormal patterns to persist or develop. Perhaps the difficulties in dissecting the venous system at autopsy or the acceptance of many more "normal variations" preclude detection and description.

ARTERIOVENOUS MALFORMATIONS

Arteriovenous malformations (AVM) within the skull encompass a spectrum of morphologic types. The pathogenesis of these lesions

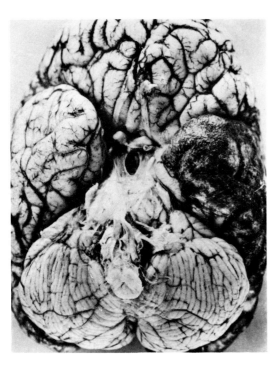

FIG. 20–8. Ventral view of the brain of a patient with Sturge–Weber syndrome. Only a portion of the angioma is shown in the left temporal region.

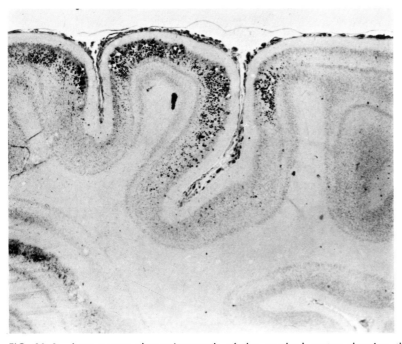

FIG. 20–9. Low power photomicrograph of the cerebral cortex showing the anomalous vessels in the left occipital cortex and leptomeninges exercise from a patient with Sturge–Weber syndrome. Combined Nissl–von Kossa stain. (#D-427)

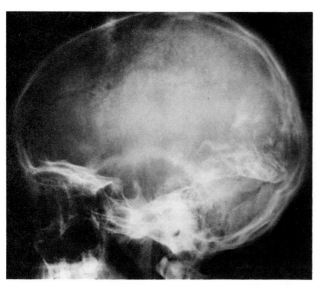

FIG. 20–10.   Lateral radiograph of the skull showing intracranial calcification in the occipital lobe in Sturge–Weber syndrome.

is still not entirely clear, but Padget[45] has presented two important considerations: 1) the developing arteries and veins frequently cross each other at right angles, and although they are in direct contact with each other, this angulation of blood flow probably tends to prevent AVM from occurring and 2) most of the malformations probably occur before 40-mm CR length; *i.e.*, before the arterial walls thicken. Between 20- and 40-mm CR length, opportunities for AVM may result from an abnormal arterial influx into a relatively large vein via a communicating sinusoidal channel that then becomes a fistula. The amount of arterial influx will determine whether the resulting venous coils remain relatively localized or progressively spread to other areas. The primary fistula between the artery and vein may result in secondary dilatations elsewhere, and the primary fistula may regress after initiating the secondary anomaly. Depending on whether regression occurs, there may be shifting and reversals of current in the blood flow. In some cases the malformations have a predilection for certain regions (*e.g.*, Sturge–Weber syndrome, where the terminal embryonic plexuses are drained chiefly by the marginal sinus at a point where several cerebral arteries meet).

The classifications of AVM vary somewhat due in part to differences in clinical and pathologic findings. There seems to be agreement that the mildest degree of these lesions is represented by simple telangiectasias, which grossly present as small, sharply or ill-defined areas of red discoloration resembling a cluster of petechial hemorrhages.[35] Microscopically, they are composed of thin-walled capillaries or small sinusoids of varying sizes with no smooth muscle or elastic tissue. Although the surrounding parenchyma is usually normal, it can become gliotic and mineralized. Telangiectasias represent approximately 3% of AVM[48] and are usually "incidental" findings at autopsy. Although they may be found in any part of the CNS, the central pontine, deep cerebral white and cerebellar cortex are the most frequent locations.[1]

Large telangiectasias, which may also be termed *capillary and venous angiomas*, represent 23% of AVM.[48] These lesions are of the type found in the Sturge–Weber syndrome and are of more clinical concern than the small telangiectasias noted above. The Sturge–Weber syndrome consists of cutaneous (facial) angioma, seizures, hemiparesis, intracranial calcification, mental retardation and glaucoma.[62] Although familial cases exist, the hereditary basis is unclear.[37] There is evidence of a nosologic relationship between the Sturge–Weber and Klippel–Trénaunay–Weber syndrome, the latter of

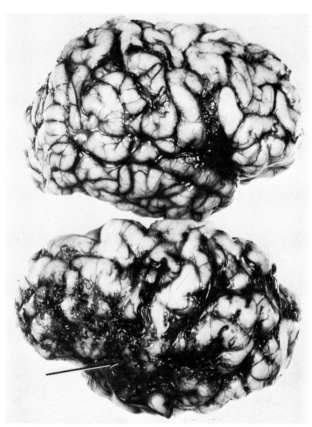

FIG. 20–11. An arteriovenous malformation in the distribution of the left middle cerebral artery (*arrow*) in a newborn. The right side (above) is normal. (#JD A-57-448)

which has more-widespread angiomatous lesions.[19] Neuropathologic findings include a capillary or venous angioma over the cerebral cortex, mainly involving the leptomeninges but sometimes extending into the cerebral cortex (Figs. 20–8 and 20–9). The track-like calcifications (Fig. 20–10), resembling large vessels in cranial x rays , are really sulcal patterns produced by the intracortical calcifications, usually of laminar necrosis of cortex and not usually of the vessels. There is usually an associated port-wine hemangioma over the ipsilateral side of the face, in one or another division of the trigeminal nerve distribution.

The most common type (70%) of AVM is an aggregation of dilated arteries and veins (Fig. 20–11) with one or more communications.[48] These lesions may be found in all parts of the nervous system, but the larger ones most frequently occur in areas supplied by the middle cerebral artery[11, 35] and appear less frequently in the posterior fossa.[36, 40, 63] These can present as expanding lesions extending from the meninges into the brain parenchyma (Figs. 20–12 and 20–13); they frequently are calcified. The microscopic appearance is variable, ranging from well-defined arteries and veins to hyaline vessels of undefinable nature. Parenchymal degeneration around an AVM is common, as is evidence of recent and old hemorrhage.[35] The age at the time of diagnosis varies, in most cases being between 20 and 50 years.[47] In one study involving 13 children with AVM, the average age at diagnosis was 15.5 years, but the average age of onset of clinical manifestations was 7.5 years, the youngest being 1 year.[31] Occasional cases are seen incidentally at autopsy at any age, from newborn to adult.

Aneurysms of the great vein of Galen are another type of AVM, in that the dilated vein is directly fed by branches from either the carotid or basilar arteries.[33, 55] Clinically

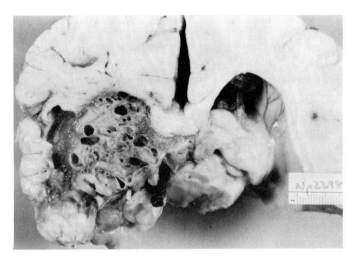

FIG. 20–12. Arteriovenous malformation in the left occipitoparietal lobe in a 52-year-old mentally retarded, epileptic woman. The lesion was fed predominantly by the posterior cerebral artery, but also by the middle cerebral artery. (#Np 2298)

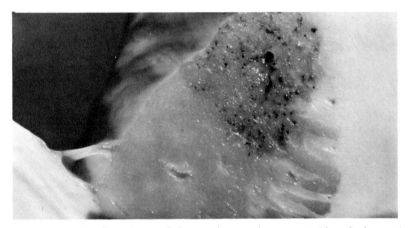

FIG. 20–13. Small angioma of the caudate nucleus, an incidental observation at autopsy of an 81-year-old man. (#HH A-60-110)

the picture may be quite variable: 1) the aneurysm can cause aqueductal stenosis (and hydrocephalus) by pressure over the midbrain; 2) because a large amount of blood may be shunted, congestive heart failure may be the major problem, and this may lead the clinician to overlook examination of the head. Such failure may occur with other types of intracranial AVM,[27, 48] but it is especially common in cases of aneurysms of the great vein of Galen becoming symptomatic near the time of birth. In some cases the dilated vein of Galen is only a small aspect of a more extensive AVM involving midline vessels around the caudal thalamus and midbrain[33] or over the occipital lobes. Because of this, O'Brien and Schechter[42] feel that the term "arteriovenous malformations involving the Galenic system" is more appropriate, even for isolated aneurysms of the vein of Galen (Figs. 7–10 and 20–5).

Although rare, true congenital fistulas have been reported between the internal carotid artery and internal jugular vein,[18, 30] but the most common cause of carotid–cavernous or carotid-jugular fistulas is trauma to the base of the skull or neck. Anomalous connections between branches of the external carotid artery and emissary veins have also been noted.[60]

REFERENCES

1. Aronson SM: Vascular malformations. Pathology of the Nervous System, vol II. Edited by J Minckler. New York, McGraw-Hill, 1971, pp. 1884–1897

2. Austin JH, Stears JC: Familial hypoplasia of both internal carotid arteries. Arch Neurol 24: 1–10, 1971

3. Bast TH: Blood supply of the otic capsule of a 150 mm (CR) human fetus. Anat Rec 48: 141–151, 1931

4. Battacharji SK, Hutchinson EC, McCall AJ: The Circle of Willis—the incidence of developmental abnormalities in normal and infarcted brains. Brain 90:747–758, 1967

5. Bergström K, Lodin H, Ottander HG: Normal topography of the cerebral vessels in childhood. Acta Radiol [Diagn] 8:146–160, 1969

6. Blain JG, Logothetis J: The persistent hypoglossal artery. J Neurol Neurosurg Psychiatry 29:346–349, 1966

7. Bremer JL: Congenital aneurysms of the cerebral arteries. An embryologic study. Arch Pathol 35:819–931, 1943

8. Calabro A, Palmieri A: Anomalous duplication of the posterior part of the internal cerebral vein and the great vein of Galen. J Neurosurg 36:646–648, 1972

9. Congdon ED: Transformation of the aortic-arch system during development of the human embryo. Contrib Embryol 14:47–110, 1922

10. Crawford T: Some observations of the pathogenesis and natural history of intracranial aneurysms. J Neurol Neurosurg Psychiatry 22: 259–266, 1959

11. Crawford JV, Russell DS: Cryptic AV malformations and venous hematomas of the brain. J Neurol Neurosurg Psychiatry 19:1–11, 1956

12. Dandy WE: Intracranial Arterial Aneurysms. Ithaca, NY, Comstock Publishing Co., 1947

13. Evans HM: The development of the vascular system. Manual of Human Embryology, vol II. Edited by F Keibel and FP Mall. Philadelphia, JB Lippincott, 1912, pp. 570–709

14. Fallon JT, Stehbens WE: The endothelium of experimental vascular aneurysms of the abdominal aorta in rabbits. Br J Exp Pathol 54:13–19, 1973

15. Fields WS: The significance of persistent trigeminal artery: carotid-basilar anastomosis. Radiology 91:1096–1101, 1968

16. Finley EB: The development of the subcutaneous vascular plexus of the head of the human embryo. Contrib Embryol 14:155–161, 1922

17. Forbus WD: On the origin of miliary aneurysms of the superficial cerebral arteries. Bull Johns Hopkins Hosp 47:239–284, 1930

18. Fraser GR: Congenital internal carotid-internal jugular fistula. J Pediatr 79:343–344, 1971

19. Furukawa T, Igata A, Toyokura Y, Ikeda S: Sturge–Weber and Klippel–Trénaunay syndrome with nevus of Ota and Ito. Arch Dermatol 102:640–645, 1970

20. Gabriele OF, Bell D: Ophthalmic origin of the middle meningeal artery. Radiology 89:841–844, 1967

21. Gibbs EL, Gibbs FA: The cross section areas of the vessels that form the torcular and the manner in which flow is distributed to the right and to the left lateral sinus. Anat Rec 59:419–426, 1934

22. Gillilan LA: The arterial and venous blood supplies to the forebrain (including the internal capsule) of primates. Neurology (Minneap) 18:653–669, 1968

23. Glynn LE: Medial defects in the circle of Willis and their relation to aneurysm formation. J Pathol Bacteriol 51:213–222, 1940

24. Hackett ER, Wilson CB: Congenital external carotid-vertebral anastomosis. A case report. Am J Roentgenol Radium Ther Nucl Med 104: 86–89, 1968

25. Harvey FH, Alvord EC Jr: Juvenile cerebral arteriosclerosis and other cerebral arteriopathies of childhood: Six autopsied cases. Acta Neurol Scand 48:479–509, 1972

26. Hills J, Sament S: Bilateral agenesis of the internal carotid artery associated with cardiac and other anomalies: case report. Neurology (Minneap) 18:142–146, 1968

27. Holden AM, Fyler DC, Shillito J Jr, Nadas AS: Congestive heart failure from intracranial arteriovenous fistula in infancy. Pediatrics 49:30–39, 1972

28. Kaplan HA: The transcerebral venous system. Arch Neurol 1:148–152, 1959

29. Kaplan HA, Aronson SM, Browder EJ: Vascular malformations of the brain: an anatomical study. J Neurosurg 18:630–635, 1961

30. Lagos JC, Riley HD Jr: Congenital internal carotid-internal jugular fistula. J Pediatr 77: 870–872, 1970

31. Lagos JC, Riley HD Jr: Congenital intracranial vascular malformations in children. Arch Dis Child 46:285–290, 1971

32. Lie TA: Congenital Anomalies of the Carotid Arteries. New York, Excerpta Medica, 1968, pp. 1–143.

33. Litvak J, Yahr MD, Ransohoff J: Aneurysms of great vein of Galen and midline cerebral arteriovenous anomalies. J Neurosurg 17:945–954, 1960

34. Mall FP: On the development of the blood vessels of the brain in the human embryo. Am J Anat 4:1–18, 1904

35. McCormick WF: The pathology of vascular ("arteriovenous") malformations. J Neurosurg 24:807–816, 1966

36. McCormick WF, Hardman JM, Boulter TR: Vascular malformations ("angiomas") of the brain with special reference to those occurring in the posterior fossa. J Neurosurg 28:241–251, 1968

37. McKusick VA: Mendelian Inheritance in Man, ed 3. Baltimore, Johns Hopkins Press, 1971

38. Moffat DB: The embryology of the arteries of the brain. Ann R Coll Surg Engl 30:368–382, 1962

39. Morris ED, Moffat DB: Abnormal origin of the basilar artery from the cervical part of the internal carotid and its embryological significance. Anat Rec 125:701–711, 1956

40. Newton TH, Weidner W, Greitz T: Dural arteriovenous malformation in the posterior fossa. Radiology 90:27–35, 1968

41. Newton TH, Young DA: Anomalous origin of the occipital artery from the internal carotid artery. Radiology 90:550–552, 1968

42. O'Brien MS, Schechter MM: Arteriovenous malformations involving the Galenic system. Am J Roentgenol Radium Ther Nucl Med 110:50–55, 1970

43. Padget DH: The development of the cranial arteries in the human embryo. Contrib Embryol 32:205–261, 1948

44. Padget DH: Designation of the embryonic intersegmental arteries in reference to the vertebral artery and subclavian stem. Anat Rec 119:349–356, 1954

45. Padget DH: The cranial venous system in man in reference to development, adult configuration and relation to the arteries. Am J Anat 98:307–355, 1956

46. Padget DH: The development of the cranial venous system in man, from the viewpoint of comparative anatomy. Contrib Embryol 36:81–140, 1957

47. Perret G, Nishioka H: Arteriovenous malformations. J Neurosurg 25:467–490, 1966

48. Pool JL, Potts DG: Aneurysms and Arteriovenous Anomalies of the Brain. New York, Harper & Row, 1965

49. Riggs HE, Rupp C: The pathologic anatomy of ruptured cerebral aneurysms. Proc First International Congress Neuropathol, Rome. 2:206–214, 1952

50. Sarkari NBS, Holmes JM, Bickerstaff ER: Neurological manifestations associated with internal carotid loops and kinks in children. J Neurol Neurosurg Psychiatry 33:194–200, 1970

51. Seydel HG: The diameters of the cerebral arteries of the human fetus. Anat Rec 150:79–88, 1964

52. Smith DE, Windsor RB: Embryologic and pathogenic aspects of the development of cerebral vascular aneurysms. In Pathogenesis and Treatment of Cerebrovascular Disease. Edited by WS Fields, Springfield, Ill, Charles C Thomas Publishers, 1961, pp 367–386

53. Stehbens WE: Medial defects of the cerebral arteries of man. J Pathol Bacteriol 78:179–185, 1959

54. Stehbens WE: Experimental production of aneurysms by microvascular surgery in rabbits. Vasc Surg 7:165–175, 1973

55. Stehbens WE, Saligal KK, Nelson L, et al: Aneurysms of vein of Galen and diffuse meningeal angiectasia. Occurrence in a neonate with cardiac failure. Acta Pathol 95:333–335, 1973

56. Streeter GL: The development of the venous sinuses of the dura mater in the human embryo. Am J Anat 18:145–178, 1915

57. Streeter GL: The developmental alterations in the vascular system of the brain of the human embryo. Contrib Embryol 8:5–38, 1918

58. Streeter GL: Developmental Horizons in Human Embryos. Age group XI–XXIII. Embryology Reprint, vol II. Washington DC, Carnegie Inst Wash, 1951

59. Suzuki J, Takaku A: Cerebrovascular "Moyamoya" disease. Disease showing abnormal netlike vessels in base of brain. Arch Neurol 20:288–299, 1969

60. Takekawa SD, Holman CB: Roentgenologic diagnosis of anomalous communications between the external carotid artery and intracranial veins. Am J Roentgenol Radium Ther Nucl Med 95:822–825, 1965

61. Turnbull I: Agenesis of one internal carotid artery. Neurology (Minneap) 12:588–590, 1962

62. Warkany J: Congenital Malformations. Chicago, Year Book Med Publ, 1971

63. Zingesser LH, Schechter MM, Kier EC, O'Brien MS: Vascular malformations of the posterior fossa including the tentorial hiatus. Am J Roentgenol Radium Ther Nucl Med 105:341–347, 1969

chapter 21

ANTERIOR PITUITARY

NORMAL DEVELOPMENT*

PARS DISTALIS, TUBERALIS AND INTERMEDIUS

The normal development of the human anterior pituitary gland (adenohypophysis) has been studied by Atwell,[3] Covell,[8] Tilney,[28] Wislocki,[30] Streeter[27] and Falin.[12] Because the posterior pituitary gland (neurohypophysis) has no functional relationship with the adenohypophysis and has a different derivation, its development is discussed separately in Chapter 6.

During stage XIII (4- to 6-mm CR) of embryonic development, a shallow diverticulum known as Rathke's pouch appears on the roof of the foregut (Fig. 21–1). This is the first indication of the adenohypophysis; the position is just rostral to the notochord. Rathke's pouch deepens in stages XIV and XV (5- to 9-mm CR) and makes contact with the floor of the diencephalon in the midline at the level of the tuber cinereum. Late in stage XVI (8- to 11-mm CR), the first indications of the lateral lobes are found and referred to as the tuberal processes, which will differentiate into the pars tuberalis. An evagination on the floor of the diencephalon, the infundibulum, marks the first indication of the neural hypophysis during this stage. Whether or not there is any inductive relationship between the infundibulum and the formation of the tuberal processes is not known. Between the lateral lobes and the diencephalon is a small zone of mesenchyme that will later differentiate into the blood vessels serving the pituitary gland. Tilney[28] labeled this the "vascular groove."

* See Chapter 1 for background information on embryologic development and staging system.

Two distinct changes occur in stage XVII (11- to 14-mm CR): 1) the elongated stalk-like attachment of Rathke's pouch with the oral epithelium begins to constrict in places such that there is no longer a continuous lumen and 2) the tuberal processes surround the infundibulum laterally. These changes begin to give some definition to the primordium of the anterior pituitary gland. During stage XVIII (13- to 17-mm CR), those midline anterior lobe cells that are in close approximation with the infundibulum (which can now be called the *neural hypophysis,* or *posterior lobe*) mark the primordium of the pars intermedia. The fact that the pars intermedia later grows laterally around the posterior lobe in stage XIX (16- to 18-mm CR) can cause it to be confused with the bilateral tuberal processes during this period. Atwell[3] clarifies this point:

Developmentally, the pars intermedia may be defined as that portion of the wall of Rathke's pouch which early comes in contact with the neural lobe, remains relatively thin and epithelium-like, faces the residual lumen, and does not become strongly vascularized. The pars tuberalis . . . arises at the opposite end of Rathke's pocket, near the attachment of the pouch to the mouth epithelium, from a pair of lateral lobes.

With the pars intermedia and the primordia of the pars tuberalis now delineated developmentally, the pars distalis can be regarded as comprising the remainder of the epithelial adenohypophysis.

The absorption of the epithelial stalk, occurring between stages XIX and XXIII (16- to 31-mm CR), is useful in staging embryos.[27] As noted above, constrictions in the stalk are found in stage XVII (11- to 14-

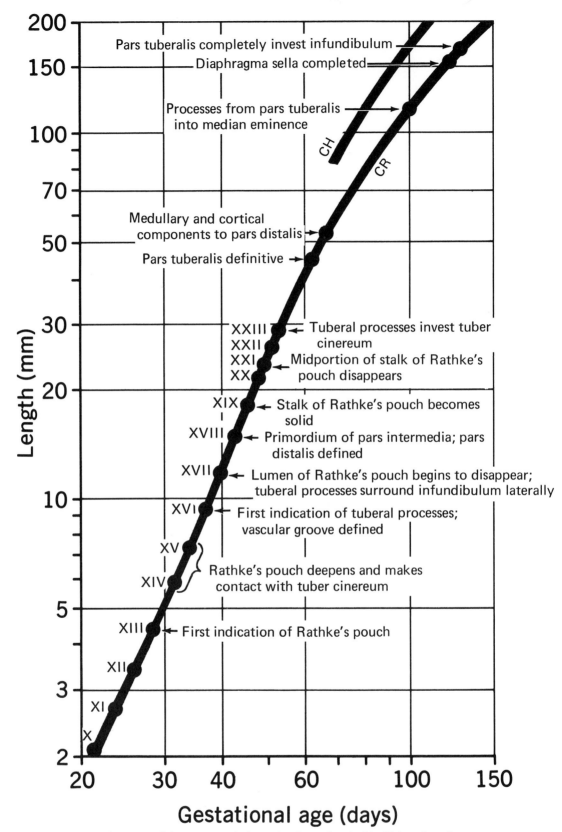

FIG. 21–1. Development of the anterior pituitary gland correlated with CR length and gestational age.

mm CR). During stage XIX, the stalk becomes quite solid and thick with only a remnant of the lumen remaining. Following this, the stalk becomes slender in stage XX and threadlike in stage XXI, and the middle portion completely disappears.[28] By stage XXII, only a remnant of the stalk is found at each end. The cranial remnant disappears during stage XXIII as the sphenoid cartilage ablates the original track. The remnant of Rathke's pouch (stalk) persists in the posterior nasopharynx throughout life as the "pharyngeal pituitary."[6, 21]

During stage XXI (22- to 24-mm CR), the pars distalis of the anterior lobe begins to thicken in the midline dorsally. At the same time, the floor of the third ventricle broadens, and the vascular grooves between it and the tuberal processes deepen. The tips of the bilateral tuberal processes begin to curve medially and by the end of stage XXIII (27- to 31-mm CR) meet in the midline just behind the optic chiasm; with progression caudally, they come to invest the median eminence of the tuber cinereum. By 45-mm CR length this relationship is completed, and the pars tuberalis is a definitive structure.

At 55-mm CR length, the pars tuberalis is fused with the median eminence but is still separated from the pars distalis by the vascular grooves. The mesenchyme of the vascular grooves is now differentiated into blood vessels that penetrate the pars tuberalis and pars distalis, both of which have become glandular tissue (as has the pars intermedia). The presence of vascular tissue in the pars distalis provides distinction between its medullary and cortical components. The cavity between these portions of the pituitary gland and the pars intermedia will gradually reduce in size, but a small component will remain as a residual lumen of Rathke's pouch, which is now termed Rathke's cleft.[14]

By 120-mm CR length, several processes extend from the pars tuberalis into the median eminence. The pars distalis is still separated from the pars intermedia by the residual lumen. Histologically, the pars distalis has two regions of glandular tissue separated by fenestrated vascularized connective tissue (derived from the vascular groove). The medullary portion has large acini with moderate-size intercellular spaces, whereas the cortical portion has small acini

and large intercellular spaces. The pars intermedia is characterized by coarse dense acini, small intercellular spaces and much less vascularity than the other portions of the anterior lobe.[28]

Between 120- and 170-mm CR length, the pars tuberalis grows caudally such that it completely invests the infundibulum.[3, 28] The major gross changes in the hypophysis during the remainder of the gestational period consist of a deepening of the gland into the sella tursica, an increasing angulation of the hypophyseal axis relative to the floor of the third ventricle and an increasing attenuation of the pars intermedia. Cytologic differentiation of the acidophil cells was studied by Porteous and Beck,[24] who found staining activity for human growth hormone beginning at from 4 1/2 to 5 gestational months and reaching adult levels by birth.

RELATIONSHIP OF MENINGES

The relationship of the development of the meninges to the pituitary gland has been studied by Wislocki.[30] Between stages XVII and XIX (11- to 18-mm CR), the mesenchyme that will later form the meninges around the pituitary gland is loose and unorganized. However, rostral, caudal, and lateral to this area the primordia of the pia mater and dura mater can be identified as small cellular concentrations. The future subarachnoid space is present between the pia and dura, and gradually forms around the pituitary stalk by 60-mm CR length. The subarachnoid space usually does not gain access to the gland itself, being limited by the overlying dura mater, which forms a collar around the pituitary stalk. This collar, termed the *diaphragma sella,* normally completes development by 160-mm CR length. In some cases, the diaphragma sella is incomplete, and a subarachnoid space is present around the pituitary gland.

ABNORMAL DEVELOPMENT

ABSENCE AND HYPOPLASIA

Absence or hypoplasia of the entire pituitary gland is associated with hypoplasia of the adrenal and may be associated with other abnormalities. Blizzard and Alberts[5] found complete absence associated with a small sella tursica that was covered by a diaphragma sellae with no opening. Reid[25] reported absence of the pituitary in a case with a normal-size sella tursica with no opening to indicate that a pituitary stalk had ever been present. In both cases, the adrenal glands were hypoplastic.

Brewer[7] reports a premature infant (case 1) with bilateral cleft lip and a deficiency in the anterior palate. Necropsy revealed an infundibular stalk attached to a small knob of tissue that histologically resembled normal neurohypophysis. No trace of the adenohypophysis was found despite a careful microscopic search. There was associated adrenal hypoplasia.

Edmonds[10] describes absence of the pituitary gland in three cyclopic fetuses. There was associated absence of the sella tursica and optic nerves, as well as hypoplasia of the adrenal glands. The pituitary was present in two additional cases of cyclopia, each of which had a normal-appearing sella tursica, a single optic nerve and normal adrenal glands. The pituitary was absent in case 2 of Brewer,[7] which had cyclopia and an encephalocele. Cyclopia is the severest form of a continuum of anomalies known as holoprosencephaly (see Chapter 14). Cebocephaly, another type included in this spectrum, is also sometimes associated with complete[16] or partial[15] absence of the pituitary gland.

Mosier[23] reports a case with hypoplasia of the pituitary gland with associated adrenal hypoplasia. There were no acidophil cells, and chromophobes and basophils were present in an equal percentage. Ehrlich[11] found a hypoplastic pituitary gland ectopically located anterior and inferior to the optic chiasm. Most of the cells were chromophobes; there were moderate numbers of basophils, but only a few acidophils. The adrenals were hypoplastic. The diagnosis of pituitary hypoplasia can be suspected in patients with a small sella tursica who have associated growth or endocrine problems.[13, 20] The diagnosis cannot be firmly established until autopsy since the gland might be in an ectopic position and may be dysfunctioning for other reasons.

ANENCEPHALY

The pituitary gland is usually present, but abnormal in anencephalics.[1, 9] The sella tursica is usually absent or markedly hypoplastic, and the diaphragma sellae is lacking. The gland itself is flattened, but it may appear enlarged during the midgestational period. Most of this enlargement is due to vascular engorgement, and when this factor is corrected for, the gland is nearly of normal weight.[9] The anterior lobe is always present, but the pars intermedia and posterior lobe are frequently missing.

PITUITARY DUPLICATION

Morton[22] reports duplication of the pituitary gland in a newborn with a cleft palate and other oral malformations. In addition, accessory anterior lobe masses were present in the roof of the pharynx. Warkany[29] shows a photograph of two pituitary glands occurring in a cephalothoracopagus type of conjoined twin.

ANOMALOUS CRANIOPHARYNGEAL CANAL

A canal corresponding to the previous tract of Rathke's pouch is found in 9% of newborns and in 0.4% of older people.[2] The typical canal extends from the sella tursica to a point where the wings of the vomer meet the body of the sphenoid. The contents of the canal vary; connective tissue, blood vessels and accessory pituitary tissue have been described. The fact that the canal corresponds to the previous course of Rathke's pouch once led some to speculate that it was a persistence of this structure, but a careful study by Arey[2] showed this concept to be erroneous; instead it appears to be a channel formed during bone development by blood vessels connecting with the marrow spaces. His views have been supported by the more recent study of Lowman et al.[19] The craniopharyngeal canal is formed during development of the chondrocranium "when vessels come to connect with the marrow spaces by erupting into the dissolving cartilage and developing bone, from the young periosteal tissue."[2]

PITUITARY CYSTS AND TUMORS

Shanklin[26] observed cilia-lined asymptomatic cysts of the pituitary gland in 22 out of 100 autopsies (ages ranging from 2 days to 83 years). These were classified as microfollicular (9 cases), macrofollicular (8 cases), cystic clefts (3 cases), multilocular (1 case) and hypophyseal stalk cyst (1 case). Such cysts are derived from Rathke's cleft in contrast to the usual craniopharyngioma, which is thought to be derived from cells from the original tract of Rathke's pouch and pars tuberalis (see Chapter 23).[14] Some cysts are symptomatic[4] in a manner similar to that of the more-solid pituitary tumors.

A different entity, known as the "empty sella tursica," can be confused with pituitary cysts. The pituitary is flattened at the bottom of the sella and covered by subarach-noid space. The basic defect seems to be either primary or secondary hypoplasia or absence of the diaphragma sellae.[17]

DYSTOPIA OF THE POSTERIOR PITUITARY

The normal development of the posterior pituitary, which is a derivative of ependyma, is presented in Chapter 6. Dystopia of the neurohypophysis is an unusual anomaly that consists of the pars nervosa lying between the infundibulum and the diaphragma sellae. Its connection to the anterior lobe is by a stalk of pars tuberalis.[18]

REFERENCES

1. Angevine DM: Pathologic anatomy of hypophysis and adrenals in anencephaly. Arch Pathol 26:507–518, 1938

2. Arey LB: The craniopharyngeal canal reviewed and reinterpreted. Anat Rec 106:1–16, 1950

3. Atwell WJ: The development of the hypophysis cerebri in man with special reference to the pars tuberalis. Am J Anat 37:159–193, 1926

4. Baar HS: Dysontogenic pituitary cysts: pituitary cachexia in childhood. Arch Dis Child 22:118–127, 1947

5. Blizzard RM, Alberts M: Hypopituitarism, hypoadrenalism and hypogonadism in the newborn infant. J Pediatr 48:782–792, 1956

6. Boyd JD: Observations on the human pharyngeal hypophysis. J Endocrinol 14:66–77, 1956

7. Brewer DB: Congenital absence of the pituitary gland and its consequences. J Pathol Bacteriol 73:59–67, 1957

8. Covell WP: Growth of the human prenatal hypophysis and the hypophyseal fossa. Am J Anat 38:379–422, 1927

9. Covell WP: A quantitative study of the hypophysis of the human anencephalic fetus. Am J Pathol 3:17–28, 1927

10. Edmonds HW: Pituitary, adrenal and thyroid in cyclopia. Arch Pathol 50:727–735, 1950

11. Ehrlich RM: Ectopic and hypoplastic pituitary with adrenal hypoplasia; case report. J Pediatr 51:377–384, 1957

12. Falin LI: The development of human hypophysis and differentiation of cells of its anterior lobe during embryonic life. Acta Anat (Basel) 44:188–205, 1961

13. Ferrier PE, Stone EF Jr: Familial pituitary dwarfism associated with an abnormal sella tursica. Pediatrics 43:858–865, 1969

14. Frazier CH, Alpers BJ: Tumors of Rathke's cleft (hitherto called tumors of Rathke's pouch). Arch Neurol Psychiatr 32:973–984, 1934

15. Gorlin RJ, Yunis J, Anderson VE: Short arm deletion of chromosome 18 in cebocephaly. Am J Dis Child 115:473–476, 1968

16. Haworth JC, Medovy H, Lewis AJ: Cebocephaly with endocrine dysgenesis; report of 3 cases. J Pediatr 59:726–733, 1961

17. Kaufman B: The "empty" sella tursica—a manifestation of the intrasellar subarachnoid space. Radiology 90:931–941, 1968

18. Lennox B, Russell DS: Dystopia of the neurohypophysis: Two cases. J Pathol Bacteriol 63:485–490, 1951

19. Lowman RM, Robinson F, McAllister WB: The craniopharyngeal canal. Acta Radiol [Diagn] (Stockh) 5:41–53, 1966

20. Lundberg PO, Gemzell C: Dysplasia of the sella tursica; clinical and laboratory investigations in three cases. Acta Endocrinol (Kbh) 52:478–488, 1966

21. Melchionna RH, Moore RA: The pharyngeal pituitary gland. Am J Pathol 14:763–771, 1938

22. Morton WRM: Duplication of the pituitary and stomatodaeal structures in a 38 week male infant. Arch Dis Child 32:135–141, 1957

23. Mosier DH: Hypoplasia of the pituitary and adrenal cortex. Report of occurrence in twin siblings and autopsy findings. J Pediatr 48:633–639, 1956

24. Porteous IB, Beck JS: The differentiation of the acidophil cell in the human foetal adenohypophysis. J Pathol Bacteriol 96:455–462, 1968

25. Reid JD: Congenital absence of the pituitary gland. J Pediatr 56:658–664, 1960

26. Shanklin WH: Incidence and distribution of cilia in the human pituitary with a description of micro-follicular cysts derived from Rathke's cleft. Acta Anat 11:361–382, 1951

27. Streeter GL: Developmental Horizons in Human Embryos: Age Groups XI to XXIII. Embryology Reprint, vol II. Washington DC, Carnegie Inst Wash, 1951

28. Tilney F: The development and constituents of the human hypophysis. Bull Neurol Inst NY 5:387–436, 1936

29. Warkany J: Congenital Malformations. Chicago, Year Book Med Publ, 1971

30. Wislocki GB: The meningeal relations of the hypophysis cerebri. II. An embryological study of the meninges and blood vessels of the human hypophysis. Am J Anat 61:95–129, 1937

section **VI**

RELATED CONSIDERATIONS

chapter 22

CONGENITAL TUMORS OF THE NERVOUS SYSTEM

INTRODUCTION

An understanding of neoplasms of the nervous system occurring in infancy and childhood can only be derived from many disciplines, including oncology, pathology and teratology. Indeed, some understanding of cancer in general may eventually be found in the further elucidation of cellular control mechanisms which are so readily evident in normal embryogenesis and ever so slightly out of control in certain malformations and tumor-like conditions in which cellular proliferation is not yet truly neoplastic.

A tumor may be considered to be congenital either because it is obviously present at the time of birth or because its genesis is thought to have taken place *in utero*. Congenital tumors of the nervous system (Table 22–1) may originate from cells normally present at the site of occurrence (*i.e.*, autologous) or may originate from cells which are not normally found in that site (*i.e.*, heterologous). Among heterologous tumors, some (*e.g.*, germinomas) are thought to have originated from germ cells, which Witschi,[165] and Mintz and Russell[97] have shown to migrate widely throughout the early embryo before arriving at their destination—the gonads. Other heterologous tumors (*e.g.*, epidermoids) consist of tissues which could have been displaced in later stages of development. Thus, Van Gilder and Schwartz[156] were able to produce spinal epidermoid cysts by direct implantation of skin homografts into the epidural and subarachnoid spaces of immature animals. The very slow growth of these tumors may be a reflection of their origin from relatively normal cells.

Carcinogenesis is both dose- and time-dependent[124] and may be affected by cocarcinogens as well as by stimuli of cell proliferation and growth. Druckrey *et al.*[43] have shown that gestational age is also a significant factor. Any particular agent may be both teratogenic and oncogenic, as clearly indicated by DiPaolo and Kotin,[41] and as suggested for many years by observations linking cancer with congenital defects.[96] Thus consideration of the causes of a tumor or malformation must include evaluation of the agent (dose, origin, specificity and duration of action), the biologic system (age, sensitivity) and many other related factors. Of these factors, the individual genetic make-up is obviously of considerable significance, for the newer theories allow interaction of carcinogens, either viral or chemical, with the gene system.[2] All in all, the number of combinations and permutations of such interactions is enormous in any particular case.

That the mechanisms involved must also be quite variable is supported by the nonspecificity of the chemical agent resulting in carcinogenesis.[41] From a purely morphologic view, it is suggested that some, if not all, mechanisms underlying congenital malformations are applicable to tumors of all types, although it is obvious that there is a time (termination period) after which a potentially teratogenic insult can no longer produce a specific malformation. However, acting over a longer period of time, a given agent may produce tumors, perhaps requir-

TABLE 22–1. ETIOPATHOGENETIC CLASSIFICA-
TIONS OF CONGENITAL TUMORS
OF THE NERVOUS SYSTEM

I. *Cell of Origin*
  A. Autologous
    1. Malformation, e.g., hemangiomas,
      Sturge–Weber disease
    2. Hamartomas, e.g., tuberous sclerosis
    3. Neoplasms, e.g., gliomas, medulloblas-
      tomas
  B. Heterologous
    1. Ectopias
      a. Displaced early in embryogenesis:
        teratomas, germinomas
      b. Displaced later in embryogenesis:
        epidermoids, ependymal cysts
    2. Embryonic rests, e.g., craniopharyngi-
      oma, chordomas, neuroepithelial cysts
II. *Inciting Agent* (Teratogenic and Oncogenic)
  A. Virus
  B. Genes
    1. Oncogene
    2. Protovirus
    3. Chromosomal anomalies
  C. Chemicals (drugs)
  D. Ionizing radiation
III. *Mechanisms*
  A. Arrest in development
  B. Excessive development (abnormally in-
    creased development)
  C. Anomalous structural development
  D. Anomalous functional development
  E. Degeneration

ing a greater dose. Such a pattern of events may include the entire life of the organism since it is not birth or the causative agent that is unique, but the state of the biologic system.

From the biologic point of view, it is the growth rate of the tumor which is most important (Collins *et al.*[29]). It is generally believed that rapidly growing tumors usually possess other characteristics of malignancy (invasiveness and the tendency to metastasize), whereas slowly growing tumors do not, but the available evidence is remarkably scanty and at least the most recent findings are somewhat against this view (see below). Unfortunately growth rates vary widely for tumors of the same histologic appearance, and are difficult to define for most primary and many metastatic neoplasms. Where they have been defined, it seems clear that each patient's neoplasm has its own constant growth rate, a simple exponential doubling rate (Fig. 22–1), which may be the same or different for the primary as compared to its metastases (possibly related to the particular

internal milieu of each site), but which nevertheless is characteristic of that particular neoplasm. It seems clear that neoplasms of multicentric origin will be rare, since the most rapidly growing will dominate the picture, and only occasionally will two or more clones of neoplastic cells have practically the same growth rate. One should keep in mind that the apparent "recurrence" of a tumor may actually be due to the late appearance of the more slowly growing one after the first has been cured.

From this concept of simple exponential growth one can define "Collins' law", namely that the slowest rate of growth of a tumor would be obtained on the assumption that the tumor had grown over the longest possible time, *i.e.*, it had originated at conception. A patient must be considered at risk for recurrence until he has survived free of tumor for a time equal to his "total age" at diagnosis, *i.e.*, his age plus 9 months gestation. This "period of risk" is based on the assumption that symptoms or signs of the recurrence will occur after the same number of doublings of the neoplastic cells, *i.e.*, when the same mass of tumor has regrown as was initially diagnosable. Since most tumors recur within the first 2 years after diagnosis, it is obvious that most tumors do not actually begin anywhere near the time of conception. Furthermore, the classic 5-year survival index can be quite misleading in comparisons made of patients with "histo-

TABLE 22–2. GROWTH RATES OF NEOPLASMS

Growth Rate	Time To Double Volume	Time To Early Diagnosis (30 Doublings, 1g)* (in years)	Time To Late Death (45 Doublings, 32 Kg)† (in years)
Rapid	6–25 days	0.5–2	0.75–3
Moderate	25–75 days	2–6	3–9
Slow	75–180 days	6–15	9–22
Very slow	0.5–1.5 yr	15–45	22–67
Negligible	2–3 yr	60–90	90–135

* Assuming cuboidal cells 10 μ on each edge.
† Assuming either that the primary is not excised or that the ultimately fatal metastases developed about the same time as the primary. Alternatively, the time to death may be considered the additional time beyond diagnosis, assuming a single cell remains after excision of the primary.

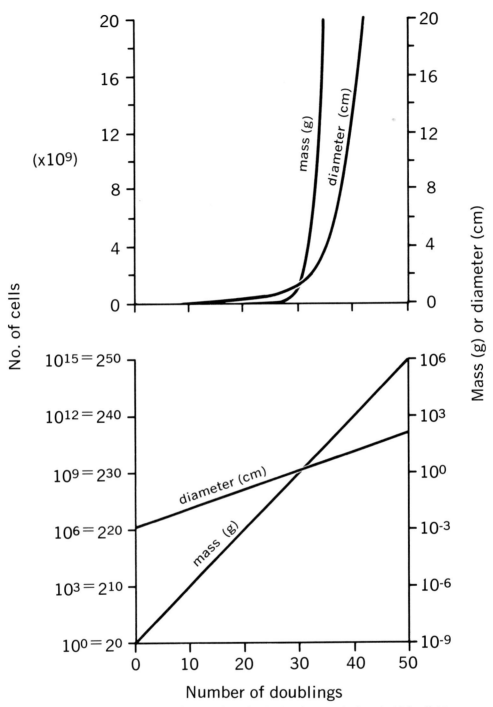

FIG. 22–1. Hypothetical growth of a neoplasm beginning from a single cuboidal cell 10μ on each edge and doubling at a constant rate. (Redrawn from Collins et al., 1956)

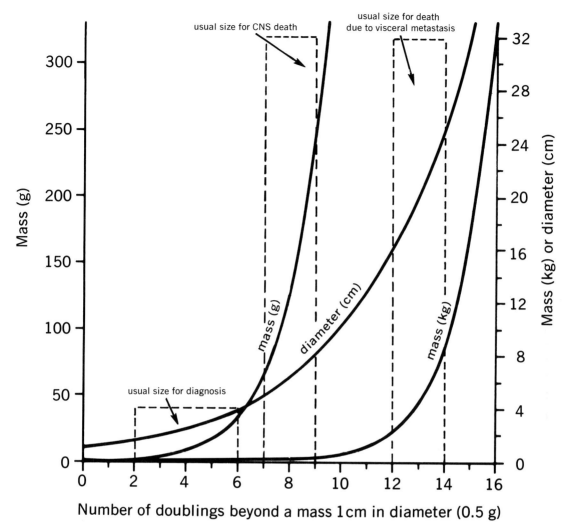

FIG. 22–2. Approximate times of diagnosis and death in the natural history of a neoplasm. Note the 1000-fold change in mass scales (g or Kg). Time is expressed as numbers of doublings of the volume (mass) after the tumor has reached 1 cm in diameter. Placing the origin at this size (0.5 g) eliminates the necessity for consideration of the average size of the tumor cells or the number of doublings after the onset of the neoplasm, but would correspond to doubling number 29 in Fig. 22–1.

logically the same" tumors occurring significantly before or after the age of 5 years.

Collins et al.[29] pointed out that the first 20 doublings of a tumor (beginning from a cuboidal cell about 10 μ on each edge) would result in a mass of about 1 cu mm, just at the threshold of clinical detectability in special circumstances, e.g., by chest x rays. A mass of about 1 g, 1.26 cm in diameter would result after 30 doublings and another 6 doublings would result in a mass of about 64 g, about 5 cm in diameter. These

are the ranges of the usual sizes clinically diagnosed, perhaps the most common size being about 2.5 cm in diameter, corresponding to 33 doublings (Fig. 22–2).

In the study of Collins et al.[29] metastatic neoplasms to the lung from various sources were observed to grow at doubling rates of 11–164 days, a remarkably wide range which others have extended even further. One can make several arbitrary groups (Table 22–2) with estimates of the duration to diagnosis and to death.

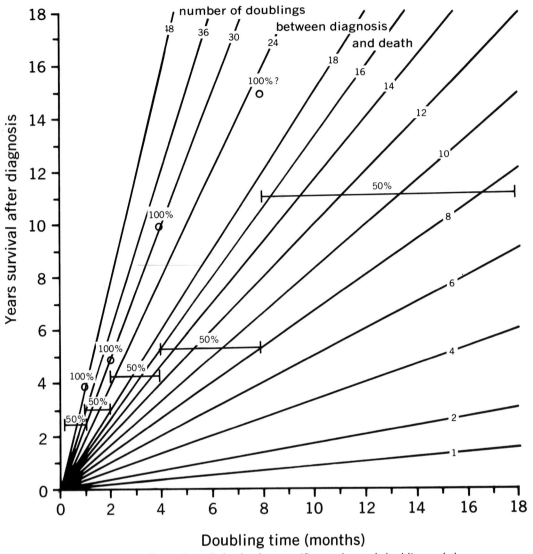

FIG. 22–3. Times between diagnosis and death after specific numbers of doublings of the mass of tumors which are doubling at particular rates. Also indicated are 50% survival times and 100% mortality times for groups of patients with ranges of doubling times of the primary tumor actually measured preoperatively. (This example of the best studied human neoplasm, carcinomas of the breast, was reported by Kusama et al., 1972)

Kusama et al.[86] reported similar ranges for primary carcinomas of the breast, which required from 0.2–18 months or more to double in size. They correlated the growth rates with the duration of survival after radical mastectomy. From their observations one can easily measure 50% survival times, and one can even estimate when 100% of the deaths from that neoplasm have occurred. By plotting these times on Fig. 22–3, where

lines have been drawn indicating the time between diagnosis and death in terms of the numbers of doublings for tumors doubling at various rates, one can begin to estimate when the ultimately fatal metastases originated. Replotting these data with reference to the origin of the metastases at or before the time of excision of the primary neoplasm (Fig. 22–4) leads to the rather surprising conclusion that the metastases must have

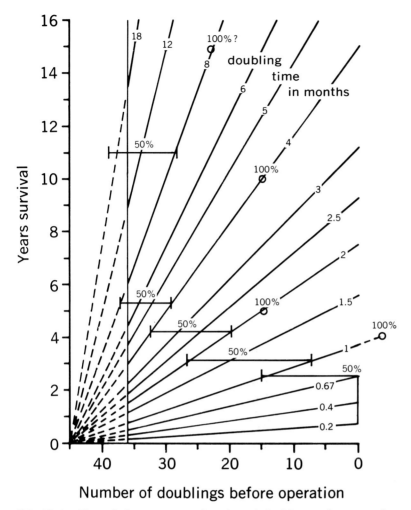

Number of doublings before operation

FIG. 22–4.   Times before treatment (number of doublings) when a single metastasis could have occurred to give the 50% and 100% mortality times (from Kusama et al., 1972) for carcinomas of the breast which were doubling at the ranges of doubling times indicated for each group of patients. An arbitrary maximum of 45 doublings is assumed (c.f., Fig. 22–1). If 1,000 (2^{10}) metastases occurred, the number of doublings before treatment would be reduced by 10. If 1,000,000 (2^{20}) metastases occurred, the number of doublings would be reduced by 20.

occurred very late (about the time of diagnosis and treatment) in the rapidly growing cases and very early (about the time of onset) in the slowly growing ones. These calculations assume a single metastasis as being ultimately fatal, but one can easily see that for 2^{10} metastases (about 1,000) 10 doublings can be subtracted, for 2^{20} metastases (about 1,000,000), 20 doublings. It seems likely that 1,000,000 metastases are far more than any patient actually has, but even so, the most slowly growing neoplasms must have metastasized early, long before the

primary was diagnosable. As far as we can discover, this is the only neoplasm for which such correlations have been made and from which such deductions can be drawn. Needless to say, further work needs to be done since growth rates may not remain constant. Necrosis is common late in the course of rapidly growing neoplasms and may well contribute to an apparent slowing of the growth rate. In the opposite direction, one may speculate that the late development of blocking serum factors[61] may contribute to an apparent increase in the growth rate.

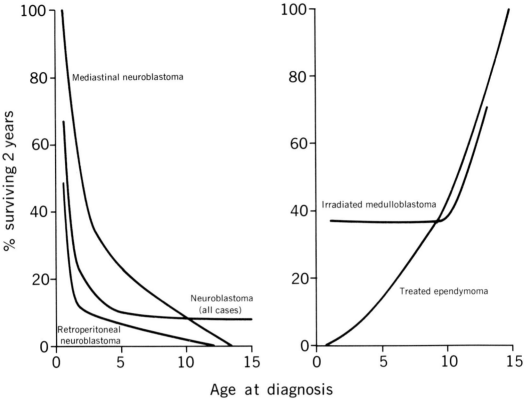

FIG. 22–5.   Two-year survival rates for neuroblastomas of various sites, irradiated medulloblastomas and ependymomas diagnosed at various ages. It should be noted that survival for
2 years is practically synonymous with cure for neuroblastomas but not for medulloblastomas
or ependymomas. (From de Lorimier *et al.*, 1969, Breslow and McCann, 1971, Bloom *et al.*,
1969, and Shuman *et al.*, 1975)

Even in many tumors of adults there is some tendency for a correlation of growth rates with the age of the patient; but, as Collins *et al.*[29] pointed out, young people can only have rapidly growing neoplasms, whereas old people can have rapidly or slowly growing ones. For example, a tumor doubling every two months would require 5 years to reach even 1 cm in diameter and, therefore, could not be diagnosed before age 4 years and 3 months. Thus, all neoplasms appearing in childhood must be relatively rapid in growth. For certain tumors characteristically occurring in children, specifically medulloblastomas[18] and ependymomas,[132] there is strong evidence that growth rates are proportionate to age; but for certain other tumors, specifically neuroblastomas[21, 92] and Wilms' tumors,[141] quite different behavior is noted, with few survivors in older children (Fig. 22–5). One of the difficulties with

studies such as these is that "the same" neoplasm arising in different sites may behave quite differently (see Ependymomas and Neuroblastomas below), so that lumping all cases by histologic appearance regardless of the site of origin may confuse the issue—but these specific details can more appropriately be considered below with each type of tumor.

TUMORS OF INFANCY AND CHILDHOOD

The first major obstacle to a coherent discussion of congenital tumors and other tumors of infancy and childhood is the array of terms used by different authors with their different connotations or implications. The second obstacle, related to the first, arises from attempts at too rigorous a categorization of

TABLE 22–3. CHILDHOOD TUMORS OF THE NERVOUS SYSTEM

Tumor	Cases	Male	Female
Neuroblastoma	83	47	36
Retinoblastoma	28	13	15
Ependymoma:			
4th ventricle	24	15	9
cerebrum	7	4	3
spinal cord (cauda equina)	3	2	1
Medulloblastoma	32	20	12
Astrocytoma:			
cerebellum	26	15	11
cerebrum	26	15	11
brain stem	19	13	6
optic nerve and chiasm	14	5	9
spinal cord	6	2	4
Craniopharyngioma	9	5	4
Meningioma	2	0	2
Hemangioblastoma	1	0	1
Pinealoma (germinoma)	4	2	2
Teratoma	1	1	0
Leptomeningeal sarcoma	1	1	0
Choroid plexus papilloma	1	0	1
Choroid plexus hemangioendothelioma	1	1	0
Undetermined	1	1	0
Tuberous sclerosis:			
surgical	2	0	2
autopsy	3	3	0
Epidermoid (autopsy)	1	0	1
Neurofibromatosis	10	5	5
Totals	305	170	135

From Children's Orthopedic Hospital and Medical Center, Seattle, Washington, 1952–1971.

the different tumors. It is difficult, if not impossible, to separate the neoplastic, the hamartomatous and the malformational aspects of many tumors. Some are clearly neoplastic, demonstrating a growth rate that exceeds and is uncoordinated with that of the normal tissues. Others are clearly hamartomatous (*i.e.*, tumor-like but essentially non-neoplastic malformations) and are characterized by an abnormal mixture of tissues indigenous to the site. Hamartomas generally grow considerably slower than true neoplasms and generally do not display the well recognized potential for malignancy. Unfortunately, the two conditions are difficult to separate in certain diseases, *e.g.*, neurofibromatosis. Classification, therefore, must remain flexible and for the moment rather arbitrary.

For the purposes of brevity and simplicity, the following categories of tumors will be considered:

A. Neoplasms:
 Teratomas and germinomas
 Gliomas (astrocytomas, medulloblastomas, ependymonas, etc.)
 Neuroblastomas and retinoblastomas
B. Ectopias and embryonic rests:
 Epidermoid cysts
 Dermoid cysts
 Craniopharyngiomas
 Colloid cysts
 Cartilaginous tumors
 Lipomas
 Chordomas
 Leptomeningeal and other cysts
C. Malformations:
 Arteriovenous malformations
 Sturge–Weber syndrome
 Nasal glioma
D. Genetic and/or hamartomatous conditions:
 Von Recklinghausen disease (neurofibromatosis)
 Bourneville disease (tuberous sclerosis)
 Von Hippel–Lindau syndrome
 Lipomatous conditions

NEOPLASMS

Intracranial tumors in infancy and childhood are surprisingly common[45, 94] but, as Anderson[5] notes, the special interests of the hospital and the different classifications of tumors

TABLE 22–4. TUMORS OCCURRING BEFORE 6 MONTHS OF AGE

Tumor	Total Cases	Cases Occurring At Birth
Neuroblastoma	19	0
Retinoblastoma	7	0
Medulloblastoma	2	0
Ependymoma	2	0
Germinoma	1	0
Papilloma of choroid plexus	1	0
Glioma	1	0
Tuberous sclerosis	4	2
Neurofibromatosis	2	1
Teratoma	1	0
Total	40	3

Data from all University-affiliated hospitals in Seattle, Washington.

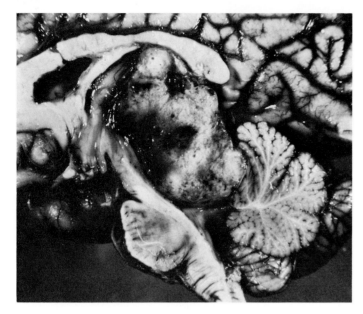

FIG. 22–6

FIG. 22–7

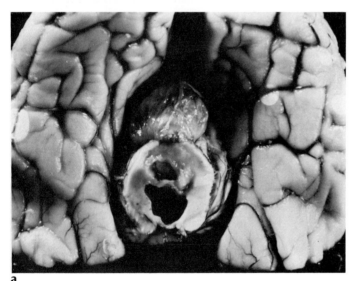

a

b

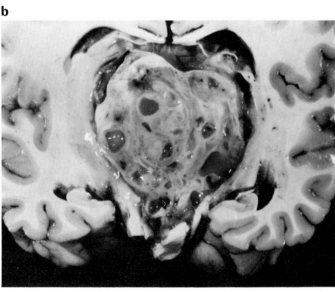

FIG. 22–6. Midsagittal section of the brain from a 20-year-old man with a pineal teratoma compressing the midbrain and caudal diencephalon. A small remnant of a postchiasmatic mass can be seen and was probably responsible for the panhypopituitarism and diabetes insipidus which characterized his early course. (#Np 652)

FIG. 22–7. **a.** Basal view of the brain of a 5-year-old boy with hydrocephalus, ataxia and Parinaud syndrome due to a pineal teratoma. **b.** Coronal section of the same brain. (#Np 2650)

FIG. 22–8. **a.** Photomicrograph of a representative area of a pineal teratoma containing glandular structures secreting mucus. **b.** Midsagittal section of the same brain showing compression of the midbrain by the pineal teratoma. The patient was a 6-year-old boy with precocious puberty and Parinaud syndrome. (#Np 3037)

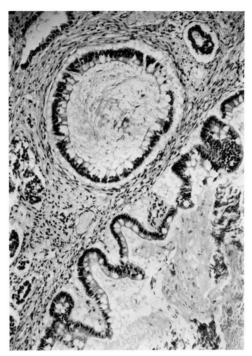

a

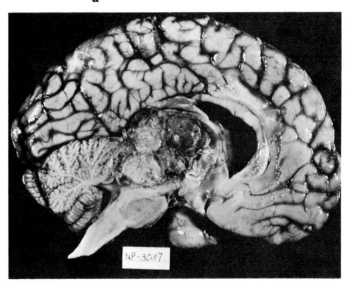

b

seriously bias many reports. For example, Dargeon[36] reported only 14 examples of CNS neoplasms during 30 years, while Matson[94] had 750 cases for approximately the same period of time. Our experience is summarized in Table 22–3. Further difficulty is encountered because different sites (*e.g.*, intracranial, spinal cord and peripheral nervous system) are included or excluded as different authors choose. We shall try to consider the entire spectrum of tumors and their biologic characteristics, where they have been defined, but we would caution the reader not to confuse biology with histology!

TABLE 22–5. OTHER POSSIBLY CONGENITAL TUMORS

Case (Np #)	Tumor	Site	Age (yr)	Sex	Additional Features
3190	Teratoma	Cerebellopontine angle	7/12	F	None
3037	"	Pineal	5	M	None
3200	"	3rd ventricle	9	M	Hamartoma of hypothalamus
161	"	Olfactory ridge	56	M	None
3623	"	Nasopharynx	0	M	Olfactory hamartoma & encephalocele
3172	"	Sacrococcygeal	0	F	None
416	Epidermoid	Cerebellar	2	F	"
931	"	Pineal	69	M	"
2636	"	Interpeduncular fossa	54	M	"
3102	"	Ventral medulla	71	M	"
380	Colloid cyst	3rd ventricle	68	M	"
774	" "	" "	20	F	"
836	" "	" "	93	F	"
1042	" "	" "	82	M	"
2152	" "	" "	78	M	"
2500	" "	" "	84	F	"
3340	" "	" "	13	M	"

Data from all University-affiliated hospitals in Seattle, Washington.

Congenital Neoplasms

Congenital neoplasms, those present at birth or occurring within the first six months of life, are quite uncommon in the nervous system. Solitaire and Krigman[137] listed only 26 cases as definitely congenital and 19 more as probably or possibly congenital. Of the total, one-third were teratomas, one-third were gliomas, and the remaining one-third included a heterogeneous group of neoplasms representing the variety of tumors seen at later ages.[6, 40, 52, 91, 98, 107, 116, 125] Our experience is summarized in Tables 22–4 and 22–5.

TERATOMAS AND GERMINOMAS. Teratomas vary greatly in size, even replacing the entire brain. They occur in many sites, characteristically in the midline, and particularly near the pineal gland (Figs. 22–6 to 22–9) or sacrococcygeal region (Figs. 22–10 and 22–11) and elsewhere (Fig. 22–12).[52, 68] Teratomas may be considered well differentiated forms of germinomas,[50, 78, 134] which are thought to arise from germ cells migrating from the germinal ridge during the embryonic period.[97, 165] Germinomas occur most commonly in the gonads, as one would expect, and are truly malignant neoplasms. Those occurring in the region of the pineal gland (Fig. 22–9) or optic chiasm

(the favorite site of "ectopic pinealomas") differ in no way from those occurring in the gonads, retroperitoneum, or mediastinum. There is no reason to continue discussing them as "pinealomas" except for the frequency of their occurrence in the pineal, and their frequent association (in about 11% of cases) with precocious puberty, 95% occurring in males. Those occurring in the suprasellar region characteristically present with diabetes insipidus, visual disturbances and hypopituitarism during the first two decades of life.[26]

Childhood Tumors

After birth there is a progressive increase in the incidence of intracranial tumors, reaching a peak between the ages of 5 and 8 years.[94] On the whole, there are about equal numbers of supratentorial and infratentorial tumors in children, the ratio varying from 43%–54%.[37, 89, 94] In the reviews of both Matson[94] and Dargeon,[36] and in agreement with our own observations (Table 22–3), astrocytomas (of all sites) are the most frequent type of tumor, with medulloblastomas occurring next most frequently. The frequency of occurrence of other types of tumors varies in the experience of different reporters. Ependymomas are common in our

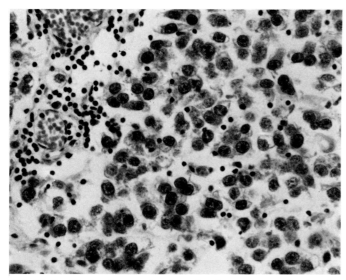

FIG. 22–9. Photomicrograph of a pineal germinoma having large polygonal tumor cells and stromal lymphocytes. The patient was a 46-year-old man with diabetes insipidus for 8 months and obstructive hydrocephalus due to numerous intraventricular metastases. (#Np 1308)

FIG. 22–10. Sacrococcygeal teratoma appearing as a small sacral mass. (From Lemire et al., 1971)

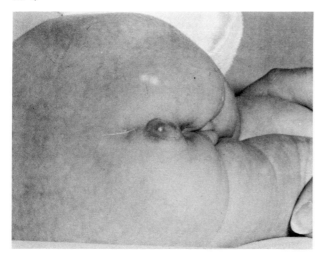

experience[132] (about equal to medulloblastomas), but relatively much less common in the series of Dargeon[36] and Matson[94] and others.[33, 89, 93]

ASTROCYTOMAS. The most frequent tumor in this age group, astrocytomas occur in several different sites: The cerebellum, either solid or cystic (Fig. 22–13); the brain stem (Fig. 22–14); the optic chiasm (Figs. 22–15 and 22–16) and the optic nerves (Fig. 22–17). The biology of astrocytomas is quite variable, some of the ones in the optic nerve[42, 47, 63, 64, 145, 167] and cerebellum[25] being self-limited and not requiring total excision for a cure. Others in the same site, however, are slowly progressive, extend beyond the grossly apparent limits defined at

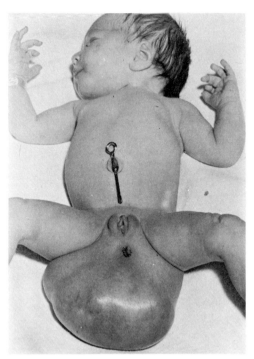

FIG. 22–11. Massive sacrococcygeal teratoma displacing pelvic contents.

operation and are practically incurable. At the present time, unfortunately, we see no way to differentiate one from the other. Cystic astrocytomas of the cerebellum are especially easy to cure by excision of the mural nodule, but when occurring in other sites are notorious for recurring and "transforming" or progressing into malignant neoplasms (glioblastoma multiforme). Cerebral astrocytomas frequently progress into glioblastoma multiforme, whereas cerebellar astrocytomas practically never do. Brain stem gliomas, practically never biopsied early to determine whether a histologic change occurs, include the entire range of astrocytomas from grade 1 (slow growing, "benign") to grades 3–4 (glioblastoma multiforme). There is just no substitute for "knowing the territory"—the logic, if any, escapes us!

MEDULLOBLASTOMAS. Medulloblastomas are highly undifferentiated and malignant neoplasms usually occurring in the cerebellar vermis (Fig. 22–18). Although controversy[71] persists about their origin from postulated

bipotential cells,[7, 8] external granule cells[139] or cell rests in the posterior medullary velum,[113] we have seen individual cases which "have matured into" astrocytoma, neuroblastoma or even fibrous sarcoma. We have learned the hard way, from personal experience, not to use the term *cerebellar sarcoma,* since neurosurgeons and radiotherapists may be misled into thinking it a different tumor. The term was introduced about 25 years ago in an attempt to account for tumors which usually developed off the midline in older individuals. They were characterized by marked proliferation of reticulin about reticulin-free nodules of neoplastic cells. This last feature should have been the tip-off that these were not sarcomas. As Rubinstein and Northfield[123] have pointed out, the term sarcoma should be discontinued and these neoplasms more accurately referred to as sclerosing or desmoplastic medulloblastomas, since the reticulin is clearly reactive to the neoplasm and usually derived from the leptomeninges, not from the tumor cells themselves. In spite of this reaction by the host, the biology of

FIG. 22–12. Basal view of the brain of a 56-year-old man with an olfactory teratoma obscuring the orbital regions of the frontal lobes. (#Np 161)

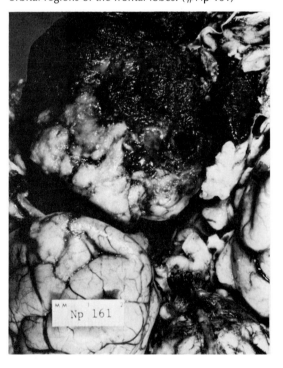

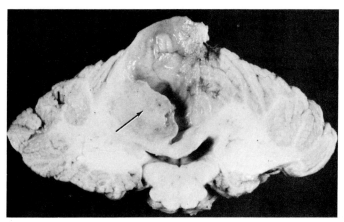

FIG. 22–13. Horizontal section of the cerebellum and medulla of a 15-year-old boy who died unexpectedly while waiting in the emergency room. There is a cystic astrocytoma of the vermis with a mural module of tumor present in the left wall (*arrow*). (#D-312)

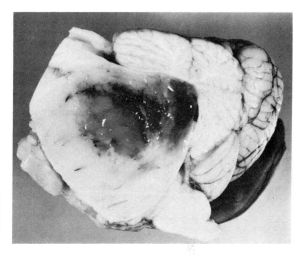

FIG. 22–14. Midsagittal section of the brain stem and cerebellum of a 4-year-old girl showing a cystic and gelatinous glioblastoma multiforme of the brain stem. The fourth ventricle is obliterated by the tumor. (#Np 2344)

FIG. 22–15. Coronal section of the cerebral hemispheres of a 9-year-old girl showing a massive glioma of the optic chiasm. (#Np 685)

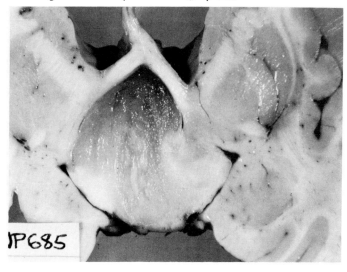

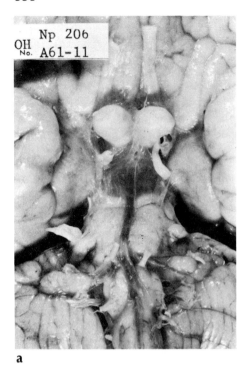

a

b

FIG. 22–16. **a.** Basal view of the brain of a 21-month-old boy showing bilateral gliomas of the optic nerves. Several *cafe au lait* spots 1–2 cm in diameter and "xanthomas" up to 1.4 cm in diameter were present in the skin as evidence of neurofibromatosis. **b.** Close-up view of the same brain showing that the optic nerve gliomas extend to the chiasm. (#Np 206)

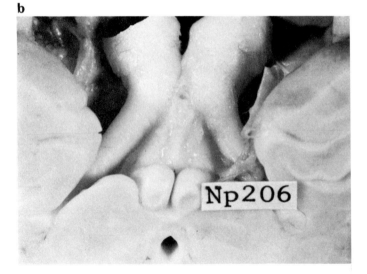

these neoplasms seems to follow that of the ordinary nonsclerosing medulloblastomas, especially when one corrects for any differences in age, and they certainly require whole axis irradiation.

The biology of medulloblastomas has been well summarized by Bloom *et al.*[18] who noted that males are affected twice as commonly as females, that 80% of medulloblastomas occur in children under 15 years of age with two minor peaks at 3–4 and 8–9

years, and that medulloblastomas account for 20% of intracranial neoplasms in children and 4% of intracranial neoplasms at all ages. Applying Collins' "law" as a criterion, Bloom *et al.*[18] reported 14 cures (plus up to 6 more possible cures of patients who have not been followed for sufficient periods of time) out of 82 cases irradiated (17%–24%). Using the classic 5-year survival rate, they obtained 38% success (broken down to 31–33% for children under 4 years or over 10 years of

TABLE 22–6. BIOLOGIC FEATURES OF EPENDYMOMAS

Site	Number	Median Age (yrs)	M/F
Lateral Ventricle	18	6	1/1
Fourth Ventricle	50	2	2/1
Cauda Equina	6	14	5/1

age at the time of diagnosis). They recommended surgical excision of as much tumor as possible without markedly increasing the operative risk, followed by high doses of X-irradiation to the cerebellum: 4000–4500 r in 6–7 weeks for children under 3 years and 4500–5000 r for children over 3 years of age, 3000–4000 r to the rest of the brain and 2000–2500 r to the spinal cord. From their data it is possible to define a simple straight line y = 0.15x, where x = the "total" age at diagnosis and y = the average time to recurrence in those who are not cured. This is remarkably similar to the lines y = 0.15x derived by Shuman et al.[132] for unirradiated ependymomas and y = 0.52x for adequately irradiated ependymomas, but quite different from the behavior of neuroblastomas (see below).

EPENDYMOMAS. Shuman et al.[132] have recently defined the biology of ependymomas occurring in childhood. These tumors occur in 3 sites: lateral ventricles, fourth ventricle (Figs. 22–19 to 22–21) and cauda equina. The spinal cord itself may be involved (Fig. 22–22), but none of our patients has been in the pediatric age range. The frequency,

usual age at diagnosis and the sex incidence vary remarkably with the site (Table 22–6). Of the 50 ependymomas occurring in the fourth ventricle, 5 occurred within the first year of life and at a median age of 2.3 years for the entire group.

Regardless of their site of origin the prognosis was grim (Figs. 22–23 and 22–24) with no survivors if operation was not followed by irradiation. The effectiveness of radiotherapy has been investigated, taking advantage of Collins' "law" and correcting for the effect of age by utilizing a ratio,

$$R = \frac{\text{symptom-free time}}{\text{total age at diagnosis,}}$$ in order to com-

pare the outcome in cases treated only operatively with those treated also with postoperative irradiation. Fig. 22–24 shows that no unirradiated case has passed the "risk threshold" (R = 1), that lightly irradiated cases have died at similarly short intervals and that practically the only surviving cases have been subjected to 4500 r (tumor dose), or more. Tables 22–7 and 22–8 confirm these observations, the adequately irradiated cases living twice as long (either as actual years or as R values) as the unirradiated or inadequately irradiated cases, a pattern that is true for ependymomas occurring at each of the three sites.

Tumors in Infancy

Between the most common intracranial gliomas (astrocytomas, medulloblastomas and ependymomas) having a peak incidence at

TABLE 22–7. RESULTS OF X-IRRADIATION OF EPENDYMOMAS ARISING IN VARIOUS SITES

	Median Symptom-free Interval (years)			Median Symptom-free Ratio R*		
	No X Ray Rx	Intermediate X Ray Rx†	Adequate X Ray Rx‡	No X Ray Rx	Intermediate X Ray Rx†	Adequate X Ray Rx‡
Lateral ventricle	0.5	0.0	2.4	0.1	0.1	0.3
Fourth ventricle	0.4	0.8	1.8	0.1	0.1	0.3
Cauda equina	3.1	12.4	7.0	0.4	0.8	0.5

* $R = \dfrac{\text{symptom-free interval}}{\text{age} + 9 \text{ months}}$

† Less than 4500 rads in 60 days.

‡ More than 4500 rads in 60 days.

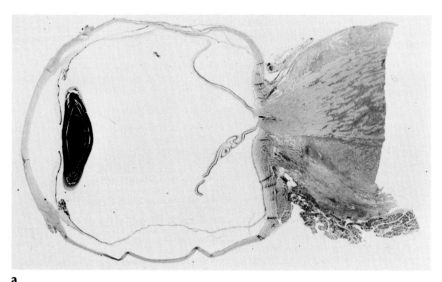

a

b   c

FIG. 22–17. **a.** Low power photomicrograph of a glioma of the optic nerve beginning just behind the globe. The patient, a 5-year-old girl, showed progressive proptosis for 4 months as well as a surprisingly late decrease in visual acuity. **b.** Macroscopically, the posterior extent of the longitudinally sectioned tumor appears to stop just short of the optic foramen; microscopically, however, pleomorphic astrocytes could be seen intracranially even at the level of the optic chiasm. **c.** Cross section through the middle of the tumor. **d.** Higher magnification of the tumor showing prominent Rosenthal fibers near the stromal margins. **e** and **f.** Photomicrographs showing extensions of the tumor into the subarachnoid spaces and marked proliferation of the leptomeninges. (#Np 4260)

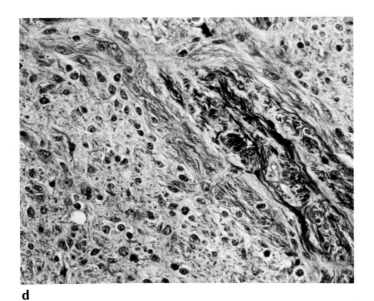

d

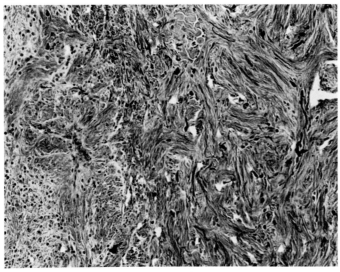

e

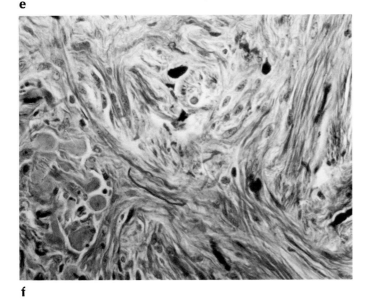

f

361

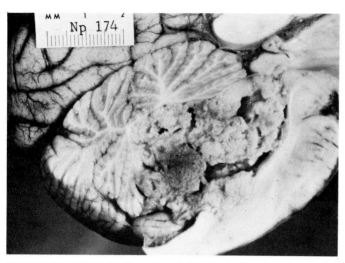

FIG. 22–18. Midsagittal section of the cerebellum and brain stem of a 5-year-old girl with medulloblastoma arising in the posterior vermis and filling the fourth ventricle. (#Np 174)

5–8 years of age and the least common intracranial neoplasms (teratomas) occurring congenitally, there is an intermediate group of neurogenic tumors (neuroblastoma and retinoblastoma) which usually occur extracranially in the first two years of life.

NEUROBLASTOMAS. Neuroblastomas are actually the most common type of solid tumor of childhood[38], rarely appearing at birth,[83, 111, 159] but nearly half the cases re-

ported occur in the first two years of life.[15, 53] They arise from undifferentiated cells of neural crest origin and, therefore, may arise in many sites, including sympathetic ganglia,

FIG. 22–19. An ependymoma of the fourth ventricle is seen through the posterior medullary velum at craniectomy.

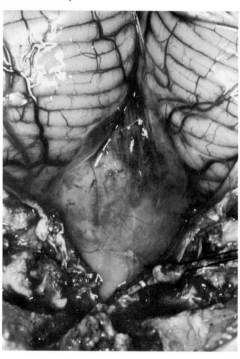

TABLE 22–8. RESULTS OF X-IRRADIATION OF EPENDYMOMAS, ALL SITES COMBINED

	No or Inadequate Irradiation*	Adequate Irradiation†
Mean age at diagnosis	4.60 ± 0.54‡	8.90 ± 1.26
Mean symptom-free interval (years)	1.00 ± 0.25‡	4.20 ± 1.07
Mean symptom-free ratio R§	0.16 ± 0.03‡	0.52 ± 0.10
Number living and well	1/47¶	11/20

* For intracranial ependymomas less than 4500 rads in 60 days; for cauda equina ependymomas no irradiation.

† For intracranial ependymomas more than 4500 rads in 60 days; for cauda equina ependymomas more than 1700 rads in 60 days.

‡ p is less than 0.01 by student's t-test.

§ $R = \dfrac{\text{symptom-free interval}}{\text{age} + 9 \text{ months}}$

¶ p = 1.13 × 10⁻⁶ by Fisher's exact test.

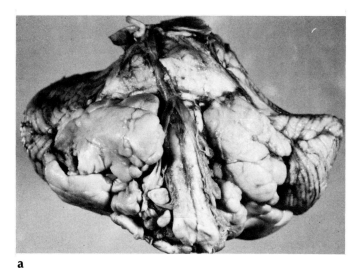

a

FIG. 22–20. **a.** Basal view of the brain stem and cerebellum of a 2-year-old boy who died unexpectedly at home. The multinodular tumor was a mixed ependymo–astrocytoma arising subependymally from the roof of the fourth ventricle and extending through the foramina of Luschka. **b.** Midsagittal view of the same brain, showing tumor filling the entire fourth ventricle and extending through the foramen of Magendie to fill the cisterna magna. (#Np 744)

b

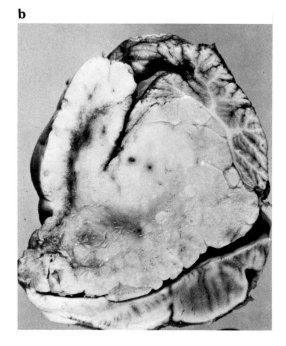

dorsal root ganglia, parasympathetic ganglia and paraganglia.[10] Turkel and Itabashi[154] reported neuroblastic nodules in all fetal adrenal glands, with a peak in number and size at 17–20 weeks gestation and with subsequent regression. It would appear that many of these represent normal variations rather than incipient malignancies, but the possibility remains that at least some represent spontaneously regressing neoplasms (see below).

As Mäkinen[92] and deLorimier et al.[39] pointed out, the site of origin is very important in defining the prognosis. Neuroblastomas of the thorax or mediastinum are relatively rare but have the best prognosis (Fig. 22–5), whereas those of the commonest sites, adrenal and retroperitoneum, have the poorest prognosis. Furthermore, as noted above, the age at the time of initial diagnosis determines the prognosis; most of the survivors come from the group under 1 year of age at diagnosis, and practically none from the group over 3 years of age. Mäkinen[92] emphasized the importance of any histologic evidence of differentiation of the neuroblasts into neurons in improving the prognosis, and

Breslow and McCann[21] emphasized the importance of the clinical stage or extent of the disease in determing the prognosis. Unfortunately, no study has yet separated all three of these variables (site of origin, evidence of histologic differentiation and age), each of which contributes heavily to the prognosis.

One of the most striking features of neuroblastomas is that patients diagnosed before 1 year of age have a good prognosis, with 80% survival if local disease (or even regional metastasis) is present and 50% survival even if distant metastases are present.[141] Such

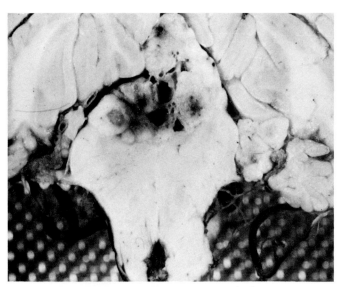

FIG. 22–21. On horizontal section of the medulla and cerebellum of this 76-year-old man, an incidental "subependymal astrocytoma," "subependymoma," or ependymoma of the fourth ventricle is seen extending into the subarachnoid space via the foramina of Luschka. (#Np 171)

"spontaneous remissions" have been attributed to the development of resistance (by sensitized lymphocytes) unimpeded by the development of blocking antibodies which enhance the growth of the tumor at the expense of the host.[60, 61]

Hellstrom and Hellstrom[60, 61] have indicated that lymphocyte-mediated hyersensitivity to tumor-associated antigens of many tumors, including neuroblastoma, can specifically destroy the tumor cells, are regularly detectable in all tumor patients, but can be thwarted by "blocking" factors (probably antigen–antibody complexes or occasionally free antigens) in the serum of patients with progressing tumors. "Unblocking" serum factors can be detected in many patients free of tumor, and the disappearance of unblocking factors can be detected before the blocking factors appear as the tumor recurs. "Potentiating" serum factors may appear during remission and increase the cytotoxic effects of the immune lymphocytes, and "arming" serum factors may cause nonimmune lymphocytes to become cytotoxic, both of these phenomena being shown with dilute sera, whereas unblocking activity quickly diminishes on dilution. It is quite likely that the

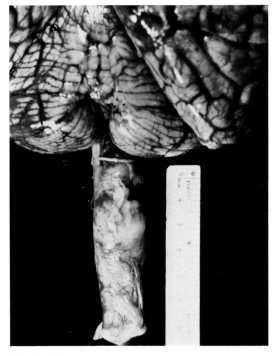

FIG. 22–22. An ependymoma distends the mid-cervical region of the spinal cord.

different components of these complex immunologic mechanisms may mature at different rates, so that the age-related phenomena observed may be illustrating the maturation of the various immunologic systems: approximately 50–100 times as many

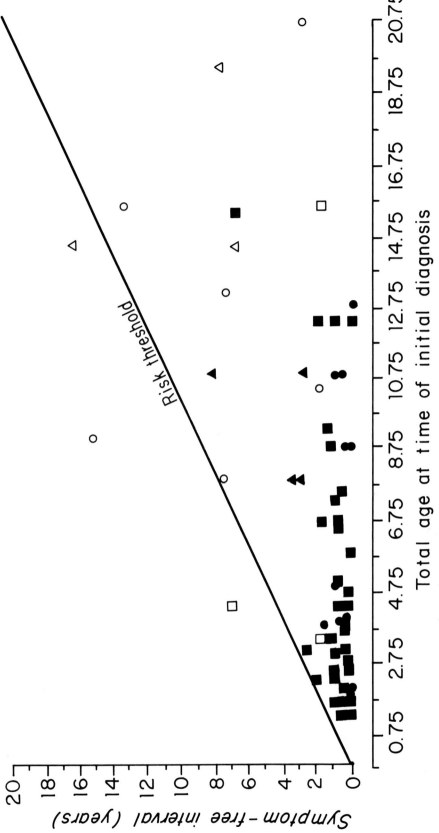

FIG. 22–23. Postoperative survivors of ependymomas: the symptom-free interval after operation for each case is plotted against the child's total age at which the diagnosis was first established. *Circles* include 18 cases with supratentorial tumors; *squares*, 42 cases of fourth ventricular tumors; *triangles*, 5 cases of cauda equina tumors. The *open symbols* indicate patients who are alive and well; *solid symbols*, patients who are either alive with recurrent tumor or dead. *Total age* is the age at diagnosis plus 9 months. *Risk threshold* is y = x, based on Collins' "law."

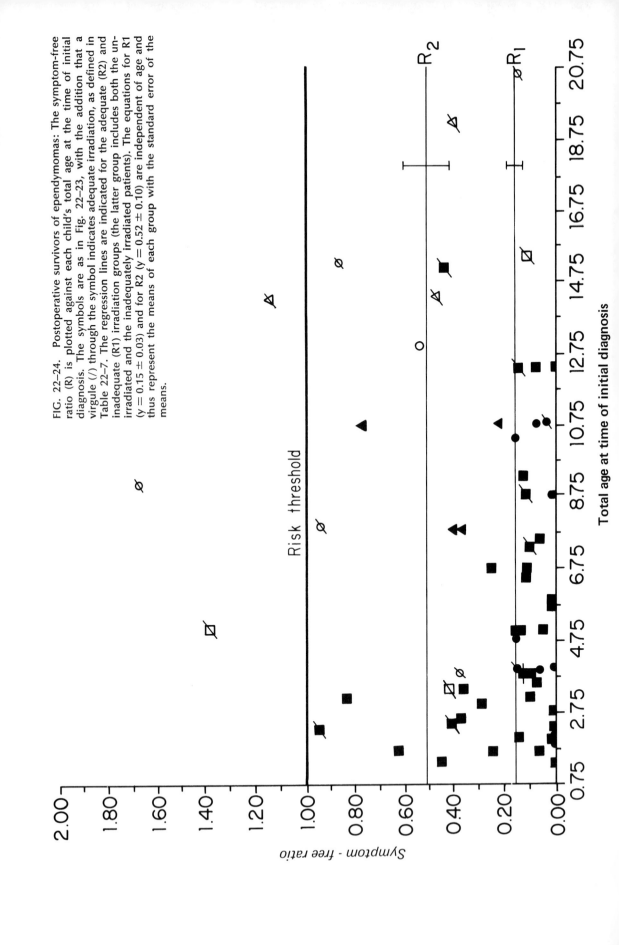

FIG. 22–24. Postoperative survivors of ependymomas: The symptom-free ratio (R) is plotted against each child's total age at the time of initial diagnosis. The symbols are as in Fig. 22–23, with the addition that a virgule (/) through the symbol indicates adequate irradiation, as defined in Table 22–7. The regression lines are indicated for the adequate (R2) and inadequate (R1) irradiation groups (the latter group includes both the un-irradiated and the inadequately irradiated patients). The equations for R1 (y = 0.15 ± 0.03) and for R2 (y = 0.52 ± 0.10) are independent of age and thus represent the means of each group with the standard error of the means.

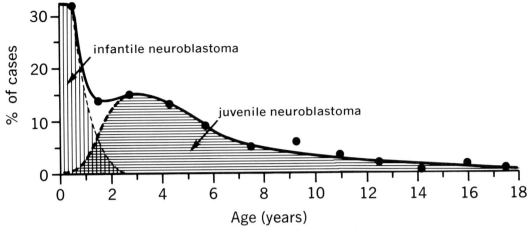

FIG. 22–25. Distribution of neuroblastomas by age at diagnosis. (From de Lorimier et al., 1969; Breslow and McCann, 1971)

FIG. 22–26. Survival rates for children with neuroblastomas diagnosed after 2 years of age. (From Sutow et al., 1970) It would appear that the disease progresses from local to metastatic stages in about 0.2 year and to death in another 0.6 year in the median patient.

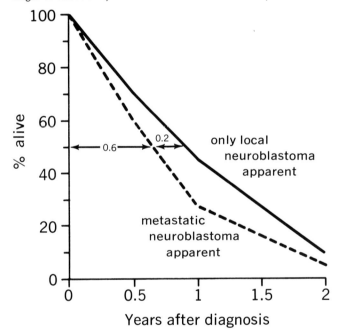

in situ neuroblastomas are seen in infants autopsied under age 3 months as develop clinically overt neuroblastomas later, spontaneous regressions of neuroblastomas occur relatively commonly in children under age 2 years and very rarely later. The "differentiation" of neuroblastoma may be only apparent, the more malignant cells being actively killed by the lymphocytes, the presence of which in biopsies or in peripheral blood also correlates with a better prognosis.

There is evidence that resistance is increasingly abrogated in older children, so that 90% of children over 2 years of age at the time of diagnosis of neuroblastoma die within 2 years.[141] This is true even if the

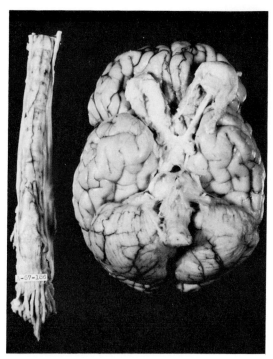

FIG. 22–27. Basal view of the brain and spinal cord of a 6-year-old boy with retinoblastoma diffusely invading the leptomeninges. The left eye had been removed 8 months before death. (#JDH A-57-186)

disease is relatively localized. One can readily imagine that an individual's ability to produce blocking antibodies develops later in life than the ability to produce sensitized lymphocytes, so that one is prompted to ask the question, when do neuroblastomas begin?

Let us begin by dividing the cases into two groups, *infantile*—those appearing before 1 year of age (about 30% of the total)— and *juvenile*—those appearing after 2 years of age (about 55% of the total). Indeed, the bimodal age distribution[39] shown in Fig. 22–25 suggests that the 15% appearing between 1 and 2 years of age are an almost equal mixture of the two major groups.

For an infantile neuroblastoma to appear before 1 year of age (21 months maximally available) would require doubling times of less than 0.7 months (29 doublings, 1 cm in diameter) and more likely less than 0.6 months (36 doublings, 5 cm in diameter). If the infant's lymphocytes are destroying the neuroblastoma, the rates would be even faster. In any event, it seems quite logical,

indeed inevitable, that these neoplasms must have begun *in utero*, and probably very early in gestation. The common incidental neuroblastoma found at autopsy in infants under 3 months of age (50–100 times more often than expected for cases clinically diagnosed)[11,153] and the occasional "maturation" or "differentiation" of neuroblastoma into ganglioneuroma could represent the great effectiveness of the infant's lymphocytes in destroying malignant immature cells, leaving the benign mature ones. The rare "recurrence" of neuroblastoma many years after the end of the usual "period of risk"[39] could be explained as relapses of the same primary (or more likely the appearance of a second primary) due to the late production of blocking antibodies.

As for those "juvenile" neuroblastomas appearing after 2 years of age, one need not worry about the tumoricidal effects of sensitized lymphocytes decreasing the growth rate: statistically speaking, these lymphocytes are completely prevented from attacking the tumor by blocking antibodies, since over 90% of the children die within 2 years. This prognostic factor is surprisingly independent of age.[39] About one-third of the patients appear with local disease, but still the median patient dies in about 0.8 year.[141] About two-thirds of the children appear for diagnosis with distant metastases, and the median patient dies in about 0.6 year (Fig. 22–26). It would appear that we are witnessing the progression of the disease in the median patient from local to metastatic disease in about 0.2 year and to death in another 0.6 year. Neoplasms doubling every 0.8–1.2 months would reach the stage of 31–35 doublings (local disease) within 2.0–3.5 years after onset, the stage of 34–37 doublings (metastatic disease) within 2.2–3.7 years after onset and the stage of 43 doublings (death with 8 Kg of neoplasm, about half the weight of the median child of 5 years) within 2.8–4.3 years after onset. It thus appears quite possible that even the youngest child in this group could have developed his neuroblastoma late in gestation or even at birth, and that almost certainly a child 4 or more years old at the time of diagnosis developed his neuroblastoma after birth.

The biologic differences between the two groups of cases of neuroblastomas, infantile

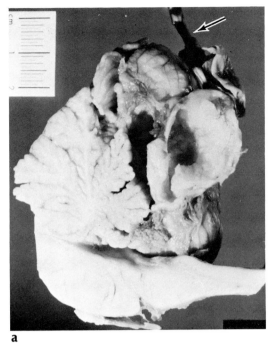
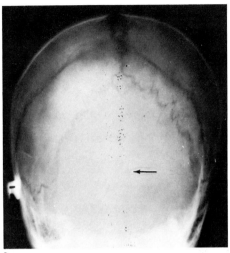

a   b

FIG. 22–28. **a.** Midsagittal section of the brain stem and cerebellum from a 21-month-old girl who had had 3 episodes of purulent meningitis. Only terminally was the head shaved and a pinpoint sized opening found in the skin at the tip of the occipital prominence. A congenital epidermal sinus (*arrow*) is seen to connect with a large epidermoid cyst which compresses the vermis of the cerebellum posteriorly. **b.** Radiograph showing a defect (*arrow*) in the midline of the skull, through which ran the congenital epidermal sinus. This defect was unfortunately overlooked until autopsy revealed the congenital sinus shown in Fig. 22–28**a.** (#D-414)

and juvenile, would fit the phylogenetic pattern of development of certain basic immunologic mechanisms. Cellular hypersensitivity is more primitive, develops early and effectively kills off infantile neuroblastoma cells developing early *in utero,* whereas humoral blocking antibodies develop later and effectively protect the late-arising juvenile tumors rather than the patients. It is as though immunologic tolerance preventing formation of humoral antibodies is easier to establish in the younger individual than is tolerance preventing formation of cellular immunity (or hypersensitivity).

RETINOBLASTOMA. Retinoblastoma (Fig. 22–27) is an uncommon neoplasm of primitive neurons of the retina with capability for differentiation into photoreceptor cells.[150, 151, 152] It is a tumor of prenatal origin, occurring in about 1 out of every 23,000 births, and having a peak age of diagnosis soon after birth. The peak in mortality occurs between 2–3 years of age,[74] especially due to extension through the optic nerve. During that period negroes have a mortality rate 2.5 times greater than whites, a difference probably reflecting the delayed diagnosis.[102]

Most cases are sporadic, hereditary cases accounting for as few as 4% of all cases.[157] In the inherited cases, the disease is due to an autosomal dominant with at least 80% penetration.[157] New mutations involving a dominant gene probably account for no more than 15% of sporadic cases with other possibilities including dominant genes of low penetration, recessive genes, environmental agents acting postzygotically or combinations of such factors.[74] Retinoblastomas involve both eyes in 25% of cases, occurring simultaneously or at different times. In families with hereditary retinoblastomas, at least 60% show bilateral involvement, whereas only 25% of sporadic cases have bilateral involvement.

Retinoblastomas may be associated with

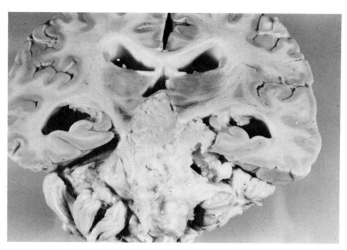

FIG. 22–29. A pearly-white epidermoid tumor covers and distorts the brain stem, elevates the floor of the third ventricle and produces internal hydrocephalus. This was a 54-year-old man who had had symptoms for three years, beginning with tic-like pains in his left face but progressively involving most of his cranial nerves and long tracts. (#Np 2636)

normal chromosomes or a variety of chromosomal abnormalities, including partial deletions of the long arm of 13 (one of the D group), trisomy 21 and XXX.[49, 112, 146, 163] Taylor[146] found that 55% of reported Dq— cases had retinoblastomas whereas none of the reported Dr cases had a retinoblastoma. An excess of mental retardation in cases of retinoblastoma was noted by Jensen and Miller[74] and the associated malformations suggested a D— deletion syndrome. The deleted chromosome has been identified as number 13.[163] Features of this syndrome include mental retardation, retinoblastoma, aplastic or hypoplastic thumbs (in about one-quarter of the reported cases) and other findings, such as microcephaly, trigonocephaly, protruding upper teeth, low set ears, cleft or highly arched palate, micrognathia and retarded growth and development.[163]

Although most infants survive, radiotherapy may be associated with osteosarcoma, soft-tissue neoplasms and carcinoma of the skin.[74] Primary tumors of other organs may occur in affected infants. Spontaneous regression of a retinoblastoma may occur but is rare, occurring before the age of 6 years.[140]

ECTOPIAS AND EMBRYONIC RESTS

Ectopias develop in situations where their cells of origin are not normally found. They are a heterogeneous group, but most are cystic. Some have been considered neoplastic, others hamartomatous, and others maldevelopmental. It is difficult to know if their growth potential exceeds that of similar but normally placed tissues.

Epidermoid and Dermoid Tumors

Epidermoid tumors and dermoid cysts (Figs. 22–28 to 22–30) probably arise through epithelial misplacement during embryogenesis.[148] The traumatically-induced lesions of Van Gilder and Schwartz[156] are of significance more because they indicate that such misplaced cells can survive and produce tumors than because they are strictly traumatic. Metaplasia as a possible mechanism seems less necessary. Dermoid cysts contain all layers of the skin and are initially symptomatic within the first two decades of life. They are usually associated with a congenital dermal sinus and have a predilection for certain sites: occipital (cerebellum and fourth ventricle), lumbar, orbit and anterior fontanelle (Fig. 22–28).

Epidermoid tumors contain only the superficial (epithelial) layer of the skin, usually become symptomatic between 20–50 years of age, usually are not associated with a congenital dermal sinus and are relatively uniformly distributed throughout the neuraxia, with perhaps a predilection for the ventral brain stem (Fig. 22–29).

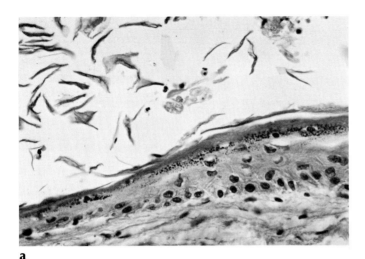

a

FIG. 22–30. **a.** Photomicrograph showing the lining of an epidermoid tumor which is composed of stratified squamous epithelium containing keratohyalin granules and sloughing off as "dry" keratin. **b.** High power microscopic view of "dry" keratin. Note the change in shape of the thin hexagonal cells as the plane of section changes.

Craniopharyngiomas

Unfortunately, Toglia *et al.*,[148] in a review that many others have considered authoritative, included craniopharyngiomas as arising from epithelial cells misplaced during embryogenesis and differing only in the type of squamous epithelium and the degree of desquamation. Such an oversimplification leads to important practical and conceptual errors, since craniopharyngiomas are not derived from epidermal cells but from mucosal cells. Thus, craniopharyngiomas never have ordinary "dry" keratin, such as the "dandruff" that epidermoids have (Fig. 22–30), rather a variety of other types of completely different epithelium, especially mucosal squamous epithelium with "wet" parakeratin (Fig. 22–31). From a practical point of view, the "wet" parakeratin characteristic of the usual craniopharyngioma is found only in the suprasellar region, whereas the "dry" keratin characteristic of epidermoid tumors may be found anywhere (theoretically also in the same suprasellar region, but actually very rarely, if ever).

Theories of the genesis of craniopharyngiomas include their derivation from remnants of the craniopharyngeal duct, from squamous rests of the pars tuberalis and from

b

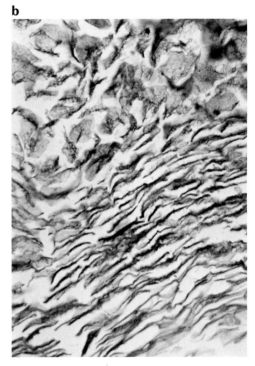

misplaced tissue of the embryonic enamel organ. These theories will be examined in detail.

As a neoplastic growth of a remnant of the craniopharyngeal duct, craniopharyngiomas become part of a spectrum that includes cysts of the sellar region. As described in Chapter 21, such cysts may have walls composed of cells of low cuboid to columnar epithelium, some of which may produce mucus; these cells probably derive from

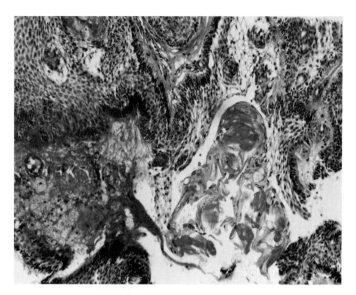

FIG. 22–31. Photomicrograph of a craniopharyngioma of a 55-year-old man showing a confluent mass of "wet" keratin within the degenerating mucosal epithelium growing from the basal columnar layer. Note the swollen globular cells characteristic of "wet" keratin and different from the shrunken cells composing "dry" keratin shown in Fig. 22–30. (#Np 2147)

Rathke's cleft.[128] Thus, mucous and clustered cells were characteristic of the microfollicular cysts found incidentally in pituitaries by Shanklin.[128] Other cysts may have walls composed of cilia-bearing cells, which are thought to be derived from ependyma (neuroepithelium).[44, 130] Depending on the type of epithelium, it is convenient to speak of cysts derived from Rathke's cleft or from the neuroepithelium, although Shuangshoti et al.[130] considered neuroepithelium histologically indistinguishable from Rathke's cleft epithelium.

Squamous rests are commonly seen in the pituitary, in 24% of adult pituitary glands according to Luse and Kernohan,[90] although none occurred in patients under 10 years of age. Thus, such rests can hardly be considered a congenital tumor, but rather must be a neoplastic alteration in autologous cells that have undergone metaplasia.

The original hypothesis relating the genesis of craniopharyngiomas to misplaced cells of the enamel organ of teeth attempted to account for a common histologic feature of craniopharyngiomas, namely, an epithelial pattern suggestive of adamantinomas. However, this is a misinterpretation of the inside and outside relationship of the epithelium: the stroma of craniopharyngiomas is derived from the outside (pia or leptomeninges), carrying blood vessels toward the basal layer of the mucosal epithelium, which keratinizes into "wet" keratin pearls and desquamates into the inside of the tumor. Thus, the basal layer is not composed of the epithelial cells of the enamel organ, nor are the other layers of the mucosa derived from the stellate reticulum of the enamel organ. However, in one interesting but unique case, a rudimentary tooth was found in a craniopharyngioma, and was interpreted by Seemayer et al.[127] as the result of the inclusion of pharyngeal endoderm with oral ectoderm during the stomatodeal evagination.

Colloid Cysts

Colloid cysts (Figs. 6–4 to 6–8) have also been considered congenital in nature even though they occur almost exclusively in adults. Their congenital nature is postulated on their origin[33] as a remnant of a vestigial embryonic structure (the paraphysis cerebri) or as an offshoot of the choroid plexus or embryonic ependyma. The origin from the paraphysis most adequately accounts for the gross location of practically all of these cysts, i.e., in the rostral superior region of the third ventricle. However, as Kappers[80] points out, the cells of the true paraphysis are not ciliated, whereas most colloid cysts are composed of ciliated columnar epithelium. To account for this discrepancy, Kappers[80] proposes that most colloid cysts arise from other evaginations of the ependyma which also occur transiently in the immediate vicinity of the paraphysis. If related to either of these transient structures, colloid cysts should be attached to the velum interpositum, immediately caudal to the foramina of Monro. In most cases it is extremely difficult to establish the exact site of attachment of the cyst in this region, but in at least one case we have been satisfied that the cyst was caudal to the choroid plexus that continued from the lateral ventricle around the cyst into the roof of the third ventricle (Fig. 6–5). The ciliated columnar epithelium of this cyst was quite different from the nonciliated cuboidal epithelium of the choroid plexus and of the ependyma of the adjacent third ventricle. The proposal of Shuangshoti et al.[131] that all such cysts are simple folded derivatives of the neuroepithelium could account for such epithelium but would require some other explanation for the overwhelming preponderance of localization to the anterior roof of the third ventricle. Ependymal cysts have been reported in sites other than the third ventricle, usually near a ventricular surface,[131] and even in sites more distant from a ventricular surface (such as the Sylvian fissure[106]), and within the subarachnoid spaces of the spinal cord.[164] But can one really call these colloid cysts? Although the "acquired" component of this hypothesis may explain the age distribution in adults (none in Table 22–3), one must recall that the growth rate remains undefined and may well approach that of normal cells.

Chondromas

Rare examples of intracranial cartilaginous tumors[168] have been thought to arise from misplaced cells, but simple metaplasia of mesodermal elements cannot be excluded.

Lipomas

Lipomas of the CNS have a predilection for the corpus callosum, midbrain and other midline sites (Figs. 22–32 and 22–33). They are rarely symptomatic, except in the spinal cord, and have been found in all age ranges.[158, 170] The pathogenesis of such lipomas is unknown beyond the fact that the fat cells develop in the pia, probably from the mesodermal elements contributing to the pia. The occasional association of lipomas with other malformations of the brain, such as agenesis of the corpus callosum,[170] suggests that they are malformations rather than neoplasms. Lipomas of the lumbosacral region are frequently attached to the spinal cord or cauda equina and are commonly seen in cases of spina bifida occulta.[75, 87, 88] Such lipomas may be both extradural and intradural, having attachments to the cauda equina, conus medullaris and spinal cord. Other abnormalities have been reported, including a bifid spinal cord[69] and diastematomyelia.[87] Ingraham and Swan[70] utilize the term lipomyelomeningocele when nerve elements are found. There were 18 such cases in their study, in addition to 14 examples of lipomeningocele (a lipomatous tumor associated with a meningeal sac) and 13 lipomas associated with spina bifida occulta without other abnormalities. Neurologic symptoms may include abnormal reflexes, poor sphincter tone, abnormal sensation in the lower extremities, paresis or spasticity and foot deformities.[9, 24, 69, 87] There have been few adequate neuropathologic examinations of such cases since the mortality rate is low. Bassett[9] reported finding cartilaginous and aberrant neural elements in one case.

Examination of two autopsied cases presently under study in our laboratory revealed the direct continuity of the pia mater of the lumbar spinal cord with the lipoma. The dura mater and arachnoid were lost in the tumor and a well defined herniation of meninges could not be demonstrated. The spinal cord was quite abnormal, in both cases demonstrating a dorsal kink and bulbous termination containing a presumed terminal ventricle. Such findings suggest that the syndrome cannot be viewed simply as an association of a subcutaneous lipoma with spina bifida. We would view the two as an integral part of a developmental, possibly hamartomatous, malformation. As such, lipomeningoceles constitute a distinct pathoanatomic entity with a spectrum of findings relating it to meningoceles and meningomyeloceles.

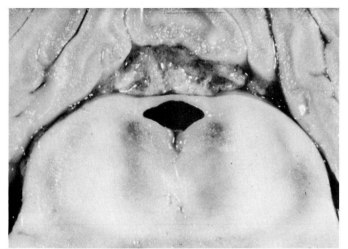

FIG. 22–32. Horizontal section of the ponto-mesencephalic junction of a 72-year-old woman showing an incidental lipoma which lies between the anterior vermis and the anterior medullary velum. Microscopically this tumor was attached to, and infiltrated, the inferior colliculus. (#MH-N-58-216)

FIG. 22–33. Photomicrograph of a lipoma adherent to the mammillary bodies, an incidental observation at autopsy of a 58-year-old man. (#Np 1361)

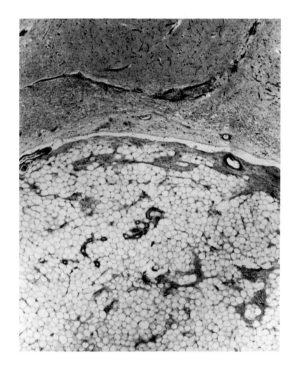

A lipomatous condition with extensive abnormalities of the CNS has been presented by Haberland and Perou,[57] who noted extensive cutaneous and viseral lipomatosis, multiple circumscribed lipomas of the nervous system, meningeal lipoangiomatosis, and cerebral malformations which included polymicrogyria of one hemisphere and glial heterotopias. As with so many of the tumors under discussion, it is difficult to separate the neoplastic, hamartomatous and maldevelopmental aspects of such a case.

Chordomas

Chordomas, like colloid cysts, are another example of a "congenital" tumor occurring late in life, having its peak incidence in the sixth decade and rarely being found in the first two decades. It is a relatively uncommon neoplasm believed to arise from remnants of the primitive notochord, which forms the nucleus pulposus.[30, 35, 99, 138] Malignant, locally aggressive tumors, chord-omas show a predilection for the ends of the spinal column, 80% or more occurring in either the sacrococcygeal or sphenooccipital bones, and uncommonly in the cervical, thoracic and lumbar spine.[34]

The malignant neoplasm must be differentiated from the benign notochordal remnants or excrescences on the clivus found in 1–2% of autopsies and designated as ecchordosis physaliphora (Fig. 22–34).[30, 138] Such

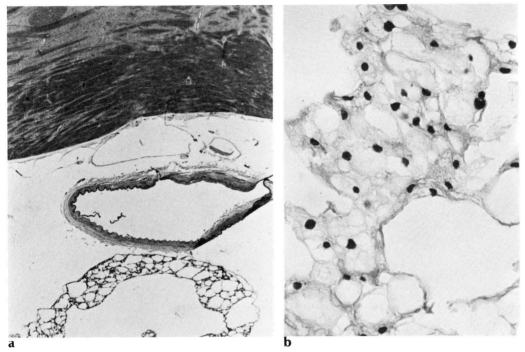

a   b

FIG. 22–34. **a.** Low power photomicrograph of an ecchordosis physaliphora attached to the basilar artery, an incidental observation in a 51-year-old man. (#Np 2607) **b.** High power photomicrograph showing the foamy physaliphorous cells.

remnants are very likely related to collections of similar cells found along the original tract of the notochord.

Cysts

In addition to the solid epidermoid and dermoid cysts and colloid cysts which are discussed separately, there are a number of fluid-filled cysts in or near the nervous system for which no adequate classification has yet been attempted. These occur in a variety of sites (Tables 22–9 and 22–10), and most are considered congenital in origin. They are distinctly uncommon and histologically have walls composed either of fibrous tissue, usually interpreted as arachnoid or leptomeningeal in type, or composed of epithelial cells, usually interpreted as ependymal or neuroepithelial. Epithelium-lined cysts also include those in the sellar region, which have been interpreted as derivations of Rathke's cleft, and those in the spinal canal, considered ectopic or teratomatous in nature.

The clinical presentation of such cysts usually reflects the site of origin, with symptoms of spinal cord compression, seizures, hydrocephalus, or hypothalamic dysfunction. An unusual neurologic finding is that of head-bobbing associated with third ventricular cysts.[12, 95, 103]

Cysts occurring within the vertebral canal may be intra- or extradural and occasionally intraspinal. The extradural cysts usually have fibrous walls[56, 67] and are frequently considered congenital, although some appear to be acquired, such as the synovial cyst reported by Sypert *et al.*[143] Intraspinal intradural cysts include those of the arachnoid,[155] and an unusual form of teratomatous tumor with epithelium resembling respiratory or intestinal mucosa.[62, 82, 119] The teratomatous cysts lie mostly posterior or posterolateral to the spinal cord. They are benign lesions and may be associated with other malformations such as spina bifida. According to Matson,[93, 94] such neurenteric cysts occur most commonly at the level where the primitive lung bud arises from the foregut, in the low cervical or upper thoracic region.

Spinal arachnoid cysts[67, 155] usually occur

TABLE 22–9. CYSTS OF THE NERVOUS SYSTEM

I. Peripheral nervous system
  Nerve root (dorsal)
    meningeal diverticulum[109, 135]
    perineural cyst[144]
  Peripheral nerve
    mucoid or traumatic cystic degeneration[56]
II. Intraspinal
  Extradural
    meningeal[67]
    ganglion[79]
    synovial[143]
  Intradural
    arachnoid[155]
    teratomatous (neurenteric, epithelial and
      gastrocytoma)[62, 72, 82, 119]
    ependymal[164]
  Intramedullary cyst of conus medullaris[101]
III. Intracranial
  Intracerebellar or posterior fossa
    arachnoid[13, 103]
    meningoencephalocele[3, 59]
  Paracollicular or cisterna ambiens
    arachnoid[1, 55, 65, 81, 85, 120]
    ependymal[58, 85]
    meningoencephalocele[3]
  Temporal fossa–Sylvian fissure
    arachnoid[13, 73, 120]
    ependymal[106]
  Parasagittal or interhemispheral
    arachnoid[73, 120]
    cyst of cavum
    veli interpositi
  Third ventricle
    arachnoid[95]
    ependymal[23]
  Intracerebral
    arachnoid[13]
    ependymal[20, 73]
    meningoencephalocele[114]
    glial
    unknown[59]
IV. Colloid cyst[58, 105]
V. Sellar cysts[48, 100, 128, 130, 164]
VI. Choroid plexus cyst
VII. Related but different conditions
    cyst of cavum septi pellucidi and cavum
      Vergae[66, 129]
    diencephalic cyst[22, 104]
    ependymal fusion[84]
    acquired leptomeningeal cyst[54, 120]

in young patients and are commonly situated posteriorly in the midthoracic region. Communication with the subarachnoid space has been demonstrated in a number of cases, suggesting they are acquired diverticula and not congenital tumors,[155] a mode of origin more readily accepted for those cysts morphologically similar but arising in a sacral root.[109, 144] Cystic dilatation of the central canal of the conus medullaris may occur[101]

and clinically may simulate syringomyelia, tumor or herniated nucleus pulposus.

Intracranial arachnoid cysts are commonly found in the temporal fossa or Sylvian fissure[13, 73, 120] and the cisterna ambiens or paracollicular region.[1, 55, 65, 81, 85, 120] Those occurring in the temporal fossa are commonly associated with a malformed or poorly developed temporal lobe, with few clinical signs, whereas those in the paracollicular region are commonly associated with compression of the aqueduct resulting in hydrocephalus. Epithelial or ependymal cysts have been reported in the Sylvian fissure[106] and the paracollicular region.[58, 85] Arachnoid cysts may occur in other sites, including the cerebellum,[13] the third ventricle[95] and the parasagittal or interhemispheral location.[73, 120] Ependymal cysts have also been reported in the third ventricle.[23]

Cysts occurring within the cerebral parenchyma include those with fibrous walls,[13] ependyma-lined walls[20, 73] and others with walls containing choroid plexus, ependyma and fibrous tissue.[114] We have seen two cases of intracerebral cysts with only glial tissue composing the wall (Fig. 15–23). Some intracerebral cysts have been reported without histologic descriptions.[59]

Cysts in the region of the sella may also be lined with epithelial cells or fibrous tissue. The former are considered derivations of Rathke's pouch[48, 100, 128] or of neuroepithelium,[130] whereas the latter are considered arachnoid in origin.[126] Some of these may involve the floor of the third ventricle or possibly even protrude into the third ventricle.[103]

Aside from the well-defined leptomeningeal cysts and perhaps some of the teratoma-

TABLE 22–10. PROPOSED ORIGINS OF BRAIN CYSTS

1. leptomeningeal
2. teratomatous: notochordal–endodermal interaction
3. dilatation of spinal cord
4. ventricular or neuroepithelial diverticulum
5. paraphysis
6. choroid plexus
7. Rathke's cleft
8. acquired: encephaloclastic or hemorrhagic processes, viral infection
9. unknown
10. epithelial or ependymal rest

tous cysts of the spinal canal, we know very little of the exact origins of most brain cysts (Table 22–10). Even the leptomeningeal cysts may be acquired,[67, 120] but their time of origin is usually unknown. The long-standing controversy regarding the origin of colloid cysts and their relationship to other brain cysts is well known, but unresolved. Diverticula of the ventricular wall or primitive neuroepithelium may account for many cysts, including some in the third or fourth ventricles, cerebral or cerebellar parenchyma, or paracollicular region.[3, 59, 105, 114] Both encephaloclastic and hemorrhagic processes *in utero* may also play a role. Intraparenchymal arachnoid cysts may indeed be true arachnoid cysts; however, it is quite possible that inadequate sampling of the cyst wall would reveal an area denuded of epithelium and reveal a fibrous scar resulting from an encephaloclastic process which had occurred in the distant past.

Other possible cysts include those of the cavum septi pellucidi or Vergae,[66, 129] diverticula of the roof of the third ventricle resulting from agenesis of the corpus callosum and appearing as interhemispheral cysts[22, 104] or ependymal fusions resulting in the appearance of intracerebral cysts.[84]

MALFORMATIONS

Vascular anomalies, *e.g.*, hemangiomas, arteriovenous malformations (AVM) and the Sturge–Weber syndrome (Figs. 20–8 to 20–10), are considered to be malformations recapitulating certain stages of the vascular network in its embryologic development,[122] and representing an abnormal retention of a primitive configuration into adult life. As described in Chapter 20, vascular malformations are exceedingly variable in size and morphology.[32, 115] They may occur in almost any site and may become symptomatic at any age because of the complications that may occur, usually hemorrhage and seizures.[118, 142, 149] They are frequently found incidentally at autopsy. Their classification remains unsettled,[117] but neoplastic transformation is extremely rare.

Hemangioblastomas

Hemangioblastomas are vascular neoplasms that, because of their association with a variety of conditions, have been generally included among the hamartoses. They may occur as part of an hereditary disorder in which there are congenital cysts of the pancreas, kidneys or other organs and occasional hypernephromas. Such cases are examples of the Lindau syndrome, or when associated with retinal vascular tumors, of the von Hippel–Lindau syndrome. Hemangioblastomas are uncommonly associated with other abnormalities, and in our experience only one of six well-documented cases of hemangioblastoma was part of another syndrome. Five of these were adults and only one was a child, age 13 (Table 22–3). The simultaneous occurrence of pheochromocytoma with hemangioblastoma has been used as an indication for the relationship of the von Hippel–Lindau syndrome to neurofibromatosis.[27] However, pheochromocytomas are known to be associated with a number of other types of tumors,[133] and the relationship of the various so-called neurocutaneous syndromes to a number of possible multiple endocrine tumor syndromes is still speculative.[161]

Sturge–Weber Syndrome

The Sturge–Weber syndrome (facial and ipsilateral leptomeningeal telangiectasia) is a complex malformation usually recognized in early childhood[122, 166] with abnormalities in vascular, meningeal, visceral and cerebral tissues, including heterotopias in the CNS and hyperplasia of the capsule cells of the Gasserian ganglia. The presence of the last two lesions has been used as evidence for a relationship to tuberous sclerosis and neurofibromatosis. However, the major abnormality remains the telangiectasia or angiomatous malformation, which is predominantly in the leptomeninges and is viewed as a result of incomplete involution of a transitory phase in the normal development of the vascular system.[122] The calcification is typically within the middle layers of the underlying hypoxic cerebral cortex, and the parallel lines seen on radiographs of the head represent the two lips of gyri, not vessels.

Nasal Glioma

The nasal glioma is an interesting tumorous malformation that is best considered as aris-

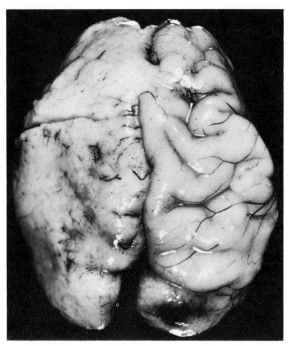

FIG. 22–35. Dorsal view of brain of a 1300 g premature infant, daughter of a 40-year-old chronic alcoholic, showing extensive and diffuse neuronal glial heterotopic infiltration of the leptomeninges over the left cerebral hemisphere and extending across the midline frontally. The corpus callosum was absent and multiple anomalies affected the nose, ears, palate, phalanges, vagina, and heart. The olfactory tracts and chromosomal studies were normal. This patient is described in detail as case 2.[76] (#Np 2825)

ing in the same fashion as an encephalocele that has lost its connection to the brain.[16, 38, 136] Herniation of such tissue is thought to occur early, at from 3–5 weeks of gestation. Clinically the tumor presents as a congenital extranasal mass at the bridge of the nose. Many names have been applied to nasal gliomas, e.g., ganglioma, fibroglioma, encephalochoristoma and encephaloma. Such tumors are relatively rare and generally benign, although examples with recurrence have been reported.[16]

Glial Heterotopias

An unusual tumor consisting of heterotopic brain tissue in the pharynx, is probably related to nasal gliomas and encephaloceles in its mode of origin. Most of the cases have

presented in newborn infants manifesting respiratory distress.[28] Smith et al.[136] mentioned other heterotopic glial tumors being found in the cheek, occiput and scalp, probably arising in the same fashion.

Small heterotopic glial protrusions pinched off from the neuraxis may be found in the subarachnoid space of many brains (see Chapter 17). They are rarely grossly visible and occur most frequently over the medulla oblongata and lumbosacral spinal cord. Such malformations are of interest because it has been suggested that they can give rise to subarachnoid gliomas and because they are commonly seen in individuals with other congenital abnormalities of the nervous system, such as meningomyelocele and the Arnold–Chiari malformation.[31, 110] Such microscopic subarachnoid nodules are not to be confused with brain warts or verrucose dysplasia of the cerebral cortex,[14, 51] a condition which typically has superficial cortical nodules associated with deeper, more widespread cortical abnormalities, and which is probably related to polymicrogyria (see Chapter 15).

One of the more extravagant examples of subarachnoid glial heterotopia in our series was present in a premature infant with the fetal alcohol syndrome.[76, 77] In addition to the marked leptomeningeal gliomatosis (Fig. 22–35), there were heterotopias of the subependymal, mantle and marginal regions, colpocephaly and agenesis of the corpus callosum. The role of maternal alcoholism in the production of such a malformation remains to be clarified.

GENETIC AND HAMARTOMATOUS CONDITIONS

Hamartomas are defined as tumor-like, essentially nonneoplastic malformations characterized by an abnormal mixture of tissue indigenous to the site.[162] As a purely morphologic description the term is useful for many tumors; as a unifying concept it leaves much to be desired for it has been applied all too often to the entities that are not easily separated from either malformations or neoplasms or even to combinations of both. Furthermore, there is still inadequate evidence linking the various hamartomatous or neurocutaneous disorders. The most useful characteristic has been their genetic basis. Within this group is included von Hippel–Lindau disease (discussed above), neurofibromatosis and tuberous sclerosis.

Neurofibromatosis

Neurofibromatosis (von Recklinghausen disease) is considered a primary disorder of neural crest derivatives with secondary involvement of mesenchymal elements.[46] It is transmitted as an autosomal dominant trait with variable penetrance and a high mutation rate, which is thought to explain the high frequency of a negative family history. It is commonly seen in childhood with up to 43% of the cases being manifest at birth, although such a high rate of diagnosis at birth has not been seen in our material (Tables 22–2 and 22–3). The peripheral tumors of neurofibromatosis are frequently considered hamartomas, although it is difficult if not impossible to distinguish them from true neoplasms, since malignant change does occur. In addition to the multiple peripheral nerve tumors, many other abnormalities have been well documented,[60, 70, 108, 121] including multiple tumors of the brain, spinal cord, cranial nerves (Figures 22–11 and 22–12) and meninges, endocrine tumors and syringomyelia. The presence of ganglion cells or ganglioneuromatous elements in the neurofibromas of von Recklinghausen disease has been used as evidence for a histogenetic relationship to neuroblastomas,[19] but the evidence remains inconclusive.

Tuberous Sclerosis

Tuberous (tuberose) sclerosis (Bourneville disease) is an autosomal dominant hereditary disease which is characterized by multiple organ abnormalities, including hamartomas of many organs, pathognomonic skin lesions ("adenoma sebaceum" or Pringle tumor, usually in a "butterfly" distribution on the cheeks) and occasionally polycystic kidney disease.[4, 160] The last may occur alone, or with renal angiomyolipomas, which may be of such a size as to be confused with polycystic kidneys. The lesions of tuberous sclerosis develop slowly, and the facial lesion usually does not appear until after the onset of the seizure disorder. Thus, according to

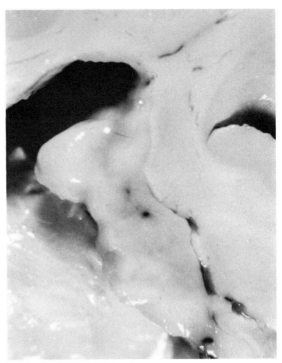

FIG. 22–36. A large white nodular "candle-guttering" is attached to the ventricular surface near the trigone of the lateral ventricle of this 3-year-old girl with tuberose sclerosis, epilepsy, mental retardation and depigmented areas (vitiligo?) on the legs. (#Np 1320)

Zaremba,[169] seizures usually begin in the first year, most of them in the first six months, whereas Pringle tumors are usually noted in the fourth year. Hence, the classic triad of mental deficiency, epilepsy and Pringle tumors obviously is not present in many patients when first seen. The cortical and subependymal tubers (Fig. 22–36) may grow sufficiently during post-natal life to obstruct the CSF circulation and may even undergo malignant transformation.[17] The tubers are best felt in the fresh brain, sometimes being detectable in the fixed brain only with difficulty. In our cases, the tubers were characteristically quite inapparent visually if the child died within the first few days of life and in one case the brain actually appeared grossly normal. Tubers have been reported in premature infants of 33 weeks gestation.[147] Among our cases of tuberose sclerosis are two examples of neoplasms, one a gemistocytic astrocytoma of the septum pellucidum and one a giant cell astrocytoma, diagnosed by surgical biopsy.

Although neurofibromatosis, tuberous sclerosis, von Hippel–Lindau disease and the Sturge–Weber syndrome are spoken of as neuroectodermal dysplasias or hamartomatous disorders, they remain individually quite distinct, and the evidence for any interrelationship is inconclusive.

REFERENCES

1. Alexander E: Benign subtentorial supracollicular cyst as a cause of obstructive hydrocephalus. J Neurosurg 10:317–323, 1953

2. Allen DW, Cole P: Viruses and human cancer. N Engl J Med 286:70–82, 1972

3. Alvord EC Jr, Marcuse PM: Intracranial cerebellar meningoencephalocele (posterior fossa cyst) causing hydrocephalus by compression at the incisura tentorii. J Neuropathol Exp Neurol 21:50–69, 1962

4. Anderson D, Tannen RL: Tuberous sclerosis and chronic renal failure. Am J Med 47:163–168, 1969

5. Anderson DH: Tumors of infancy and childhood. Cancer 4:890–906, 1951

6. Arnstein LH, Boldrey E, Naffziger HC: A case report and survey of brain tumors during the neonatal period. J Neurosurg 8:315–319, 1951

7. Bailey P, Cushing H: Medulloblastoma cerebelli. A common type of midcerebellar glioma of childhood. Arch Neurol Psychiatry 14:192–224, 1925

8. Bailey OT: Medulloblastoma. Pathology of the Nervous System. Edited by J Minckler. Vol 2. New York, McGraw-Hill, 1971, pp. 2071–2081

9. Bassett RC: The neurologic deficit associated with lipomas of the cauda equina. Ann Surg 131:109–116, 1950

10. Beckwith JB, Martin RF: Observations on the histopathology of neuroblastomas. J Pediatr Surg 3:106–110, 1968

11. Beckwith JB, Perrin EV: In situ neuroblastomas: A contribution to the natural history of neural crest tumors. Am J Pathol 43:1089–1104, 1963

12. Benton JW, Nellhaus G, Huttenlocher PR, Ojemann RG, Dodge PR: The bobble-head doll syndrome. Neurol 16:725–729, 1966

13. Berkman YM, Brucher J, Salmon JH: Congenital arachnoid cysts. Am J Roentgenol Radium Ther Nucl Med 105:298–304, 1969

14. Bertrand I, Gruner J: The status verrucosus of the cerebral cortex. J Neuropathol Exp Neurol 14:331–347, 1955

15. Bill AH Jr: The regression of neuroblastoma. J Pediatr Surg 3:103–106, 1968

16. Black BK, Smith DE: Nasal glioma. Arch Neurol Psychiatry 64:614–630, 1950

17. Blackwood W, McMenemey WH, Meyer A, Norman RM, Russell DS: Greenfield's Neuropathology. Baltimore, Williams & Wilkins, 1963

18. Bloom HJG, Wallace ENK, Henk JM: The treatment and prognosis of medulloblastoma in children: A study of 82 verified cases. Am J Roentgenol Radium Ther Nucl Med 105:43–62, 1969

19. Bolande RP, Towler WF: A possible relationship of neuroblastoma to von Recklinghausen's disease. Cancer 26:162–175, 1970

20. Bouch DC, Mitchell I, Maloney AFJ: Ependymal-lined paraventricular cerebral cysts: Report of 3 cases. J Neurol Neurosurg Psychiatry 36:611–617, 1973

21. Breslow N, McCann B: Statistical estimation of prognosis for children with neuroblastoma. Cancer Res 31:2098–2103, 1971

22. Brocklehurst G: Diencephalic cysts. J Neurosurg 38:47–51, 1973

23. Buchsbaum HW, Colton RP: Anterior third ventricular cysts in infancy. J Neurosurg 26:264–266, 1967

24. Buckner WM: Spina bifida occulta. Am J Med Sci 155:473–502, 1918

25. Bucy PC, Thieman PW: Astrocytomas of the cerebellum, a study of a series of patients operated upon over 28 years ago. Arch Neurol 18:14–19, 1968

26. Camins MB, Mount LA: Suprasellar atypical teratoma. Presented at Am Assoc Neurol Surg, 1973

27. Chapman RC, Diaz-Perez R: Pheochromocytoma associated with cerebellar hemangioblastoma. JAMA 182:1014–1017, 1962

28. Cohen AH, Abt AB: An unusual cause of neonatal respiratory obstruction: Heterotopic pharyngeal brain tissue. J Pediatr 76:119–122, 1970

29. Collins VP, Loeffler RK, Tivey H: Observations on growth rates of human tumors. Am J Roentgenol Radium Ther Nucl Med 76:988–1000, 1956

30. Congdon CC: Benign and malignant chordomas. Am J Pathol 28:793–810, 1952

31. Cooper IS, Kernohan JW: Heterotopic glial nests in the subarachnoid space: Histopathologic characteristics, mode of origin and relation to meningeal glioma. J Neuropathol Exp Neurol 10:16–29, 1951

32. Courville CB: Morphology of small vascular malformations of the brain. J Neuropathol Exp Neurol 22:274–284, 1963

33. Coxe WS, Luse SA: Colloid cyst of the third

ventricle. J Neuropathol Exp Neurol 23:431–445, 1964

34. Dahlin DC: Bone Tumors. Springfield, Ill, Charles C. Thomas, 1970, pp. 222–233

35. Dahlin DC, MacCarty CS: Chordoma. Cancer 5:1170–1178, 1952

36. Dargeon HW: Tumors of Childhood. New York, Hoeber Medical, 1960

37. Davis CH, Woodhall B: Brain tumors in children. Pediatrics 18:856–861, 1956

38. Davis EW: Gliomatous tumors in the nasal region. J Neuropathal Exp Neurol 1:312–319, 1942

39. DeLorimier A, Bragg KU, Linden G: Neuroblastoma in childhood. Am J Dis Child 118:441–450, 1969

40. DeSaussure RL, Miller JH, Strickland CE: Brain tumors in the newborn. South Med J 53:918–921, 1960

41. DiPaolo JA, Kotin P: Teratogenesis–oncogenesis: A study of possible relationships. Arch Pathol 81:3–23, 1966

42. Dodge HW Jr, Love JG, Craig WM, Dockerty MB, Kearns TP, Holman CB, Hayles MB: Gliomas of the optic nerves. Arch Neurol Psychiatry 79:607–621, 1958

43. Druckrey H, Preussmann R, Ivankovic S: N-nitroso compounds in organotropic and transplacental carcinogenesis. Ann NY Acad Sci 163:676–696, 1969

44. Fager CA, Carter H: Intrasellar epithelial cysts. J Neurosurg 24:77–81, 1966

45. Fessard C: Cerebral tumors in infancy. Am J Dis Child 115:302–308, 1968

46. Fienman NL, Yakovac WC: Neurofibromatosis in childhood. J Pediatr 76:339–346, 1970

47. Fowler FD, Matson DD: Gliomas of the optic pathways in childhood. J Neurosurg 14:515–527, 1957

48. Frazier CH, Alpers BJ: Tumors of Rathke's cleft. Arch Neurol Psychiatry 32:973–984, 1934

49. Gey, W: Dq–, multiple Missbildungen und Retinoblastom. Humangenetik 10:362–365, 1970

50. Ghatak NR, Hirano A, Zimmerman HM: Intrasellar germinomas: a form of ectopic pinealoma. J Neurosurg 31:670–675, 1969

51. Grcevic N, Robert F: Verrucose dysplasia of the cerebral cortex. J Neuropathol Exp Neurol 20:399–411, 1961

52. Greenhouse AH, Neuberger KT: Intracranial teratomata of the newborn. Arch Neurol 3:718–724, 1960

53. Gross RE, Farber S, Martin CW: Neuroblastoma sympathicum. Pediatrics 23:1179–1191, 1959

54. Gruber FH: Posttraumatic leptomeningeal cysts. Am J Roentgenol Radium Ther Nucl Med 105:305–307, 1969

55. Gruszkiewicz J, Peyser F: Supratentorial arachnoid cyst associated with hydrocephalus. J Neurol Neurosurg Psychiatry 28:438–441, 1965

56. Gurdjian ES, Larsen RD, Lindner DW: Intraneural cyst of the peroneal and ulnar nerves. J Neurosurg 23:76–78, 1965

57. Haberland C, Perou M: Encephalocraniocutaneous lipomatosis. Arch Neurol 22:144–155, 1970

58. Hamby WB, Gardner WJ: An ependymal cyst in the quadrigeminal region. Arch Neurol Psychiatry 33:391–398, 1935

59. Handa H, Bucy PC: Benign cysts of the brain simulating brain tumor. J Neurosurg 13:489–499, 1956

60. Hellstrom KE, Hellstrom I: Immunity to neuroblastomas and melanomas. Ann Rev Med 23:19–38, 1972

61. Hellstrom KE, Hellstrom I: Lymphocyte-mediated cytotoxicity and blocking serum activity to tumor antigens. Adv Immunol 18:209–277, 1974

62. Hirano A, Ghatak NR, Wisoff HS, Zimmerman HM: An epithelial cyst of the spinal cord. An electron microscopic study. Acta Neuropathol 18:214–223, 1971

63. Hoyt WF, Baghdassarian SA: Optic glioma of childhood. Natural history and rationale for conservative management. Br J Ophthalmol 53:793–798, 1969

64. Hoyt WF, Meshel LG, Lessell S, Schatz NJ, Suckling RD: Malignant optic glioma of adulthood. Brain 96:121–132, 1973

65. Huckman MS, Davis PO, Coxe WS: Arachnoid cyst of the quadrigeminal plate. J Neurosurg 32:367–370, 1970

66. Hughes RA, Kernohan JW, Craig WM: Caves and cysts of the septum pellucidum. Arch Neurol Psychiatry 74:259–266, 1955

67. Hyndman BR, Gerber WF: Spinal extradural cysts, congenital and acquired. J Neurosurg 3:474–486, 1946

68. Ingraham FD, Bailey OT: Cystic teratomas and teratoid tumors of the central nervous system in infancy and childhood. J Neurosurg 3:512–532, 1946

69. Ingraham FD, Lowery JJ: Spina bifida and cranium bifidum. III. Occult spinal disorders. N Engl J Med 228:745–750, 1943

70. Ingraham FD, Swan H: Spina bifida and cranium bifidum. I. A survey of five hundred and forty-six cases. N Engl J Med 228:559–563, 1943

71. Jacobson M: Developmental Neurobiology. New York, Holt, Rinehart and Winston, 1970

72. Jackson, FE: Neurenteric cysts. J Neurosurg 18:678–682, 1961

73. Jakubiak P, Dunsmore RH, Beckett RS: Supratentorial brain cysts. J Neurosurg 28:129–136, 1968

74. Jensen RD, Miller RW: Retinoblastoma: Epidemiologic characteristics. N Engl J Med 285:307–311, 1971

75. Johnson A: Fatty tumour from the sacrum of

a child, connected with the spinal membranes. Trans Pathol Soc Lond 8:16–18, 1857

76. Jones KL, Smith DW: Recognition of the fetal alcohol syndrome in early infancy. Lancet 2: 999–1001, 1973

77. Jones KL, Smith DW, Ulleland CN, Streissguth AP: Patterns of malformation in offspring of chronic alcoholic mothers. Lancet 1:1267–1271, 1973

78. Kageyama N: Ectopic pinealoma in the region of the optic chiasm. J Neurosurg 35:755–759, 1971

79. Kao CC, Uihlein A, Bickel WH, Soule EH: Lumbar intraspinal extradural ganglion cyst. J Neurosurg 29:168–172, 1968

80. Kappers JA: Development of paraphysis cerebri in man with comments on its relationship to the intercolumnar tubercles and its signficance for the origin of cystic tumors in the third ventricle. J Comp Neurol 102:425–509, 1955

81. Katagiri A: Arachnoidal cyst of the cisterna ambiens. Neurology (Minneap) 10:783–786, 1960

82. Knight G, Griffiths T, Williams I: Gastrocytoma of the spinal cord. Br J Surg 42:635–638, 1955

83. Kouyoumdjian AV, McDonald JJ: Association of congenital adrenal neuroblastoma with multiple anomalies, including an unusual oropharyngeal cavity (imperforate buccopharyngeal membrane?). Cancer 4:784–788, 1951

84. Kozlowski P, Dymecki J: Deformation of the lateral ventricle of the brain due to ependymal fusions. Acta Radiol [Diagn] (Stockh) 9:187–192, 1969

85. Kruyff E: Paracollicular plate cysts. Am J Roentgenol Radium Ther Nucl Med 95:899–916, 1965

86. Kusama S, Spratt JS Jr, Donegan WL, Watson FR, Cunningham C: The gross rates of growth of human mammary carcinoma. Cancer 30:594–599, 1972

87. Lassman LV, James CCM: Lumbosacral lipomas: Critical survey of 26 cases submitted to laminectomy. J Neurosurg 30:174–181, 1967

88. Lemire RJ, Graham CB, Beckwith JB: Skin-covered sacrococcygeal masses in infants and children. J Pediatr 79:948–954, 1971

89. Low NL, Correll JW, Hammill JF: Tumors of the cerebral hemisphere in children. Arch Neurol 13:547–554, 1965

90. Luse SA, Kernohan JW: Squamous cell rests of the pituitary gland. Cancer 8:623–628, 1955

91. Luse SA, Teitelbaum S: Congenital glioma of the brain stem. Arch Neurol 18:196–201, 1968

92. Mäkinen J: Microscopic patterns as a guide to prognosis of neuroblastoma in childhood. Cancer 29:1637–1646, 1972

93. Matson DD: Benign intracranial tumors of childhood. N Engl J Med 259:330–337, 1958

94. Matson DD: Neurosurgery of Infancy and Childhood, 2d ed. Springfield, Charles C Thomas, 1969

95. Mayher WE, Gindin RA: Head bobbing associated with third ventricular cyst. Arch Neurol 23:274–277, 1970

96. Miller RW: Relations between cancer and congenital defects in man. N Engl J Med 275:87–93, 1966

97. Mintz B, Russell ES: Gene-induced embryological modification of primordial germ cells in the mouse. J Exp Zool 134:207–237, 1957

98. Moragas A, Vidal M-T: Giant congenital intracranial teratoma. Helv Paediatr Acta 24:106–110, 1969

99. Murad TM, Murthy MDN: Ultrastructure of a chordoma. Cancer 25:1204–1215, 1970

100. Naiken VS, Tellem M, Meranzo DR: Pituitary cyst of Rathke's cleft origin with hypopituitarism. J Neurosurg 18: 703–708, 1961

101. Nassar SI, Correll JW, Housepian EM: Intramedullary cystic lesions of the conus medullaris. J Neurol Neurosurg Psychiatry 31:106–109, 1968

102. Newell GR, Roberts JD, Baranovsky A: Retinoblastoma: Presentation and survival in Negro children compared with whites. J Natl Cancer Inst 49:989–992, 1972

103. Obenchain TM, Becker DP: Head bobbing associated with a cyst of the third ventricle. J Neurosurg 37:457–459, 1972

104. Oftedal S: Anomalies of the mid-line structures of the brain. Acta Psychiatr Scand 34:451–467, 1959

105. Parkinson D, Childe AE: Colloid cyst of the fourth ventricle. J Neurosurg 9:404–409, 1952

106. Patrick BS: Ependymal cyst of the Sylvian fissure. J Neurosurg 35:751–754, 1971

107. Pearce RJ: A congenital neoplasm of the brain of a newborn infant. Am J Clin Pathol 24:1272–1275, 1954

108. Pearce J: The central nervous system pathology in multiple neurofibromatosis. Neurology 17:691–697, 1967

109. Plewes JL, Jacobson I: Sciatica caused by sacral-nerve-root cysts. Lancet 2:799–802, 1970

110. Popoff N, Feigin I: Heterotopic central nervous tissue in subarachnoid space. Arch Pathol 78:533–539, 1964

111. Potter EL, Parrish JM: Neuroblastoma, ganglioneuroma and fibroneuroma in a stillborn fetus. Am J Pathol 18:141–152, 1942

112. Pruett RC, Atkins L: Chromosome studies in patients with retinoblastoma. Arch Ophthalmol 82:177–181, 1969

113. Raaf J, Kernohan JW: Relation of abnormal collections of cells in posterior medullary velum of the cerebellum to origin of medulloblastoma. Arch Neurol Psychiatry 52:163–169, 1944

114. Rand BO, Foltz EL, Alvord EC Jr: Intracranial telencephalic meningo-encephalocele containing choroid plexus. J Neuropathol Exp Neurol 23:293–305, 1964

115. Raskin N: Angiomatous malformation of the brain. J Neuropathol Exp Neurol 8:326–337, 1949

116. Raskind R, Beigel F: Brain tumors in early infancy—probably congenital in origin. J Pediatr 65:727–732, 1964

117. Raynor RB, Kingman AF: Hemangioblastoma and vascular malformations as one lesion. Arch Neurol 12:39–48, 1965

118. Reuter JR, Newton TH, Greitz T: Arteriovenous malformations of the posterior fossa. Radiology 87:1080–1088, 1966

119. Rewcastle WB, Francoeur J: Teratomatous cysts of the spinal canal. Arch Neurol 11:91–99, 1964

120. Robinson RH: Congenital cysts of the brain: Arachnoid malformations. In Progress in Neurological Surgery. Edited by H Krayenbühl, PE Maspes, WH Sweet. Basel, S Karger 4:133–174, 1971

121. Rodriguez HA, Berthrong M: Multiple primary intracranial tumors in von Recklinghausen's disease. Cancer 26:162–175, 1966

122. Roizin L, Gold G, Berman HH, Bonafede VI: Congenital vascular anomalies and their histopathology in Sturge–Weber–Dimitri syndrome. J Neuropathol Exp Neurol 18:75–97, 1959

123. Rubinstein LJ, Northfield DWC: The medulloblastoma and the so-called "arachnoidal cerebellar sarcoma," a critical re-examination of a nosological problem. Brain 87:379–412, 1964

124. Ryser H J-P: Chemical carcinogenesis. N Engl J Med 285:721–734, 1971

125. Sandbank V: Congenital astrocytoma. J Pathol Bacteriol 34:226–228, 1962

126. Sansregret A, Ledoux R, Duplantis F, Lamoureux C, Chapdelaine A, Leblanc P: Suprasellar subarachnoid cyst. Am J Roentgenol Radium Ther Nucl Med 105:291–297, 1969

127. Seemayer TA, Blundell JS, Wiglesworth FW: Pituitary craniopharyngioma with tooth formation. Cancer 29:423–430, 1972

128. Shanklin WM: The incidence and distribution of cilia in the human pituitary with a description of micro-follicular cysts derived from Rathke's cleft. Acta Anat (Basel) 11:361–382, 1951

129. Shaw CM, Alvord EC Jr: Cava septi pellucidi et Vergae: Their normal and pathological states. Brain 92:213–224, 1969

130. Shuangshoti S, Netsky MG, Nashold BS: Epithelial cysts related to sella turcica. Arch Pathol 90:444–450, 1970

131. Shuangshoti S, Roberts MP, Netsky MG: Neuroepithelial (colloid) cysts. Arch Pathol 80:214–224, 1965

132. Shuman RJ, Alvord EC Jr, Leech RW: The biology of childhood ependymomas. Arch Neurol 1975 (in press)

133. Siegelman SS, Zavod R, Hasson J: Hypernephroma, pheochromocytoma and thyroid carcinoma. J Urol 102:402–405, 1969

134. Simson LR, Lampe I, Abell MR: Suprasellar germinomas. Cancer 22:533–544, 1968

135. Smith DT: Cystic formations associated with human spinal nerve root. J Neurosurg 18:654–660, 1961

136. Smith KR, Schwartz HG, Luse SA, Oguera JH: Nasal gliomas: a report of five cases with electron microscopy of one. J Neurosurg 20:968–982, 1963

137. Solitaire GB, Krigman MR: Congenital intracranial neoplasm. J Neuropathol Exp Neurol 23:280–292, 1964

138. Spjut HJ, Luse SA: Chordoma: An electron microscopic study. Cancer 17:643–656, 1964

139. Stevenson L, Echlin F: Nature and origin of some tumors of the cerebellum. Arch Neurol Psychiatry 31:93–109, 1934

140. Steward JK, Smith JLS, Arnold EL: Spontaneous regression of retinoblastoma. Br J Ophthalmol 40:449–461, 1956

141. Sutow WW, Gehan EA, Heyn RM, Kung FH, Miller RW, Murphy ML, Traggis DG: Comparison of survival curves, 1956 versus 1962, in children with Wilms' tumor and neuroblastoma. Report of the Subcommittee on Childhood Solid Tumors, Solid Tumor Task Force, National Cancer Institute. Pediatrics 45:800–811, 1970

142. Svien HJ, McRae JA: Arteriovenous anomalies of the brain. J Neurosurg 23:23–28, 1965

143. Sypert GW, Leech RW, Harris AB: Posttraumatic lumbar epidural true synovial cyst. J Neurosurg 39:246–248, 1973

144. Tarlov IM: Cysts (perineural) of the sacral roots. JAMA 138:740–744, 1948

145. Taveras JM, Mount LA, Wood EH: The value of radiation therapy in the management of glioma of the optic nerves and chiasm. Radiology 66:518–528, 1956

146. Taylor AI: Dq—, Dr and retinoblastoma. Humangenetik 10:209–217, 1970

147. Thibault JH, Manuelidis EE: Tuberous sclerosis in a premature infant. Report of a case and review of the literature. Neurology 20:139–146, 1970

148. Toglia JV, Netsky MG, Alexander E Jr: Epithelial (epidermoid) tumors of the cranium. J Neurosurg 23:384–393, 1965

149. Troupp H, Marttila I, Halonen V: Arteriovenous malformations of the brain. Acta Neurochir (Wien) 22:125–128, 1970

150. Ts'o MOM, Fine BS, Zimmerman LE: The Flexner–Wintersteiner rosettes in retinoblastoma. Arch Pathol 88:664–671, 1969

151. Ts'o MOM, Fine BS, Zimmerman LE: The nature of retinoblastoma. H. Photoreceptor differentiation: An electron microscopic study. Am J Ophthalmol 69:350–359, 1970

152. Ts'o MOM, Zimmerman LE, Fine BS: The

nature of retinoblastoma. I. Photoreceptor differentiation: A clinical and histopathologic study. Am J Ophthalmol 69:339–349, 1970

153. Tubergen DG, Heyn RM: In situ neuroblastoma associated with an adrenal cyst. J Pediatr 76:451–453, 1970

154. Turkel SB, Itabashi HH: The natural history of neuroblastic cells in the fetal adrenal gland. Am J Pathol 76:225–244, 1974

155. Ü KS, Baloh RW, Weingarten S: Intradural arachnoid cyst presenting with cord compression. Bull Los Angeles Neurol Soc 37:178–183, 1972

156. Van Gilder JC, Schwartz HG: Growth of dermoids from skin implants to the nervous system and surrounding spaces of the newborn rat. J Neurosurg 26:14–20, 1967

157. Vogel F: Genetic prognosis in retinoblastoma. Modern Trends in Ophthalmology. Edited by A. Sorsby. London, Butterworth, 1967, pp. 34–42

158. Vonderahe AR, Niemer WT: Intracranial lipoma. J Neuropathol Exp Neurol 3:344–358, 1944

159. Well HG: Occurrence and significance of congenital malignant neoplasms. Arch Pathol 30:535–601, 1940

160. Wenzl JE, Lagos JC, Alvers DD: Tuberous sclerosis presenting as polycystic kidneys and seizures in an infant. J Pediatr 77:673–676, 1970

161. Werchart RF: The neural ectodermal origin of the peptide-secreting endocrine glands. Am J Med 49:232–241, 1970

162. Willis RA: The Borderland of Embryology and Pathology. London, Butterworth, 1962

163. Wilson MG, Towner JW, Fujimoto A: Retinoblastoma and D-chromosome deletions. Am J Hum Genet 25:57–61, 1973

164. Wisoff HS, Ghatak NR: Ependymal cyst of the spinal cord: Case report. J Neurol Neurosurg Psychiatry 34:546–550, 1971

165. Witschi E: Migrations of the germ cells of human embryos from the yolk sac to the primitive gonadal folds. Contrib Embryol 32:67–80, 1948

166. Wohwill FJ, Yakovlev PI: Histopathology of meningo-facial angiomatosis (Sturge–Weber's disease). J Neuropathol Exp Neurol 16:341–364, 1957

167. Wong, IG, Lubow M: Management of optic glioma of childhood: A review of 42 cases. In Neuro-ophthalmology, vol 6. Edited by JL Smith. St. Louis, CV Mosby, 1972, pp 51–60

168. Wu WZ, Lapi A: Primary non-skeletal intracranial cartilaginous neoplasms: Report of a chondroma and a mesenchymal chondrosarcoma. J Neurol Neurosurg Psychiatry 33:469–475, 1970

169. Zaremba J: Tuberous sclerosis: A clinical and genetic investigation. J Ment Defic Res 12:63–80, 1968

170. Zettner A, Netsky MG: Lipoma of the corpus callosum. J Neuropathol Exp Neurol 19:305–319, 1960

chapter 23

ENVIRONMENTAL AGENTS PRODUCING MALFORMATIONS OF THE NERVOUS SYSTEM

GENERAL CONSIDERATIONS

Warkany has traced the development of teratology from a "science dealing with monstrosities" to one dealing with the "production of congenital malformations." It would seem only a short step to separate those last two words, even to eliminate the word congenital (meaning *present at birth*), especially when considering malformations of the nervous system, because as Norman[25] has noted, "the act of birth marks no particular milestone in the development of the human brain." By thus dissociating the temporal connotations implied by the almost constant coupling of "congenital" and "malformations," one becomes free from certain conceptual restraints and can more nearly equate "malformations of the nervous system" with "diseases of the developing nervous system."

Such freedom from restraint allows one immediately to recognize a continuity of the spectrum between two extremes, one of classic and obvious malformations (including some due to abnormal genes or choromosomes, as discussed in Chapter 24) and the other of classic and obvious destructive lesions recognizable by necrosis, inflammation and healing with scar formation (gliosis). Simply stated, as one example only, if astrocytes do not develop until the last quarter of gestation, they cannot react if a destructive lesion occurs during the first three-quarters of gestation, and since the brain is actively growing for many years, small scars of lesions produced during the last quarter of gestation or even during the first month after birth can be difficult to de-

tect at autopsy many months or years later.

The present chapter considers more specifically those agents that are considered to be of environmental origin, *i.e.,* not related to genetic factors. While the main emphasis will be on humans, a few examples of agents found to be teratogenic in subhuman species will be included.

MECHANISMS OF TERATOGENESIS

In recent years there have been at least three classifications of potential mechanisms of teratogenesis. Zwilling[45] bases his classification on inductive and morphologic relationships with the intent to be "provocative rather than definitive" and states that his classification should not be considered final. Zwilling's classification includes:

1. Abnormal initial stimulus—in which the initial stimulus could be absent, deficient or excessive
2. Abnormal response of reacting tissues—in which the response might be absent, partial, incomplete or excessive or in which something could mechanically interfere with the response
3. Abnormality of both stimulus and response
4. Abnormal differentiation of component tissues
5. Abnormal growth of structures
6. Degenerative processes—in which the degeneration might be abnormal, absent or in excess of what occurs normally
7. Abnormal functional activity

385

Patten[26] illustrates his classification with specific examples in humans. While the concept of a developmental arrest is important, he feels that it has been overemphasized and so adds other mechanisms:

1. Too little growth—synonymous with an arrest in development
2. Too little resorption
3. Too much resorption
4. A resorptive process normal in character but occurring in an abnormal location
5. A growth process normal in character but in an abnormal location
6. Too much growth of a structure or tissue

While the classifications of Zwilling and Patten have some similarities, Wilson[40] provides further elaboration and a new approach. He believes that "it is prudent to apply the term mechanism of teratogenesis tentatively to the earliest recognizable event thought to have played a primary role in abnormal development." Using this concept, he suggests the following classification:

1. Mutation
2. Chromosomal aberrations
3. Mitotic interference
4. Altered nucleic acid synthesis and function
5. Lack of precursors, substrates and coenzymes for biosynthesis
6. Altered energy sources
7. Enzyme inhibition
8. Osmolar imbalance
9. Changed membrane characteristics

Regardless of one's preference regarding a classification of the mechanisms of teratogenesis, the concept of "termination and determination periods" is an important factor. Warkany[38] discusses this at length. A "termination period" is a time in the development of a given structure or organ after which a specific malformation cannot occur by any teratogenic mechanism. A "determination period" is a time (or times) when a teratogenic influence can cause a specific malformation. Therefore, a determination period is never later than a termination period, but may precede it by hours or months. While it is sometimes possible to assign a specific time to a termination period, it is usually impossible to be very precise as to when a specific teratogenic

agent has actually caused a particular malformation.

TERATOGENIC AGENTS

RADIATION

General Effects

An organism consists of a mosaic of cells differing greatly in their sensitivity to ionizing radiations. Hematologic, gastrointestinal and neurologic syndromes are well known, but the neurologic syndrome in the adult is rarely seen because of the relatively high dose necessary. To those who work only with adults it may come as a surprise that the developing nervous system is among the most highly radiosensitive structures. Furthermore, the nervous system consists of another broad mosaic of cells of widely differing sensitivities, especially during development. The prezygotic and early embryonic periods of development are frequently mentioned as being the times when exposure to ionizing radiation produces the most devastating effects. The older embryo and fetus are generally more radioresistant and by the postnatal period are quite radioresistant. Of course, since the nervous system is so heterogeneous in cell types and stages of development, there are major exceptions to the general pattern, *e.g.*, the cerebellum lags behind the rest of the developing brain and remains relatively radiosensitive for much longer.

The effects of radiation on the developing human nervous system have been studied in three areas: 1) the atomic bombs dropped on Hiroshima and Nagasaki, Japan, in 1945, exposing adults, children, fetuses and embryos; 2) irradiation of embryos and fetuses in varying doses, either deliberately to induce abortion or inadvertently to treat maternal cancer in the pelvic region; and 3) the long-term effects of irradiation *in utero* leading to an increased risk of developing neoplasms later in life.[44]

Because of the relative simplicity of the experimental situation, these human observations can be rather easily related to the pathogenesis of radiation defects as derived from studies conducted on other species. The recent reviews of Yamazaki,[44] Hicks and D'Amato,[18] and Brill and Forgotson[4] have provided the basis for the following summary.

Pathogenesis

There are two types of radiation damage to the developing nervous system: 1) the direct damage of the nerve cells and glial cells themselves and 2) the indirect damage secondary to vascular effects. In the case of the primitive ependyma, the most sensitive period seems to be in late prophase and again immediately after mitosis, at which time there seems to be a direct effect on the chromosomes leading to "mitotic cell death." Hicks and D'Amato[18] point out that another type of cell death can occur during later fetal life, when primitive cells are not proliferating but are differentiating.

The neural cell exposed to ionizing radiation may show changes in either the size or shape of the cell body itself, including complete destruction of the cell. In other cases, the cell body may be less affected than the axons and dendrites, which can show abnormal formations that persist into postnatal life. In addition, there may be vacuolization of reticular formation cells and degeneration of microglia.

Damage to blood vessels leads to varying degrees of hemorrhage, perivascular edema and thrombi. Intimal proliferation and mitochondrial changes in the endothelial cells have been noted on electron microscopic examination. The vascular system of the neonatal rat is particularly sensitive to radiation, with perivasculitis, petechial hemorrhage and reduction in capillary proliferation.

Gross Morphologic Findings

Microcephaly has been the most common feature in humans who have been irradiated in utero, either by exposure to radiation from atomic bombs[24] or by maternal radiation therapy. Most of these subjects have also shown mental retardation; other malformations have been inconsistent. In one case irradiated on the 17th, 24th and 32nd days, there were abnormalities of the cerebral cortex (agenesis of the frontal lobes), a rudimentary corpus callosum, atresia of the aqueduct of Sylvius, anomalies of the genic-ulate bodies, microphthalmia and agenesis of the fornix and mammillary bodies.[19]

Abnormalities of the eye, especially microphthalmia, optic atrophy and coloboma, are common among humans irradiated in utero. Cataracts and chorioretinitis also have been reported.

Various other CNS anomalies have been reported in individual cases, including hydrocephalus, defects in ossification of the skull[4] and myelocele.[14] The incidence of open neural tube defects in human embryos irradiated in utero is not known, but x-irradiation of rats on the ninth gestational day results in varying forms of dysraphism of the cephalic neural tube. Undoubtedly, as with other conditions, some such embryos spontaneously abort prior to the time that the mother is even aware of being pregnant.

Numerous other malformations of the CNS are found in rodents irradiated between the tenth gestational day and birth (from 19 to 22 days). These include hydrocephalus, encephalocele, porencephaly, agenesis of the corpus collosum and various reductions or aberrations of other intracranial structures. Cerebellar hypoplasia is prominent as the irradiation is given late in gestation.

There is overwhelming evidence based on both human and experimental studies that several forms of radiation are teratogenic to the CNS. The clinician treating a potentially pregnant patient should take precautions in ordering any type of test that involves radiation (e.g., pelvic radiographs and radioisotopic studies). Unfortunately, the period during which the developing CNS is most sensitive to radiation is within the first month, at which time there is the distinct possibility of an unrecognized pregnancy.

INFECTIONS

Infections, especially viral, are a more common factor than ionizing radiations in terms of the total number of anomalies of the human CNS. Numerous studies over the past decade implicate several viruses that were previously unsuspected of having a teratogenic potential as being associated with congenital malformations. Bacteria appear to play a very minor role with respect to CNS anomalies and will not be further discussed.

Pathogenesis of Viral Infections

The most common type of viral involvement in fetal tissues is a direct effect on the cells themselves. There are two possible routes by which the virus can reach the fetus: 1) by way of the amniotic cavity following a vaginal infection and entrance through the cervix and 2) transplacentally through the bloodstream following a maternal viremia. The latter route is probably the most common since maternal viremia, increased antibody titers and isolation of viruses from the placenta (especially in rubella) are the rule. Johnson[20] has recently reviewed the mechanisms by which some viral infections cause CNS malformations in experimental animals. He found evidence for: 1) indirect effects on organogenesis, 2) selective vulnerability of specific immature cell populations and 3) primary agenesis resulting from host reactions to destruction.

One of the most distressing problems in the consideration of viruses as teratogenic agents is the fact that many of the mothers infected do not exhibit any clinical symptoms, i.e., they have subclinical or silent infections. This is well known in the case of cytomegalovirus and rubella virus and lends more credence to the possibility that several other viruses may be responsible for malformations. In addition, there is concern that some CNS diseases found in adults may be the result of slow virus infections acquired in utero.[21]

Rubella Virus

In the past 30 years, researchers identified rubella virus as a significant cause of congenital malformations,[13] cultured it in vitro and developed a now widely utilized vaccine against it. Some may regard such an interval as long, but when one considers the numerous other factors as yet unknown, this is a remarkably short chapter in medical history.

The probable mechanism by which rubella virus causes damage is by the direct invasion of sensitive organs, where it multiplies and produces a cytopathologic, necrotic and inflammatory response. The effect on the developing embryo can result in numerous anomalies, some of which occur in the CNS. These include mental retardation, microcephaly, spasticity, deafness and blindness. Blindness may be secondary to optic nerve atrophy, cataracts or both.

Neuropathologic findings[27, 28] in patients with the rubella syndrome include degeneration of blood vessels associated with ischemic necrosis of tissue (present in 65% of cases). This vascular degeneration involves one or more layers of the vessel wall and replacement of these layers by an amorphous granular material. In some cases the vessel walls are less severely affected and masses of the amorphous material are found in the pericapillary areas. These deposits, which are PAS- and Feulgen-positive, are sometimes not associated with the vessels but may appear as discrete masses in the brain. Deposits of fibrin and calcium are occasionally found in subintimal and pericapillary spaces. Micrencephaly is present in 70% of cases and is due to a decreased number of cells. Retardation of myelinization was noted in over half of the cases that survived over one month postnatally. Other cases have shown hydrocephalus, gliosis (perivascular and marginal), leptomeningitis, cysts in the white matter lined by glia, necrosis of subcortical and periventricular white matter and calcification. Subependymal cysts have been noted by Shaw[30, 31] as a gross marker of congenital viral infections, including rubella and others (see Chapter 12).

Although virtually every part of the CNS can be affected by the rubella virus, the eye is of special interest, since anomalies in the eyes of children were first related to the fact that the mother had had rubella early in the pregnancy.[13] More recently Boniuk and Zimmerman[3] studied the eyes in 19 such affected infants at autopsy. Clinical information on 17 cases revealed bilateral cataracts in 8, unilateral cataract with microphthalmia in 1, bilateral glaucoma in 1, and bilateral corneal opacifications in 1. In 6 cases the eyes were regarded as normal from the clinical viewpoint, but cataractous lens, iridocyclytis, vacuolization of iris pigment epithelium, hypoplasia of the iris and iris atrophy were found consistently microscopically. Necrosis of the ciliary body was found to be pathognomonic for the rubella virus. Other developmental defects of the eye, such as colobomata, retinal dysplasia and severe microphthalmia, were not found.

TABLE 23–1. EFFECTS OF EARLY EXPOSURE TO RUBELLA

Gestational Age (weeks)	Abnormal Lens (%)	Abnormal Inner Ear (%)
0– 4	35	12
4– 8	48	13
8–11	66	0

Rubella virus has its most devastating effects when the maternal infection occurs early in pregnancy. The cytopathologic effects in embryos have been studied by Töndury and Smith,[35] who established the following temporal relationships in Table 23–1.

In cases in which the maternal infection occurs after the 12th week, structural abnormalities are more difficult to detect since the major portion of organogenesis has been completed, but Hardy et al.[16] found a high incidence of communication deficits (decreased auditory sensitivity and delayed language development) and motor or mental retardation. These functional defects have not yet been analyzed morphologically.

Cytomegalovirus

At the present time the cytomegaloviruses (CMV) are increasingly of concern to clinicians dealing with newborns.[15, 39] Recent studies have shown that between 1% and 3% of normal newborns excrete CMV at birth.[15] Thus, CMV is probably the most common of the known fetal infections. The incidence of women infected during pregnancy is even higher, ranging between 2% and 5%.

The epidemiology and pathogenesis of CMV infections are now reasonably well defined. Several different strains exist, belonging as a group to the herpesvirus family. Although the prevalence of CMV varies in different areas of the world, a significant number of adults have been infected, usually through an inapparent infection. The subclinical form is especially true of women who acquire the infection during pregnancy. Except for the tendency to be of younger age, no other factors can be defined clinically in these women. There are two mechanisms by which the infection can be transmitted during the prenatal period: natural and iatro-

genic. Iatrogenic infections, by transfusions of infected blood, are infrequent and of less concern. The fetus seems most prone to adverse results during the second and third trimesters. Once a woman gives birth to an infant with congenital anomalies caused by CMV, a second such episode is rare.[11] After CMV gains access to the maternal bloodstream, transplacental transmission to the fetus occurs and may or may not cause damage. When CMV does gain access to the fetal cells, it forms intranuclear and cytoplasmic inclusion bodies, cytomegaly and foci of cell death. Time-lapse cinematography in vitro has shown that such cells can literally explode. Cell counts in infected organs reveal an absolute decrease in numbers of cells.

Cytomegalic inclusion disease (CID) is the term commonly used for the diagnosis of anomalies in newborns resulting from a CMV infection in utero. Characteristically these infants are "small for dates" and jaundiced, with evidence of hepatosplenomegaly, petechiae, pneumonitis and radiographic changes in the long bones. These same features can also be found in infants with the congenital rubella syndrome.

Not all of the CNS manifestations of CID are present at birth, some developing over a period of several months. Hanshaw[15] emphasizes the following cerebral abnormalities: microcephaly, microgyria, dilated ventricles, periventricular calcifications, status spongiosus, hydrocephalus, encephalomalacia, calcified cerebral arteries, cerebral cysts, cerebral cortical immaturity, cerebellar aplasia and dolichocephaly. Subependymal cysts are common[30, 31] (see Chapter 12).

In addition, deafness and ocular abnormalities have occurred in the CID syndrome, with chorioretinitis, microphthalmia, abnormal or atrophic optic discs, malformed anterior chambers, retinal calcifications and vestigial pupillary membranes. In contrast to infants with the congenital rubella syndrome, cataracts are unusual, but have been reported in CID. Seizures, blindness, motor changes and mental retardation are common manifestations of CNS involvement.

The periventricular calcifications of congenital CID are almost pathognomonic. CMV has a particular affinity for growing rapidly in the subependymal germinal matrix cells, especially those around the lateral ventricles. Calcium is subsequently deposited in these areas of necrosis in such a manner that an external cast of the ventricle is produced that is easily seen on radiographs of the skull.

At the present time serologic testing and viral cultures are available for confirmation of the diagnosis of CID, but as yet there are no known preventative measures or therapy. It is important to point out that not all infants with CID have clinically detectable neurologic deficits. Berenberg and Nankervis[2] provide follow-up data on 12 patients ranging from 4 to 12 years: 5 had severe mental retardation, 3 moderate and 1 mild, but 3 had normal intelligence. Of those 3 who were normal, 1 was described as being "awkward" and the other 2 had entirely normal neuromuscular examinations.

Other Viruses

South et al.[34] report an infant whose mother was infected with Type 2 herpesvirus during the first few weeks in pregnancy. The infant had marked microcephaly with overlapping cranial bones, microphthalmia, cloudy lenses, seizures and hypotonia. Although radiographs of the skull taken at two weeks of age were negative for intracranial calcifications, those taken at five weeks revealed periventricular casts similar to those seen in congenital CID. Microcephaly, seizures and calcification (periventricular and hippocampal) were reported by Florman et al.[12] in a patient with Type 1 herpesvirus.

Other viruses (e.g., Western equine, Saint Louis, influenza) have been shown to cross the placenta and infect the fetus, as reviewed by Brown.[5] In general, there are no data that presently implicate these viruses to the same degree of certainty as for rubella and CMV. The question of varicella being teratogenic has been raised.[29] However, with the present interest in this area and the increasing availability of diagnostic virology laboratories, these specific problems will certainly be better defined in the near future. Subependymal cysts have been emphasized[30, 31] (see Chapter 12), but one should not overemphasize the cysts themselves except as obvious markers of a disease acquired in utero and as an indicator of more-subtle and diffuse changes that are probably responsible for the mental retardation characteristic of practically every case who survives long enough to be tested clinically.

Nonviral Infections

The evidence for a role for other infectious agents, except for toxoplasmosis, in the productions of CNS malformations is negligible when compared to viruses. Toxoplasmosis is most commonly an asymptomatic infection of adults, but as an intrauterine infection it is very destructive, more so in the fetal than in the embryonic period. The affected infant can have chorioretinitis, seizures and intracranial calcifications. Warkany[38] states that approximately one-half of the cases of toxoplasmosis have hydrocephalus and microcephaly. Hydranencephaly has also resulted from in utero infection by toxoplasmosis.[1] Although there may be cerebral atrophy, the frontal lobes seem to be less affected than the rest of the cortex. Toxoplasmosis has also been reported as a coexistent infection with CMV in a microcephalic stillborn.[6]

DRUGS AND CHEMICALS

In spite of the fact that many drugs are teratogenic to the developing nervous system in lower species, they present a minor problem in humans.[32, 41] Infants born after an unsuccessful attempt at abortion with aminopterin have been found to have several anomalies, including delayed ossification of the neurocranium, hydrocephalus, encephalocele, anencephaly, cerebral aplasia and partial craniosynostosis.[38] Methotrexate has been associated with absence of the frontal bone and craniosynostosis of other sutures. Even though thalidomide was responsible for numerous malformations of other parts of the body, it has little effect on the CNS.[23, 38] Occasional malformations include hydrocephalus, microcephaly, meningomyelocele, microphthalmia and colobomata of the iris and retina.

A chemical, methyl mercury, is known to have adverse effects on the developing nervous system in the human. A significant number of the population living near Minamata bay in Japan during the 1950s acquired a neurologic illness from eating fish and shellfish which had a high content of methyl mercury. Many offspring of mothers residing in this area developed cerebral palsy post-natally and neuropathologic examinations[22] revealed that Minamata disease can be acquired transplacentally. Snyder[33] reported a newborn infant with a grossly abnormal neurologic exam and elevated urinary mercury levels whose mother had ingested methyl mercury-contaminated pork between the third and sixth month of pregnancy.

Matsumoto et al.[22] provided neuropathologic descriptions of two infants with fetal onset of Minamata disease. Both brains were very small with a reduction in size of deep nuclei and grey and white matter. The corpus callosum was very hypoplastic. There was a reduction in size and number of nerve cells in the cerebral cortex and a glial proliferation in areas where neurons were deficient. The cerebellums were small and had atrophy of the folia. There were no granule cells in one case and a decreased number in the second. Molecular and Purkinje cells were also decreased.

MALNUTRITION

The effects of nutritional deficiencies are well known in experimental teratology, and are recently under investigation in humans. Vitamin A deficiency, if severe, can cause microcephaly, microphthalmia, colobomata and retinal aplasia.[38] Severe malnutrition in children during the first year of life can be associated with decreases in brain weight, protein, RNA and DNA contents.[43] Apathy, lethargy and changes in electroencephalo-grams have been noted in severely malnourished children.[42] Ventricular dilatation has been found in children with kwashiorkor[36] and both marasmus and kwashiorkor can cause decreases in intelligence quotients.[17] Dobbing[7-10] proposes that the brain may be especially vulnerable in association with a spurt in growth that is arbitrarily defined as the period of its most rapid growth. There are numerous indices of such a growth spurt, which in the human encompasses the last three months of pregnancy and the first three to four postnatal years. Nutritional restrictions during the comparable period of brain growth in rodents has been associated with microcephaly. The consequences of malnutrition on brain growth and function in the human is one of the more important problems needing resolution at this time.

OTHER CONSIDERATIONS

Shepard[32] catalogs the numerous agents that have teratogenic potential in animals and man. Several other potential CNS teratogens exist but are not well defined at present. The question of whether hypoxia and acidosis are capable of producing malformations of the nervous system in human embryos and fetuses is the subject of considerable concern. There is certainly evidence that hypoxia–acidosis secondary to asphyxia is capable of producing cerebral damage in the premature and newborn, but the embryo and young fetus are generally thought to be quite resistant to anoxia *in utero* unless it is profound or focal (*e.g.*, encephaloclastic forms of porencephaly–hydranencephaly). Villee[37] believes that this resistance is due to a combination of metabolic factors. Warkany[38] cites several examples of cases where carbon monoxide poisoning has been associated with malformations, such as hydrocephalus, microcephaly, cortical atrophy, microgyria and softening and cavitation of the basal ganglia. Whether this is the effect of the profound anoxia or a direct effect of the carbon monoxide is not known.

REFERENCES

1. Altshuler G: Toxoplasmosis as a cause of hydranencephaly. Am J Dis Child 125:251–252, 1973
2. Berenberg W, Nakervis G: Long-term follow-up of cytomegalic inclusion disease of infancy. Pediatrics 46:403–410, 1970
3. Boniuk M, Zimmerman LE: Ocular pathology in the rubella syndrome. Arch Ophthalmol 77: 455–473, 1967
4. Brill AB, Forgotson EH: Radiation and congenital malformations. Am J Obstet Gynecol 90: 1149–1168, 1964
5. Brown GC: Recent advances in the viral aetiology of congenital anomalies. Adv Teratol 1:55–80, 1966
6. Demian SDA, Donnelly WH Jr, Monif GRG: Coexistent congenital cytomegalovirus and toxoplasmosis in a stillborn. Am J Dis Child 125: 420–421, 1973
7. Dobbing J: Vulnerable periods in brain development. Lipids, Malnutrition and the Developing Brain. Ciba Foundation Symposium, 1972, pp. 9–29

8. Dobbing J: The later development of the brain and its vulnerability. Scientific Foundations of Paediatrics. Edited by JA Davis and J Dobbing. London, Wm Heinemann, 1974, pp. 565–577.

9. Dobbing J: The later growth of the brain and its vulnerability. Pediatrics 53:2–6, 1974

10. Dobbing J, Sands J: The quantitative growth and development of the human brain. Arch Dis Child 48:757–767, 1973

11. Embil JA, Ozere RL, Haldane EV: Congenital cytomegalovirus infection in two siblings from consecutive pregnancies. J Pediatr 77:417–421, 1970

12. Florman AL, Gershon AA, Blackett PR, Nahmias AJ: Intrauterine infection with herpes simplex virus: Resultant congenital malformations. JAMA 225:129–132, 1973

13. Gregg NM: Congenital cataract following German measles in the mother. Trans Ophthalmol Soc Austral 3:35–46, 1941

14. Hammer-Jacobsen E: Therapeutic abortion on account of x-ray examination during pregnancy. Dan Med Bull 6:113–122, 1959

15. Hanshaw JB: Developmental abnormalities associated with congenital cytomegalovirus infection. Adv Teratol 4:64–93, 1970

16. Hardy JB, McCracken GH Jr, Gilkeson MR, Sever JL: Adverse fetal outcome following maternal rubella after the first trimester. JAMA 207:2414–2420, 1969

17. Hertzig ME, Birch HG, Richardson SA, Tizard J: Intellectual levels of school children severely malnourished during the first two years of life. Pediatrics 49:814–824, 1972

18. Hicks SP, D'Amato CJ: Effects of ionizing radiations on mammalian development. Adv Teratol 1:196–250, 1966

19. Johnson FE: Injury of the child by roentgen ray during pregnancy. J Pediatr 13:894–901, 1938

20. Johnson RT: Effects of viral infection on the developing nervous system. N Engl J Med 287: 599–604, 1972

21. Katz SL (Chairman): Slow Virus Infections, 64th Ross Conference on Pediatric Research, Columbus, 1973

22. Matsumoto H, Koyo G, and Takeuchi T: Fetal Minamata disease. A neuropathological study of two cases of intrauterine intoxication by a methyl mercury compound. J Neuropathol Exp Neurol 24:563–574, 1965

23. Mellin GW, Katzenstein M: The saga of thalidomide: Neuropathy to embryopathy, with case reports of congenital anomalies. N Engl J Med 267:1184–1193, 1238–1244, 1962

24. Miller RW, Blot WJ: Small head size after intrauterine exposure to atomic radiation. Lancet 2: 784–787, 1972

25. Norman RM: Malformations of the nervous system, birth injury and diseases of early life. Neuropathology. Edited by JG Greenfield, W Blackwood, WH McMenemy, A Meyer, RM Norman. London, Edward Arnold Ltd, 1958, pp. 300–407.

26. Patten BM: Varying developmental mechanisms in teratology. Pediatrics 19:734–748, 1957

27. Rorke LB: Nervous system lesions in the congenital rubella syndrome. Arch Otolaryngol 98: 249–251, 1973

28. Rorke LB, Spiro AJ: Cerebral lesions in congenital rubella syndrome. J Pediatr 70:243–255, 1967

29. Savage MO, Mossa A, Gordon RR: Maternal varicella infection as a cause of fetal malformations. Lancet 1:352–354, 1973

30. Shaw CM: Subependymal germinolysis. J Neuropathol Exp Neurol 32:153, 1973

31. Shaw CM, Alvord EC Jr: Subependymal germinolysis. Arch Neurol 31:374–381, 1974

32. Shepard TH: Catalog of Teratogenic Agents. Baltimore, Johns Hopkins Press, 1973

33. Snyder RD: Congenital mercury poisoning. N Engl J Med 284:1014–1016, 1971

34. South MA, Tomkins WAF, Morris CR, Rawls WE: Congenital malformation of the central nervous system associated with genital (type 2) herpesvirus. J Pediatr 75:13–18, 1969

35. Töndury G, Smith DW: Fetal rubella pathology. J Pediatr 68:867–879, 1966

36. Vahlquist B, Engsner G, Sjögren I: Malnutrition and size of the cerebral ventricles. Acta Paediatr Scand 60:533–539, 1971

37. Villee CA: Bioenergetic consideration in fetal and mature tissues. Brain Damage in the Fetus and Newborn from Hypoxia or Asphyxia, 57th Ross Conference on Pediatric Research. Edited by LS James, RE Myers, GE Gaull. Columbus, 1967, pp. 47–56

38. Warkany J: Congenital Malformations. Chicago, Year Book Med Publ, 1971

39. Weller TH: The cytomegaloviruses: ubiquitous agents with protean clinical manifestations. N Engl J Med 285:203–214, 267–274, 1971

40. Wilson JG: Mechanisms of teratogenesis. Am J Anat 136:129–131, 1973

41. Wilson JG: Present status of drugs as teratogens in man. Teratology 7:3–16, 1973

42. Winick M, Coombs J: Nutrition, environment and behavioral development. Annu Rev Med 23:149–160, 1972

43. Winick M, Rosso P: The effect of severe early malnutrition on cellular growth of the human brain. Pediatr Res 3:181–184, 1969

44. Yamazaki JN: A review of the literature on the radiation dosage required to cause manifest central nervous system disturbances from in utero and postnatal exposure. Pediatrics 37 (Suppl):877–903, 1966

45. Zwilling E: Teratogenesis. Analysis of Development. Edited by BH Willier, PA Weiss, V Hamburger. Philadelphia, WB Saunders, 1955, pp. 699–719

chapter 24

CNS MALFORMATIONS IN VARIOUS SPECIFIC SYNDROMES

A variety of syndromes involving the CNS are either proven or suspected to have a genetic basis. The identification and classification of these syndromes are presently undergoing rapid changes, but the works of Gorlin and Pinborg[19] McKusick,[29] Smith[47] and Warkany[57] provide outstanding discussions on clinical aspects as well as on associated factors such as pathogenesis and pathology. In addition, the recent book by McKusick[28] is an excellent resource for the identification of inheritance patterns.

NOMENCLATURE

A knowledge of the current nomenclature of chromosomes is necessary in order to understand their abnormalities. As Summit[53] noted, the normal human has a total of 46 chromosomes, 44 autosomes and two sex chromosomes, X and Y. The normal female is designated by the symbol 46,XX and the male by 46,XY. There are 22 different pairs of autosomes, which are numbered 1–22, partly on the basis of decreasing size. These pairs are divided into 7 groups (A through G) on the basis of morphologic similarity. Group A contains chromosomes 1–3; group B, 4–5; group C, 6–12; group D, 13–15; group E, 16–18; group F, 19–20; and group G, 21–22. Because of morphologic similarities, the X chromosome is usually grouped in C, and the Y in G. In situations in which autosomal anomalies are found, either the chromosome number of its group or both may be used, depending on information available.

The arms of a given chromosome, separated by the centromere, are termed short arm (designated as "p") and long arm (designated as "q"). Other symbols with which the reader should be familiar are the plus (+) and minus (−) signs, which are used to designate extra or missing pieces of a particular chromosome.

In contrast to the autosomes, extra or missing sex chromosomes are designated by extra or missing letters (e.g., Klinefelter syndrome = 47,XXY and Turner syndrome = 45,X). For simplicity, we will use XX more commonly than XY, unless the syndrome characteristically affects only males.

In most dysmorphic syndromes more than one system contains anomalies. The following presentation is limited to a discussion of malformations associated with the nervous system. In many cases neuropathologic studies have been limited, but the volume of information should expand rapidly over the forthcoming years. The following examples are intended only to provide a brief summary of this spectrum of disorders, some of which have been discussed elsewhere in the book under specific malformations.

CHROMOSOMAL ANOMALIES

4p—SYNDROME

In the 4p— syndrome, there are microcephaly, seizures, ocular hypertelorism, occasional coloboma of the iris and midline scalp defects.[18, 21, 34] With its associated psychomotor retardation, 4p— was previously confused with the cat cry syndrome (see below), from which it can be differentiated both clinically and autoradiographically.

5p— SYNDROME (CAT CRY SYNDROME)

The cat cry (cri-du-chat) syndrome involves a partial deletion of the short arm of chromosome 5 (5p−). Anomalies of the CNS are somewhat variable, but microcephaly, cortical atrophy and mental retardation are common. In addition, hypotonia, ventricular dilatation, small mammillary bodies and unilateral cerebellar hypoplasia may be found.[45, 49, 57]

TRISOMY 13 SYNDROME

The trisomy 13 syndrome (47,XX,13+) is characterized by the presence of an extra chromosome in the D group. There are numerous anomalies of many organ systems, and over half the patients die within the first six months. The incidence is between 1/5,000[47] and 1/14,500[11] live births. A slight excess of females and an increased maternal age appear to be associated with trisomy 13. Seizures, mental retardation, deafness and apneic spells are common.[48]

Malformations of the CNS are a prominent part of the syndrome and can affect nearly every portion of the brain. Probably the best known spectrum of anomalies involves the forebrain and olfactory system (see Chapter 14 for a description of holoprosencephaly and arhinencephaly). In its mildest form, there is merely an absence of the olfactory bulbs and tracts. Intermediate forms occur with arhinencephaly and agenesis of the septum pellucidum, hypoplasia or agenesis of the corpus callosum and abnormalities of gyral patterns. In the most severe cases (holoprosencephaly), hypoplasia and fusion of the frontal lobes are associated with a single ventricle representing the fused lateral and third ventricles communicating with a large cyst filling the occipital half of the cranium. Microcephaly is common. Hydrocephalus was found in 4 of 32 cases reported by Warkany et al.[58] and in some cases also involves the fourth ventricle.[37] In spite of the striking gross findings, there are relatively few microscopic abnormalities of the forebrain. The anterior commissure is frequently absent;[37] the thalami can be

fused[58] or covered by a fibrocellular membrane containing neuroglial fibers and some neurons.[37]

Ocular anomalies are extremely common and usually severe. Microphthalmia is present in approximately one-third of the cases, and anophthalmia may be found.[58] Colobomata are found in about half of the cases, and cataracts and glaucoma are common. Externally, the orbits are frequently involved in varying forms of hypotelorism, including fusion with cyclopia in the severest form.

The cerebellum has several interesting findings.[37] It is grossly abnormal in approximately 30% of cases,[58] with generalized hypoplasia, anomalous convolutional patterns and hypoplasia of the caudal vermis. Microscopic findings in the cerebellum are present in nearly all cases of trisomy 13, with heterotopic collections of nerve cells in the white matter and other cellular aggregates, including ganglion cells, granular cells and mixtures of both, found outside of their usual location. Anomalies of the dentate nucleus are common.[56]

13q— SYNDROME

The 13q− (46,XX,13q−) syndrome characteristically involves the CNS severely,[3, 57] with mental retardation, microcephaly, microphthalmia and colobomata. Allderdice et al.[3] report one case having a parietooccipital meningocele, coronal cleft lumbar vertebrae and sacral anomalies. Opitz et al.[40] present an extensive discussion of the neuropathologic findings in another case. They found absence of the sagittal sinus, an anomalous anterior cranial fossa, colobomata, a markedly distorted gyral pattern of the cerebral cortex, a common ventricle associated with a large midline cortical defect posteriorly, absence of the olfactory tracts, absence of the posterior cerebellar vermis and other defects.

TRISOMY 18 SYNDROME

The trisomy 18 syndrome (47,XX,18+) is reported to occur in 1 out of about 4,500 live births.[11] As with the trisomy 13 syndrome, the spectrum of malformations is quite severe, and life expectancy is limited. Numerous anomalies of the CNS are present, as described by Passarge *et al.*,[42] Sumi,[52] Warkany *et al.*,[58] Norman,[37] Terplan and Cohen[54] and Terplan *et al.*[55]

The gyri of the cerebral cortex can vary from normal to grossly abnormal patterns, the latter occurring in about 5% of cases. In one case described by Passarge *et al.*[42] the gyral patterns were so distorted that the occipital lobes, central sulcus and most major fissures could not be identified. Hydrocephalus, defects of the corpus callosum, encephalocele, absent olfactory nerves and meningomyelocele have been reported. Mental retardation and microcephaly are prominent features in the cases that survive infancy.

Several other CNS abnormalities should be noted: Sumi[52] reports absence of the anterior commissure in three of six cases, this being associated in two cases with hypoplasia of the corpus callosum. In another case of trisomy 18 with complete absence of the corpus callosum, he found a well-defined anterior commissure. Abnormalities of the dentate gyrus in the hippocampus can be present. Terplan *et al.*[55] found distinct neuronal heterotopias within or around the walls of the lateral ventricles in 13 of 16 cases. They were frequently surrounded by undifferentiated glial cells and primitive neuroblasts. Ocular malformations (colobomata, microphthalmia, small optic nerves and cloudy corneas) occur in over one-third of cases.

Although the cerebellum and brain stem can be normal in trisomy 18, they are usually hypoplastic and malformed. In cases with meningomyelocele, the Arnold–Chiari malformation is present. In other cases, dysplastic gyri, heterotopias and dysplastic tissue on the ventricular surface of the vermis have been found. Norman[37] found an abnormal strip of cortex bilaterally in the lateral cerebellar lobes. These contained "tubules" embedded in white matter and consisting of blood vessels surrounded by meninges, external granular layer, molecular layer, Purkinje cells and inner granular layer. Sumi[52] reports an abnormal inferior olive in all six of his cases characterized by a thick dorsal lip, a neuronal "capsule" or both.

The surrounding and supporting structures of the nervous system may also be involved in trisomy 18. Defects in the falx or skull (Lückenshädel), shallow posterior fossa, increased size of the foramen magnum, cyst of the cisterna magna and hemivertebrae have been described.

18p− SYNDROME

The 18p− syndrome is another of the many diagnoses that must be considered in newborns with multiple malformations and low birth weight for gestational age. Hypotonia and mental retardation are frequent, and approximately one-fifth of these infants have the facial and CNS features of the arhinencephaly (holoprosencephaly) spectrum.[10] In a review of 23 cases, deGrouchy[20] found increased maternal age and a female preponderance.

18q− SYNDROME

In the 18q− syndrome, Curran *et al.*[13] report mental retardation in 65% and microcephaly in 70% of a series of 17 cases. Ocular abnormalities (nystagmus, microcornea, absent anterior chamber, cloudy cornea and retinal anomalies) and ear malformations were also common. Unlike the 18p− syndrome, there does not seem to be a maternal age effect and the sex ratio is even.[20]

DOWN SYNDROME

Down syndrome (47,XX,21+), characterized by an extra 21st autosome, used to be referred to as "monogolism," but this term is being discarded because of the erroneous implications of the racial characteristic. The syndrome can occur in any race, including Mongolians. Probably no syndrome has been as extensively studied, but still the malformations of the CNS remain one of the most perplexing problems. In spite of numerous descriptive studies, there are no consistent anomalies of the nervous system that adequately explain the varying degrees of mental retardation, usually moderate, which are typically present. Microcephaly is frequent, and the brain is usually small and globular in shape with the anterior portion being less well-developed than the posterior or lateral aspects.[58] The cerebellum and brain stem are significantly smaller than the brain as a whole.[12] The most consistent finding is a small superior temporal gyrus.[5] This gyrus appears compressed into the

TABLE 24–1. FEATURES OF THE MUCOPOLYSACCHARIDOSES

Designation	Name	Features Related to the CNS
MPS I H	Hurler syndrome	Progressive mental-motor retardation; cloudy cornea; retinal degeneration; deafness; hydrocephalus with lepto-meningeal fibrosis; malformed sella tursica; scaphoceph-aly; gyral atrophy; arachnoid cysts
MPS I S	Scheie syndrome	Retinitis pigmentosa; cloudy cornea; juxtasellar arachnoid cysts
MPS I H/S	Hurler–Scheie syndrome	
MPS II A	Hunter syndrome, severe	Retinitis pigmentosa; progressive deafness
MPS II B	Hunter syndrome, mild	
MPS III A	Sanfilippo, syndrome A	Mental retardation; seizures; thickened calvarium
MPS II B	Sanfilippo, syndrome B	
MPS IV	Morquio syndrome	Cloudy cornea; progressive motor deficits secondary to spinal cord and medullary compression due to spondylo-epiphyseal dysplasia; deafness
MPS V*		
MPS VI A	Maroteaux–Lamy syndrome, classic	Cloudy cornea; abnormal sella tursica; hydrocephalus and paraplegia from atlantoaxis subluxation
MPS VI B	Maroteaux–Lamy syndrome, mild	
MPS VII	beta-glucuronidase deficiency	Mental retardation

* MPS V of the older terminology has been replaced by MPS I S.

lower bank of the lateral fissure, and the superior and medial temporal sulci are displaced superiorly. Benda also reported distortion of the fissures of the lower temporal lobe, flattened gyri recti, occasionally ectopic gray matter, increased size of the basal ganglia, loss of nerve cells, denseness of nerve cells in the cerebral cortex, shortened corpus callosum and areas of necrosis in the white matter with a "moth-eaten" appearance. In the cerebellum, the cells may have a "swollen cytoplasm," and anomalies may be found in the Purkinje and granular cell layers. In the spinal cord, he noted occasional hydromyelia and absent posterior horns. As previously mentioned, not all of the above changes are found in a given case, and the most consistent findings are the small superior temporal gyri and short frontal lobes.

In addition, evidences of premature aging are found in those cases of Down syndrome surviving 35 years or more: abundant corpora amylacea, neurofibrillary tangles and senile plaques.[15, 39] Accompanying these changes in a few cases, the additional progressive mental deterioration characteristic of Alzheimer disease can be recognized clinically.

SYNDROMES INVOLVING MUTANT GENES

In addition to syndromes with changes in chromosomes that can be documented histologically by karyotyping, many syndromes arise as a result of mutant genes which cannot yet be resolved microscopically. The best evidence includes the definition of the specific enzyme that both is lacking and typically leads to abnormal amounts of certain metabolites being excreted and/or stored. Unlike many of the chromosomal anomalies discussed above, CNS malformations are unusual, although many secondary changes in the nervous system can occur.

MUCOPOLYSACCHARIDOSES

This group of syndromes has many well-defined entities, of which the major categories are summarized in Table 24–1. More detailed discussions of the various subgroups and of other related disorders may be found in the publications of McKusick.[27, 29, 30] Most have an autosomal recessive inheritance, but Hunter syndrome (MPS IIA) is an X-linked recessive. Most are also characterized by the urinary excretion of abnormal

TABLE 24–2. NEUROPATHOLOGY OF MUCOPOLYSACCHARIDOSES

MPS	Brain weight	Leptomeninges	Hydro-cephalus	Neuronal In-volvement	Cere-bellum	Gliosis	Perivas-cular Fibrosis
I–H	variable; increased or decreased	commonly thickened; may correlate well with hydrocephalus	common	typically severe, widespread ballooning	occasional dendritic swelling	variable	almost always present, may be marked
II–A	variable	rarely mentioned to be thickened	mild or none	cerebral cortex less involved than thalamus and striatum	dendritic swellings may occur	usually not present	variable; less severe than in MPS I
III–A	decreased	may be thickened or normal	more related to loss of brain tissue	moderate to severe cortical neuronal loss	Purkinje cells reduced	usually marked	mild or none
IV, V, VI	Inadequate autopsy information						

amounts of mucopolysaccharides. On the other hand, the mucolipidoses,[50] characterized by accumulation of excessive amounts of acid mucopolysaccharides, sphingolipids and/or glycolipids in visceral and mesenchymal cells, usually do not show abnormal excretion of mucopolysaccharides. The accumulation of lipids within the neurons of the CNS probably begins prenatally, although mental retardation may not become manifest until many months after birth.

Review of the reported cases with neuropathologic examination and of 9 of our own cases representing 4 varieties of the mucopolysaccharidoses (MPS I, II, III, and a variant) demonstrates certain similarities which allow the group to be distinguished grossly and microsopically from the other storage diseases: hydrocephalus, perivascular fibrosis, and intraneuronal accumulations of LFB- and PAS-positive granules. Since many cases have not had biochemical confirmation of the particular type, only the major subdivisions of the mucopolysaccharidoses can be considered (Table 24–2).

The accumulated materials involve the cerebral cortical neurons markedly and diffusely in MPS-I-H and slightly less in MPS-II-A. Such accumulations correlate reasonably well with the degree of mental retardation. However, several cases of MPS-I-H have been reported with little cortical neuronal involvement in spite of significant mental retardation.[14,36] The lack of correlation may be due to the presence of other factors such as extensive perivascular fibrosis of the cerebral white matter (case 2, Lindsay et al.[24]). Cortical atrophy is most marked in MPS-III-A, correlating well with the cortical neuronal loss and degree of mental retardation. Such an alteration is not seen in MPS-I and MPS-II.

Hydrocephalus has been reported in many cases of MPS-I-H and correlates well with the degree of leptomeningeal fibrosis, but exceptions do occur. Probably also related to the leptomeningeal fibrosis is the formation of arachnoid cysts,[35] which may result in the sellar abnormalities recognized roentgenologically. The degree of perivascular fibrosis is variable. In some cases it appears to reflect the generalized leptomeningeal fibrosis; however, in at least one of our cases the degree of perivascular fibrosis was considerably greater than the leptomeningeal fibrosis. Thus, although the fibrous tissue is the apparent common denominator, the leptomeningeal and white matter perivascular fibrosis may be independent reactions.

An interesting observation is the frequent accumulation of LFB- and PAS-positive granules in the dendrites of Purkinje cells, forming fusiform swellings or torpedos. This alteration has been well described in MPS-I

TABLE 24–3. FEATURES OF SOME OF THE LIPIDOSES

Disease	Features Related to the CNS
Ganglioside Storage Diseases: Generalized gangliosidosis (GM$_1$, Type I)	Mental-motor retardation; cherry red spot at macula; macrocephaly
Juvenile GM$_1$ gangliosidosis (GM$_1$, Type II)	Mental-motor retardation; seizures; spasticity; ataxia
Tay–Sachs (GM$_2$, Type I)	Mental-motor retardation; cherry red spot at macula; macrocephaly; progressive decrease in cortical neurons; progressive gliosis; progressive demyelination
Sandhoff (GM$_2$, Type II)	Mental-motor retardation; macrocephaly; seizures; cherry red spot at macula
Juvenile GM$_2$ gangliosidosis (GM$_2$, Type III)	Locomotor ataxia; spasticity; seizures; optic atrophy
Other Lipidoses:	
Gaucher (infantile form)	Mental-motor retardation; focal cell loss; perivascular Gaucher cells
Niemann–Pick	Cherry red spot at macula
Krabbe (Globoid leukodystrophy)	Mental-motor retardation; absence of myelin; extensive gliosis; globoid bodies in white matter; optic atrophy
Metachromatic leukodystrophy	Mental-motor retardation; decreased nerve conduction; demyelination
Fabry	Corneal opacities

and II and also occurred in one case of MPS-III-A. No clinical significance seems to be attached to their presence alone.

Thus, from our analysis of all these cases, not only are there common pathologic features to the entire group of mucopolysaccharidoses, but there may also be sufficient anatomic evidence to suggest which variety it is. The clinico-anatomic correlation is not as perfect as one might desire, but it is clear that MPS-II-A (Hunter) shows less and MPS-III-A (Sanfilippo) more cortical involvement than MPS-1-H (Hurler). The presence of hydrocephalus, usually co-existent with leptomeningeal fibrosis, appears more characteristic of the MPS-1-H (Hurler), whereas the hydrocephalus mentioned in MPS-III-A (Sanfilippo) is more likely the result of the severe cortical atrophy, possibly complicated by a communicating obstructive hydrocephalus.

LIPIDOSES

"The lipid storage diseases are characterized by the accumulation of excessive quantities of fatty substances in various tissues with attendant malfunction of the involved organs."[7] The CNS is markedly affected in most of these disorders, as summarized in Table 24–3, with resultant mental and motor retardation.[32, 46] The ganglioside storage diseases have been discussed in detail by O'Brien.[38]

DISORDERS OF AMINO ACID METABOLISM

As in the mucopolysaccharidoses and lipidoses, mental retardation is common in many of the disorders of amino acid metabolism. The specific enzyme deficiency is usually transmitted in an autosomal recessive pattern.

Phenylketonuria

Phenylketonuria (PKU) results when absence of the enzyme phenylalanine hydroxylase prevents the conversion of phenylalanine to tyrosine. If untreated, mental retardation and microcephaly almost invariably occur. The pathologic changes in the brain are quite variable, but there seems to be a retardation in myelinization,[4] possibly a generalized progressive reduction in myelin formation or a status spongiosus of the white matter.[25] The total brain weight is usually reduced. Intense astrocytic gliosis can occur in older patients.[32] The mechanism by which the nervous system is involved biochemically is not entirely clear at this time.[26, 31-33] The offspring of mothers with

PKU can also have mental retardation and microcephaly.[16]

Homocystinuria

Homocystinuria occurs when the enzyme cystathionine synthetase is absent or inactive so that homocysteine is not converted to cystathione. The CNS is subject to thromboembolic episodes or dural sinus thromboses,[32] and about half of the patients are retarded.[57] These patients are prone to develop cataracts, downward dislocated lens and optic atrophy.

ADDITIONAL "SYNDROMES"

Wilson Syndrome

Wilson syndrome (hepatolenticular degeneration) is an inborn error affecting copper metabolism characterized by absent or deficient ceruloplasmin, a globulin that binds copper. It is transmitted as an autosomal recessive condition and has a generalized aminoaciduria but normal serum amino acids. Copper deposits may be found in the periphery of the cornea (Kayser–Fleischer ring) and in the basal ganglia, especially in the putamen, which subsequently undergoes spongy degeneration. Degenerative changes are also found diffusely, especially in the cerebral cortex, brain stem and substantia nigra.[32]

Lowe Syndrome

Lowe syndrome (oculocerebrorenal) represents an X-linked recessive disorder in which there is psychomotor retardation, seizures and aminoaciduria. Ocular findings include megalocornea, microphthalmia, cataracts and glaucoma.[1] Anomalies in the CNS are quite variable and inconsistent.[8] Richards et al.[43] describe two cases. One had pachygyria, pontine atrophy and "questionable" cerebellar hypoplasia, but definite smallness of the overall brain. The second case was normal in size and had no external anomalies except for meningeal thickening over the frontal lobes. Histologic changes in both cases consisted of "rarefaction of the molecular layer and a tendency for vacuolization of the subpial parenchyma." Richards et al.[43]

also found abnormalities in lamination of the cortex and small neurons, but in other cases, these microscopic changes have not been found.[1] Hydrocephalus and porencephaly can occur.

Tuberous Sclerosis

Tuberous sclerosis (Bourneville syndrome) is an autosomal dominant disorder in which the typical patient presents with skin lesions (adenoma sebaceum, or other "butterfly" lesions of the face, and depigmented areas), seizures and intracranial calcifications. Atypical cases (formes frustes) frequently occur without the complete triad, and the facial lesions may not develop until many years after birth. Pathologic examination of the brain reveals tubers or nodules in the cortex (palpably hard in the unfixed specimens) and in the walls of the ventricles. These intraventricular "candle gutterings" can cause obstruction of CSF flow and hydrocephalus. Histologically, the tuber is composed of giant cells, probably astrocytic, but possibly neuronal. There are cytoarchitectural alterations in the cerebral cortex, neuronal heterotopias, perivascular gliosis, calcification in the basal ganglia, demyelination and *phakomas* (glial overgrowths) in the retina.[47, 57] Some of the tubers may "degenerate" into malignant gliomas, frequently with a histologic pattern of "giant cell" astrocytoma, especially subependymally (see Chapter 22).

SYNDROMES OF UNKNOWN CAUSE

CORNELIA DE LANGE SYNDROME

In the Cornelia de Lange syndrome, numerous CNS anomalies have been described.[2,6, 17, 22] At present, the etiology is unknown. Microbrachycephaly and mental retardation are usually present. The brain is small as a whole, but the cerebellum and brain stem may be either disproportionately smaller or larger than expected as compared with the cerebrum. Other gross changes include abnormal convolutional patterns and hypoplasia of cranial nerves II, III and IV. Ocular changes sometimes include microcornea and retinal colobomata. Microscopically, there is deficient myelination, especially in the centrum semiovale and internal capsule. There may be deficient neurons and subpial astrocytic overgrowth. The pituitary gland sometimes has decreased or absent basophils, but the hypothalamus appears to be normal. Of interest is the fact that one patient with de Lange syndrome had Dandy–Walker malformation.[22]

CEREBROHEPATORENAL (ZELLWEGER) SYNDROME

The cerebrohepatorenal syndrome is probably an autosomal recessive condition that includes several changes in the CNS.[41] These consist of abnormal convolutional patterns (pachygyria or microgyria), decreased myelination, sclerotic white matter, large asymmetric medulla, ventricular dilatation, subependymal cysts, cavum septi pellucidi and cataracts.

OTHER SYNDROMES

There is an ever-increasing recognition of dysmorphic syndromes in which variable structural or cellular changes are found in the CNS and supporting structures. These include the brachycephaly, microphthalmia and cataracts in Hallermann–Streiff syndrome;[51] coloboma, megalocornea, optic atrophy, skull defects, gyral anomalies and defects of the corpus callosum in Rubinstein–Taybi syndrome;[9, 23, 44] and macrocrania, dilated ventricles and cavum septi pellucidi in cerebral gigantism or Soto syndrome.[57]

REFERENCES

1. Abbassi V, Lowe CU, Calcagno PL: Oculocerebro-renal syndrome. Am J Dis Child 115:145–168, 1968

2. Aberfeld DC, Pourfar M: De Lange's Amsterdam dwarfs syndrome. Dev Med Child Neurol 7:35–41, 1965

3. Allderdice PW, Davis JG, Miller OJ, Klinger HP, Warburton D, Miller DA, Allen FH Jr, Abrams CAL, McGilvray E: The 13q– deletion syndrome. Am J Hum Genet 21:499–512, 1969

4. Alvord EC Jr, Stevenson LD, Vogel FS, Engle RL Jr: Neuropathological findings in phenylpyruvic oligophrenia (phenylketonuria). J Neuropathol Exp Neurol 9:298–310, 1950

5. Benda CE: The Child with Mongolism. New York, Grune & Stratton, pp. 78–109, 1960

6. Berg JM, McCreary BD, Ridler MAC, Smith GF: The De Lange Syndrome. New York, Permagon Press, 1970

7. Brady RO, Johnson WG, Uhlendorf BW: Identification of heterozygous carriers of lipid storage diseases. Am J Med 51:423–431, 1971

8. Chutorian A, Rowland LP: Lowe's syndrome. Neurology (Minneap) 16:115–122, 1966

9. Coffin GS: Brachydactyly, peculiar facies and mental retardation. Am J Dis Child 108:351–359, 1964

10. Cohen MM Jr, Jirásek JE, Guzman RT, Gorlin RJ, Peterson MO: Holoprosencephaly and facial dysmorphia: nosology, etiology and pathogenesis. Birth Defects 7:125–135, 1971

11. Conen PE, Erkman-Balis B: Frequency and occurrence of chromosomal syndromes. Am J Hum Genet 18:374–398, 1966

12. Crome L, Cowie V, Slater E: A statistical note on cerebellar and brain-stem weight in Mongolism. J Ment Defic Res 10:69–72, 1966

13. Curran JP, Al-Salihi FL, Allderdice PW: Partial deletion of the long arm of chromosome E-18. Pediatrics 46:721–729, 1970

14. Dawson IMP: The histology and histochemistry of gargoylism. J Pathol Bacteriol 54:587–604, 1954

15. Ellis WG, McCulloch JR, Corley CL: Presenile dementia in Down's syndrome. Neurology 24:101–106, 1974

16. Fisch RO, Walker WA, Anderson JA: Prenatal and postnatal developmental consequences of maternal phenylketonuria. Pediatrics 37:979–986, 1966

17. France NE, Crome L, Abraham JM: Pathological features of the De Lange syndrome. Acta Paediatr Scand 58:470–480, 1969

18. Fryns JP, Eggermont E, Verresen H, van den Berghe H: The 4p– syndrome, with a report of two new cases. Humangenetik 19:99–109, 1973

19. Gorlin RJ, Pindborg JJ: Syndromes of the Head and Neck. New York, McGraw-Hill, 1964

20. de Grouchy J: The 18p–, 18q– and 18r syndromes. Birth Defects 5(5):74–87, 1969

21. Guthrie RD, Aase JM, Asper AC, Smith DW: The 4p– syndrome. Am J Dis Child 122:421–425, 1971

22. Hart MN, Malamud N, Ellis WG: The Dandy–Walker syndrome: A clinicopathological study based on 28 cases. Neurology 22:771–780, 1972

23. Johnson CF: Broad thumbs and broad great toes with facial abnormalities and mental retardation. J Pediatr 68:942–951, 1966

24. Lindsay S, Reilly WA, Gotham TJ, Skahen R: Gargoylism. Am J Dis Child 76:239–306, 1948

25. Malamud N: Neuropathology of phenylketonuria. J Neuropathol Exp Neurol 25:254–268, 1966

26. McKean CM, Peterson NA: Glutamine in the phenylketonuric central nervous system. N Engl J Med 283:1364–1367, 1970

27. McKusick VA: The nosology of the mucopolysaccharidoses. Am J Med 47:730–747, 1969

28. McKusick VA: Mendelian Inheritance in Man, ed 3. Baltimore, Johns Hopkins Press, 1971

29. McKusick VA: Heritable Disorders of Connective Tissue, ed 4. St Louis, CV Mosby Co, 1972

30. McKusick VA, Kaplan D, Wise D, Hanley WB, Suddarth SB, Sevick ME, Maumanee AE: The genetic mucopolysaccharidoses. Medicine 44: 445–483, 1965

31. Menkes JH: Cerebral lipids in phenylketonuria. Pediatrics 37:967–978, 1966

32. Menkes JH: Metabolic diseases of the nervous system (ch 6). Brennemann–Kelley Practice of Pediatrics, vol 4. Edited by VC Kelley. Hagerstown, Harper & Row, 1967

33. Menkes JH: The pathogenesis of mental retardation in phenylketonuria and other inborn errors of amino acid metabolism. Pediatrics 39:297–308, 1967

34. Miller OJ, Breg WR, Warburton D, Miller DA, deCapoa A, Allderdice PW, Davis J, Klinger HP, McGilvray E, Allen FH Jr: Partial deletion of the short arm of chromosome No. 4 (4p−): clinical studies in five unrelated patients. J Pediatr 77:792–801, 1970

35. Neuhauser EBD, Griscom NT, Gilles FH, Crocker AC: Arachnoid cysts in the Hurler-Hunter syndrome. Ann Radiol 11:453–469, 1968

36. Nisbet NW, Cupit BF: Gargoylism. Report of a case. Br J Surg 41:404–412, 1954

37. Norman RM: Neuropathological findings in trisomies 13–15 and 17–18 with special reference to the cerebellum. Dev Med Child Neurol 8:170–177, 1966

38. O'Brien JS: Ganglioside storage diseases. Adv Hum Genet 3:39–98, 1972

39. Olson MI, Shaw C-M: Presenile dementia and Alzheimer's disease in mongolism. Brain 92: 147–156, 1969

40. Opitz JM, Slungaard R, Edwards RH, Inhorn SL, Muller J, deVenecia G: Report of a patient with a presumed Dq− syndrome. Birth Defects 5(5):93–99, 1969

41. Passarge E, McAdams AJ: Cerebro-hepato-renal syndrome. J Pediatr 71:691–702, 1967

42. Passarge E, True CW, Sueoka WT, Baumgartner N, Keer KR: Malformations of the central nervous system in trisomy 18 syndrome. J Pediatr 69:771–778, 1966

43. Richards W, Donnell GN, Wilson WA, Stowens D, Perry T: The oculo-cerebro-renal syndrome of Lowe. Ann J Dis Child 109:185–203, 1965

44. Rubinstein JH, Taybi H: Broad thumbs and toes and facial abnormalities. Am J Dis Child 105: 588–608, 1963

45. Schmid W, Vischer D: Cri-du-chat syndrome. Case report. Helv Paediatr Acta 22:22–27, 1967

46. Shaw C-M, Carlson CB: Crystalline structures in globoid-epithelioid cells: An electron microscopic study of globoid leukodystrophy (Krabbe's disease). J Neuropathol Exp Neurol 29:306–319, 1970

47. Smith DW: Recognizable Patterns of Human Malformation. Philadelphia, WB Saunders, 1970

48. Smith DW, Patou K, Therman E, Inhorn SL, DeMars RI: The D_1 trisomy syndrome. J Pediatr 62:326–341, 1963

49. Solitaire GB: The cri-du-chat syndrome: neuropathologic observations. J Ment Defic Res 11: 267–277, 1967

50. Spranger JW, Wiedemann HR: The genetic mucolipidoses. Hum Genet 9:113–139, 1970

51. Steele RW, Bass JW: Hallermann–Streiff syndrome. Am J Dis Child 120:462–465, 1970

52. Sumi SM: Brain malformations in the trisomy 18 syndrome. Brain 93:821–830, 1970

53. Summit RL: Chromosome nomenclature. J Pediatr 76:314–323, 1970

54. Terplan KL, Cohen MM Jr: Cerebellar changes in association with "partial" trisomy 18. Am J Dis Child 115:179–184, 1968

55. Terplan KL, Lopez EC, Robinson HB: Histological structural anomalies in the brain in trisomy 18 syndrome. Am J Dis Child 119: 228–235, 1970

56. Terplan KL, Sandberg AA, Aceto T Jr: Structural anomalies in the cerebellum in association with trisomy. JAMA 197:557–568, 1966

57. Warkany J: Congenital Malformations. Chicago, Year Book Med Publ, 1971

58. Warkany J, Passarge E, Smith LB: Congenital malformations in autosomal trisomy syndromes. Am J Dis Child 112:502–517, 1966

INDEX

Z

75 76 77 78 79 80   10 9 8 7 6 5 4 3 2 1